# SENSORY INTEGRATION

## Theory and Practice

# SENSORY INTEGRATION

## Theory and Practice

**Anne G. Fisher, ScD, OTR**
Assistant Professor, Department of Occupational Therapy
College of Associated Health Professions
University of Illinois at Chicago
Chicago, Illinois

**Elizabeth A. Murray, ScD, OTR**
Assistant Director of Occupational Therapy
Shriver Center, Waltham, Massachusetts
and
Adjunct Assistant Professor
Department of Occupational Therapy
Sargent College of Allied Health Professions
Boston University
Boston, Massachusetts

**Anita C. Bundy, ScD, OTR**
Assistant Professor, Department of Occupational Therapy
College of Associated Health Professions
University of Illinois at Chicago
Chicago, Illinois

F.A. DAVIS COMPANY • Philadelphia

Printed in the United States of America

Last digit indicates print number: 10 9 8 7 6 5 4

NOTE: As new scientific information becomes available through basic and clinical research, recommended treatments and drug therapies undergo changes. The author(s) and publisher have done everything possible to make this book accurate, up-to-date, and in accord with accepted standards at the time of publication. The authors, editors, and publisher are not responsible for errors or omissions or for consequences from application of the book, and make no warranty, expressed or implied, in regard to the contents of the book. Any practice described in this book should be applied by the reader in accordance with professional standards of care used in regard to the unique circumstances that may apply in each situation. The reader is advised always to check product information (package inserts) for changes and new information regarding dose and contraindications before administering any drug or intervention. Caution is especially urged when using new or infrequently ordered drugs or interventions.

Library of Congress Cataloging-in-Publication Data

Sensory integration : theory and practice / edited by Anne G. Fisher,
    Elizabeth A. Murray, Anita C. Bundy.
        p.   cm. —
    Includes bibliographical references and index.
    ISBN 0-8036-3565-6 (alk. paper)
    1. Sensorimotor integration. 2. Occupational therapy for
children.  I. Fisher, Anne G., 1946–   .  II. Murray, Elizabeth A.
III. Bundy, Anita C.
RJ53.025S466 1991
616.8′515′083 — dc20                                          91-2139
                                                                CIP

*IN MEMORY OF*

A. Jean Ayres
1920 – 1988

To A. Jean Ayres, teacher, mentor, and master clinician, who changed the way we think and, in so doing, affected the lives of countless individuals.

To those many children who have contributed to the development of sensory integration theory and practice through their participation in assessment, intervention, and research.

To those adults who were able to tell us what it means to have sensory integrative dysfunction and who shared with us how intervention changed their lives.

To our clients who have provided the basis for the case descriptions included in this book and who have enabled sensory integration theory and practice to come to life.

# FOREWORD

Barber (1962), in a now-classic sociological paper, identifies several non-scientific sources of resistance to scientific discovery. While acknowledging that objectivity is the norm in scientific evaluation, he documents numerous examples of how a scientist's preconceptions, or entrenchment in certain theoretical models, methodologies, or religious views, can blind him to the merit of new ideas or research. Further, he goes on to illustrate how the relative professional standing of the scientist who makes the innovative discovery, that is his or her position as an insider or outsider in a field of specialization and whether or not he or she belongs to certain professional societies, can influence the degree of acceptance of his or her ideas. Barber demonstrates how the work of scientists of lower standing is prone to resistance by scientists of higher standing as was the case when von Nageli, from a position of higher authority, judged Mendel's work in genetics to be insignificant. After having experienced years of resistance, Lavoisier wrote in the final paragraphs of his memoirs *Reflections on Philogiston* that

> I do not expect my ideas to be adopted all at once. The human mind gets creased into a way of seeing things. Those who have envisaged nature according to a certain point of view during most of their career, rise only with difficulty to new ideas. It is the passage of time, therefore, which must confirm or destroy the opinions I have presented. Meanwhile, I observe with great satisfaction that the young people are beginning to study the science without prejudice. (cited in Barber, 1969)

During her 35-year career as a scientist, A. J. Ayres discovered a new paradigm for explaining a variety of neurological disorders in children. As an occupational therapist, she was an outsider to the medical discipline of neurology. Although the theory she proposed had educational implications, she herself was not an educator. As her work gained acceptance within her profession, resistance to it stiffened in the educational and medical communities. Indeed, during her lifetime, she was distressed by this apparent injustice, although she did not permit it to deter her from pursuing a steady program of research and scholarship. Perhaps, as had been the case with other scientists, more widespread acceptance would come in the next generation.

It is fitting that this volume is being published shortly after Dr. Ayres' death, for it clearly signifies that although A. J. Ayres is no longer among us, the theories and work she dedicated her life to developing are alive and changing. In this collection, for the first time compiled in one volume, are state-of-the-art papers that indicate that (1) sensory integration theory is being refined and further elaborated by the research and scholarship of a number of young scholars, many of whom had been A. J. Ayres' students; (2) compelling arguments have been carefully formulated that address the earlier criticisms of the theory, its related instruments, and the practice based upon it; (3) research from other disciplines is finding support for the theory;

and (4) sensory integration theory is now substantively contributing to the universe of knowledge. This collection will be useful to therapists and academics wishing to update and expand their knowledge of sensory integration theory and practice and as a text for courses on this subject. Commendably, and unlike most volumes that attempt to cover both theoretical and practice issues, neither arena is treated thinly.

In the book's first section, sensory integration theory is placed within the conceptual boundaries of the discipline of occupational science. Fisher and Murray (Chapter 1) provide a succinct but comprehensive overview of the history and current status of the theory. Although a chapter of this sort is at risk for dryness, the incorporation of stunning case studies enlivens the presentation. Especially useful to therapists and students alike will be the compelling arguments presented to correct misconceptions and counteract the criticisms that have on occasion been leveled against the theory. A systems view is elaborated to describe how sensory integration provides a foundation for self-actualization and to enable placement of the theory within the new scientific discipline of occupational science. The latter theme is further developed in Kielhofner and Fisher's discussion (Chapter 2) of mind-brain-body relationships as a single unitary system. In this chapter, some linkages between sensory integrative theory and the model of human occupation are creatively proposed. In the final chapter of this section, Bundy clarifies the relationship of sensory integration procedures to play. After describing the characteristics of play, she points out that not all play is therapeutic, and, vice versa, that not all therapy should be play. In the appropriate context, however, the coupling of therapeutic procedures and play constitutes a powerful therapeutic tool.

In the next four chapters, thoroughly researched and updated, comprehensive discussions of various kinds of dysfunction are presented. It is fortunate that the authors of Chapters 4, 5, 6, and 7, all of whom are clearly recognized as the premier researchers in occupational therapy of the disorders they address, agreed to contribute to this volume. Indeed, one feels graced with a treasure to have in one section a presentation on vestibular-proprioceptive processing deficits by Anne G. Fisher, on tactile processing and sensory defensiveness by Charlotte Royeen and Shelly Lane, on somatodyspraxia by Sharon Cermak, and on hemispheric specialization by Elizabeth Murray. In each of these chapters, cases are effectively presented to tease out the nuances that distinguish one disorder from another; the theoretical perspective of Ayres is discussed with great accuracy but is also elaborated upon through synthesis of new research; state-of-the-art instruments and tools are displayed that can readily be used in practice; and solid evidence is presented to resolve controversy and to support or refute claims. After reading these sections, one feels relieved to have in one place such a breadth of substantive information, which before this publication had appeared to be fragmented and difficult to acquire.

In the next five chapters, the focus shifts to assessment and practice issues. In Chapter 8, Ayres and Marr provide a cogent description of the content, standardization, and validity of the new Sensory Integration and Praxis Tests (SIPT) including an explanation of the computer-generated chromographs that are used in interpretation. Fisher and Bundy (in Chapter 9) then provide a detailed discussion of a case to illustrate the process of interpreting SIPT scores in relation to clinical and historical data. The interpretive process is presented here as an art form in which the therapist draws on his or her knowledge of the theory, evaluation procedures, and technology. Worksheets are presented to expedite the interpretive process.

Chapters 10, 11, and 12 concern intervention and consultation. Koomar and Bundy (in Chapter 10) provide one of the most exhaustive, exact, and imaginative descriptions of sensory integrative therapeutic procedures extant. In doing so, they are to be congratulated on avoiding the mistake of presenting a "cookbook." The case examples and descriptions in this chapter capture the essence and uniqueness of therapy in keeping with the principles of sensory integrative theory. Particularly interesting is the discussion of the therapist as a therapeutic tool. In the last three chapters in this section, Bundy (Chapters 11 and 12) offers innovative ideas on consultation and on planning and implementing intervention, and Murray and Anzalone (in Chapter 13) distinguish sensory integration from other widely used therapeutic procedures and offer examples of how various practice models can be combined.

In the final chapter, Ottenbacher assesses the problems inherent in doing sensory integrative research and suggests research designs for overcoming them. This chapter will be of great use to researchers who plan to do efficacy studies and to those who wish to evaluate the soundness of the studies already conducted.

The content of this volume is extraordinary. Not only is the book intellectually stimulating, well written, and scholarly, it is also rich with ideas and tools that can be easily applied in clinical settings. One is left convinced that sensory integration theory, research, and practice continue to be infused with vitality. The contributors should be applauded for keeping sensory integration theory and practice alive and changing.

Florence Clark, PhD, OTR, FAOTA
Professor and Chair
Occupational Therapy Department
University of Southern California

## REFERENCE

Barber, B. & Hirsch, J.W., *The Sociology of Science.* New York: The Free Press, 1962.

# PREFACE

This is a book about people who have problems with the normal processing of sensory information taken in from their environments. These people frequently have related problems in a variety of areas including psychosocial, motor, and "learning" skills. Sensory integration theory attempts to explain the relationship between these sensory processing and behavioral deficits when they cannot be attributed to frank neurological damage or abnormalities (e.g., cerebral palsy, mental retardation, traumatic brain injury, peripheral sensory loss). As such, sensory integration is a theory of brain-behavior relationships.

A. Jean Ayres developed sensory integration theory during a period that spanned three decades. Among occupational therapists, Ayres was an exemplar. She was creative, innovative, and persistent. Based on her experience, her knowledge of the neurobehavioral and developmental literature, and her intuitions, she proposed new ideas, developed new tests, and implemented research. She shared her developing theory and research findings through publications and teaching.

The decision to write a book in the area of sensory integration arose from the need for a state-of-the-art text for use in occupational therapy curricula. Ayres' most definitive works on sensory integration theory, *Sensory Integration and Learning Disorders* (1972) and *Sensory Integration and the Child* (1979), were published more than a decade ago. While her many publications provided the basis for subsequent research studies, much of the most current thinking on, and recent revisions of, sensory integration theory, both by Ayres and by other experts in the theory, have not yet been published. Therefore, this book is a logical step in the evolution of sensory integration theory in that it brings together the most current thinking and research findings of many of these experts.

This book is unique in several ways. First, many of the contributors are individuals whose involvement in sensory integration research and practice has had a significant impact on the development of the theory. They also are aware that many controversies and misconceptions surround the theory and practice of sensory integration. Against this background, contributors present their most recent perspectives on sensory integration theory and practice. They also critique some of the basic assumptions and myths of sensory integration theory and practice, and propose new hypotheses to be supported or refuted through future research.

Second, this book has been carefully designed to complement rather than duplicate major existing occupational therapy texts. For example, an entire chapter is devoted to demonstrating how and when it is appropriate to combine sensory integration theory and practice with several other occupational therapy practice models. Case studies are used to demonstrate an integrated approach to treatment across age groups and across diagnoses. Another chapter discusses the use of sensory integration theory when consulting with parents and teachers of children in need of occupational therapy services.

Third, this book is innovative in that it unites sensory integration theory with basic tenets of occupational science. One of these tenets views play as an important occupation of children; play is the primary treatment medium for the promotion of sensory integration. Another tenet maintains that participation in meaningful activity enhances both the mind and the brain-body; because the mind and the brain-body are interrelated, activity that promotes the health and development of one also promotes the health and development of the other. Two separate chapters provide detailed discussion of these tenets and their important relationships to sensory integration theory and treatment; both chapters contain the most recent theoretical work of the respective authors.

This book is divided into four parts. Part I, Theoretical Concepts, provides an overview of sensory integration theory. Included are chapters, discussed above, that address two basic tenets of occupational science and that provide the reader with the theoretical basis for understanding the role of sensory integration theory and practice within the broader context of the science and practice of occupational therapy.

Part II, Domains of Function, presents an in-depth discussion of the clinical picture; the neurobiological basis hypothesized to underlie the behavioral deficits seen in clients with sensory integrative dysfunction; and the typology, evaluation, and treatment of dysfunction in each domain.

Part III, Evaluation and Treatment, builds on Part II and provides the philosophical, ethical, and practical background necessary to interpret the results of an evaluation of sensory integrative functioning and to plan and implement comprehensive treatment of clients of varying ages and with differing patterns of sensory integrative dysfunction. Included in this section are individual chapters devoted to direct service and consultation models of service delivery.

Part IV, Research, discusses the importance of research in the development of clinical theory, test development, and the profession. Recommendations for continued research in sensory integration, as well as suggestions for research methodologies and strategies aimed toward the continued evolution of sensory integration theory and practice, are included.

This book is intended for use in entry-level and advanced professional occupational therapy education and by occupational therapists who use sensory integration theory and treatment techniques in their practice. It is appropriate for adoption in any course that covers sensory integration theory.

Anne G. Fisher, ScD, OTR
Elizabeth A. Murray, ScD, OTR
Anita C. Bundy, ScD, OTR

# ACKNOWLEDGMENTS

As with any undertaking of this magnitude, this book is the culmination of the efforts of countless people. Various drafts of individual chapters were reviewed by Kathi Baron, Kim Bryze, Janice P. Burke, Sharon A. Cermak, Ellen S. Cohn, Terry Crowe, Clare Curtin, Flo Dunlop, Winnie Dunn, Adele Germain, Barbara Hanft, Fay Horak, Gary Kielhofner, Debbie Kirking, Virgene Klein, Mary Lawlor, Lee Ann Lilly, Zoe Mailloux, Shay McAtee, Carol Ann Myers, Anita Niehues, Jane Clifford O'Brien, Mechthild Rast, Susanne Smith Roley, Barbara Sides, Linda Silber, Theresa Stevens, Catherine A. Trombly, Craig Velozo, Lisa Walsh, and G. Gordon Williamson. Three additional people reviewed the entire manuscript: Shelly J. Lane, Margaret Short-DeGraff, and Jane Case-Smith. There is no doubt in our minds that without their contributions this book would not have been possible.

We would like to express our appreciation to our editor, Jean-François Vilain, who believed in the efficacy of our skill and was there to assist and "bug" us to keep going when we needed it. Cheryl Mattingly, who has shared with us her insights into the clinical reasoning process of occupational therapists, has had a major influence on our thinking and writing. Mike Brown, Kim Watson, and their colleagues at Southpaw Enterprises generously contributed the photographs. Barbara Barlow expertly, and almost uncomplainingly, typed and retyped chapter after edited chapter. Jackie Dalton watched the animals during numerous trips to Chicago. While Bob Murray did not do anything in particular to help us, we would like to recognize him because he was in need of an acknowledgment.

Finally, we include special recognition of Anne Henderson, our mentor, teacher, colleague, and friend. Her initiative, her insight, and her creativity resulted in the development of internationally recognized occupational therapy graduate programs and educational opportunities for hundreds of occupational therapists. We were privileged to be among those who have had the opportunity to study with Anne. Anne instilled in each of us a quest for knowledge. Her goal, both for herself and for her students, was the development of occupational therapy theory and practice. This book reflects her contributions to our growth as occupational therapy educators, clinicians, and researchers.

# CONTRIBUTORS

MARIE E. ANZALONE, MS, OTR
  Instructor
  Sargent College of Allied Health
    Professions
  Boston University
  Boston, Massachusetts


A. JEAN AYRES, PhD, OTR, FAOTA
  (deceased)
  Emeritus Adjunct Associate
    Professor
  Department of Occupational Therapy
  University of Southern California
  Los Angeles, California


ANITA C. BUNDY, ScD, OTR, FAOTA
  Assistant Professor
  Department of Occupational Therapy
  College of Associated Health
    Professions
  University of Illinois at Chicago
  Chicago, Illinois


SHARON A. CERMAK, EdD, OTR, FAOTA
  Associate Professor of Occupational
    Therapy
  Sargent College of Allied Health
    Professions
  Boston University
  Boston, Massachusetts


ANNE G. FISHER, ScD, OTR, FAOTA
  Assistant Professor
  Department of Occupational Therapy
  College of Associated Health
    Professions
  University of Illinois at Chicago
  Chicago, Illinois

GARY KIELHOFNER, DrPH, OTR, FAOTA
  Professor and Head
  Department of Occupational Therapy
  College of Associated Health
    Professions
  University of Illinois at Chicago
  Chicago, Illinois


JANE A. KOOMAR, MS, OTR
  Assistant Professor of Occupational
    Therapy
  Sargent College of Allied Health
    Professions
  Boston University
  Boston, Massachusetts
  and
  Director
  Occupational Therapy Associates,
    P.C.
  Watertown, Massachusetts


SHELLY J. LANE, PhD, OTR
  Assistant Professor
  Department of Occupational Therapy
  SUNY at Buffalo
  Buffalo, New York


DIANA MARR, PhD
  Project Director
  Western Psychological Services
  Los Angeles, California
  Currently:
  Associate Measurement Statistician
  Educational Testing Service
  Princeton, New Jersey

Elizabeth "Boo" Murray, ScD, OTR
  Assistant Director of Occupational
    Therapy
  Shriver Center
  Waltham, Massachusetts
  and
  Adjunct Assistant Professor
  Department of Occupational Therapy
  Sargent College of Allied Health
    Professions
  Boston University
  Boston, Massachusetts

Kenneth Ottenbacher, PhD, OTR,
  FAOTA
  Professor and Associate Dean
  School of Health Related Professions
  State University of New York at
    Buffalo
  Buffalo, New York

Charlotte Brasic Royeen, PhD, OTR,
  FAOTA
  Research and Therapy Services
  Great Falls, Virginia
  and
  Visiting Professor in Research and
    Evaluation
  Virginia Polytechnic Institute and
    State University
  Falls Church, Virginia

# CONTENTS

# Part III. EVALUATION AND TREATMENT ...... 201

## Chapter 8. SENSORY INTEGRATION AND PRAXIS TESTS ..................... 203

### A. Jean Ayres, PhD, OTR, FAOTA and Diana B. Marr, PhD

## CHAPTER 9. THE INTERPRETATION PROCESS ............. 234

### Anne G. Fisher, ScD, OTR and
### Anita C. Bundy, ScD, OTR

## CHAPTER 10. THE ART AND SCIENCE OF CREATING DIRECT INTERVENTION FROM THEORY ...................... 251

### Jane A. Koomar, MS, OTR and
### Anita C. Bundy, ScD, OTR, FAOTA

**Elizabeth A. Murray, ScD, OTR and**
**Marie E. Anzalone, MS, OTR**

# Part *I*

## THEORETICAL CONCEPTS

# CHAPTER 1

# Introduction to Sensory Integration Theory

**Anne G. Fisher, ScD, OTR**
**Elizabeth A. Murray, ScD, OTR**

*Exactly how sensory integration occurs in the brain remains elusive, but that fact is not an excuse for avoiding an issue basic to all learning. It must be faced and dealt with in as adequate a manner as possible, with full recognition of the limitations involved and with the realization that any conceptual framework is in some respects erroneous. It will require constant revision as new knowledge unfolds.*

*A. Jean Ayres, 1968/1974b, pp. 96–97*

A. Jean Ayres developed sensory integration theory to better explain the relationship between behavior and neural functioning, especially sensory processing or integration. Her goal was to develop a theory to describe and predict the specific relationships among neural functioning, sensorimotor behavior, and early academic learning. She hoped that the emerging theory would allow her to identify specific subtypes or patterns of dysfunction among children with sensorimotor or learning problems, and to develop specific treatment intervention strategies for those subgroups of children. In fact, Ayres' primary objective in developing the theory of sensory integration was to be able to explain the underlying cause of these problems in order to determine the optimal mode of treatment (Ayres, 1972b, 1975a, 1979).

## DEFINITION OF SENSORY INTEGRATION: PROCESS AND THEORY

Sensory integration refers to both a neurological process and a theory of the relationship between the neurological process and behavior. Ayres (1972b) originally defined the sensory integration process as "the ability to organize sensory information for use" (p. 1). More recently, Ayres (1989) elaborated further, stating that

> [s]ensory integration is the neurological process that organizes sensation from one's own body and from the environment and makes it possible to use the body

**3**

effectively within the environment. The spatial and temporal aspects of inputs from different sensory modalities are interpreted, associated, and unified. Sensory integration is information processing. . . . The brain must select, enhance, inhibit, compare, and associate the sensory information in a flexible, constantly changing pattern; in other words, the brain must integrate it. (p. 11)

Sensory integration is a theory of brain-behavior relationships. Theories are provisional sets of interrelated postulates and assumptions that help us to describe, explain, and predict behavior and the relationships between observable events. Theories help us to focus our thinking and our observations, to attend to certain relevant information, and to exclude other information as irrelevant. Sensory integration theory was developed to explain an observed relationship between (a) deficits in interpreting sensory information from the body and the environment, and (b) deficits in academic or neuromotor "learning" in some individuals who demonstrate learning disabilities or clumsiness. Ayres (1989) used *learning* in a very broad sense to include both academic learning and concept formation, as well as behavior change and adaptive motor behaviors.

More specifically, within the larger group consisting of individuals with learning deficits is a subgroup whose members also display deficits in interpreting or discriminating sensory inputs from the body and the environment. These deficits are without other apparent cause (e.g., emotional problems, mental retardation, peripheral sensory loss, and neurological damage or abnormalities).

Sensory integration theory has three components. The first component pertains to development and describes normal sensory integrative functioning; the second defines sensory integrative dysfunction; and the third guides intervention programs that use sensory integration techniques. Each component, in turn, has a major, overarching postulate. The first major postulate of sensory integration theory is that learning is dependent on the ability of normal individuals to take in sensory information derived from the environment and from movement of their bodies, to process and integrate these sensory inputs within the central nervous system, and to use this sensory information to plan and organize behavior. The second postulate follows from the first. When individuals have deficits in processing and integrating sensory inputs, deficits in planning and producing behavior occur that interfere with conceptual and motor learning. Finally, the postulate that guides intervention hypothesizes that the provision of opportunities for enhanced sensory intake, provided within the context of a meaningful activity and the planning and organizing of an adaptive behavior, will improve the ability of the central nervous system to process and integrate sensory inputs, and, through this process, to enhance conceptual and motor learning.

Consistent with a theory that has components pertaining to dysfunction and intervention, sensory integration theory has associated with it an evaluation and intervention technology. Thus, when we speak of sensory integration we refer to three interrelated elements of practice: (a) the theory itself, (b) evaluation methods (i.e., the Sensory Integration and Praxis Tests [SIPT] and related clinical assessments of neuromotor behavior) (Ayres, 1989), and (c) specific sensory integration treatment techniques. The relationship between the hypothesized process of sensory integration and the three elements of practice is shown schematically in Figure 1–1.

The process of sensory integration is a theoretical construct; we are unable to *observe* central nervous system processing, sensory integration, or motor planning. We hypothesize that sensory integration does occur, based on evidence published in experimental neuroscience literature that such a process exists. However, while we

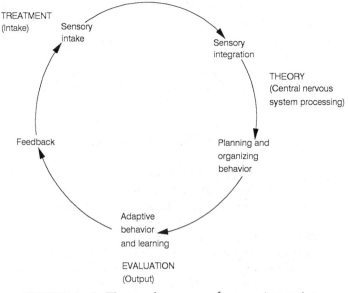

FIGURE 1-1. The circular process of sensory integration.

can observe and evaluate deficits in behavior, we can only hypothesize that these deficits are the result of poor sensory integration. Further, we can observe whether or not our intervention programs effect a change in behavior, but when behavioral changes do occur, we can only hypothesize that they are due to improved sensory integration or enhanced neural functioning.

For example, Mario has diminished tactile discrimination as indicated by problems with identifying which of his fingers is touched (Finger Identification), localizing where on his arms he was touched (Localization of Tactile Stimuli), and reproducing designs that were drawn on the back of his hand (Graphesthesia). Mario has no evidence of frank peripheral-nerve or central nervous system damage, and he is of normal intelligence. Therefore, we hypothesize that one of his problems is in processing and integrating tactile inputs within the central nervous system.

Mario also is clumsy. While other children his age are playing baseball, Mario cannot catch, throw, or bat nearly as well as his peers. Although Mario can tie his shoes and ride a bicycle, he had to practice more than other children until he learned how. Our testing indicates that Mario's ability to hop, skip, and jump are below expectations for a child of his age. He also has difficulty imitating postures (Postural Praxis) and reproducing motor action sequences that involve the use of both sides of the body (Bilateral Motor Coordination) as demonstrated by the examiner.

Again, because Mario has no evidence of frank cognitive or neurological deficits that could account for his motor incoordination, we hypothesize that his problems are related to a developmental disorder in learning new motor tasks (praxis or motor planning). Further, because empirical evidence has consistently linked diminished ability to discriminate tactile inputs with problems in motor planning, we speculate that the two problems are related. We conclude that Mario's motor learning problems are related to, and possibly caused by, his poor tactile discrimination.

We cannot directly observe tactile processing ability or the motor planning process. What we observe are the behaviors: poor tactile discrimination and motor performance skills. Speculating that the problem originated in Mario's ability to process and integrate tactile inputs within the central nervous system, we conclude that a treatment program designed to include enriched tactile experiences derived from participation in activities that Mario enjoys and finds meaningful will increase the likelihood that he will take in, process, and integrate tactile inputs as a basis for planning adaptive motor actions. While we cannot directly observe if this occurs, we can observe if Mario's motor behavior improves.

## THEORY: HYPOTHESES VERSUS FACT

Sensory integration is both a process and a theory. Theory, by definition, is not fact. We only can hypothesize about Mario's ability to integrate tactile inputs, and about the relationship between his tactile discrimination skills and his motor incoordination. All theories of human behavior are comprised of sets of interrelated postulates that have not been, and may never be, proven. As with all theories of human behavior, sensory integration theory is tentative.

The value of theory is that it helps us to provide an explanation of behavior and relationships between observable events. We also use theory to help us plan effective treatment programs, and to predict therapeutic outcomes. Finally, a theory "provides a basis for challenge of its speculative tenets or propositions and for subsequent discovery of new empirical knowledge that might explain and predict events not yet understood" (Chinn & Jacobs, 1987, p. 169). Through empirical research, theory evolves; it is continually being revised and modified to reflect new knowledge that emerges.

Thus, the value of theory in occupational therapy is that it provides a set of tenets or propositions that guide "best practice," and promotes research that adds to the basic knowledge of occupational science. The extent to which the practice of a profession is accepted as valid is related to the size and credibility of the knowledge base (research) that supports the theories that guide practice, as well as the empirical evidence that treatment based on those theories is effective. The importance of empirical research to the development of sensory integration theory and practice is discussed in more detail in Chapter 14.

## THE WORK OF A. JEAN AYRES

The theory of sensory integration is strongly rooted in neuroscience. Ayres' emphasis on neuroscience may have been the result of studying at the University of Southern California under Margaret Rood and conducting postdoctoral work at the Brain Research Institute of the University of California, Los Angeles (Sieg, 1988). Clinically, her work with children with cerebral palsy and later observations of learning-disabled children sparked an interest in exploring perceptual and motor contributions to learning. Based on a thorough review of relevant neurobehavioral literature, she formulated hypotheses about deficits in neurobiological processes that might be associated with learning disabilities. These led to the development of treatment procedures designed to enhance neural functioning (Ayres, 1964, 1968/1974b, 1972a, 1972b).

Ayres' further review of educational and neurobehavioral literature indicated a strong need for objective, standardized measures of perceptual and motor functions that could be used to test and validate her hypotheses. While her initial emphasis was on visual perception, Ayres felt that it was essential to look beyond the visual system to other sensory systems, especially vestibular, proprioceptive, and tactile, that might form a basis for learning (Ayres, 1968/1974a, 1968/1974b). As a part of her doctoral work at the University of Southern California, she began the development of tests which were eventually to become the Southern California Sensory Integration Tests (Ayres, 1972c, 1980). These tests measure not only visual perception but also tactile and kinesthetic (somatosensory) perception, and perceptual-motor function. Additionally, in 1975, the Southern California Postrotary Nystagmus Test was added as a measure of vestibular function (Ayres, 1975b). Finally, Ayres always supplemented her standardized assessment with nonstandardized observations of neuromotor maturation, such as muscle tone, the ability to extend or flex the body against gravity (prone extension and supine flexion, respectively), and balance.

In the early 1980s, recognizing the limitations of the standardization procedure of the Southern California Sensory Integration Tests, Ayres and her associates began work on a major revision and restandardization of these tests. Some tests were modified, inadequate tests were omitted, and new tests were added in an effort to better delineate the sensory integrative and related deficits in children with learning or behavioral problems. This new battery of tests, the Sensory Integration and Praxis Tests (SIPT) (Ayres, 1989), is described in Chapter 8.

Ayres was inspired by the children she sought to help (Sieg, 1988). She developed tests to be better able to understand the problems of the children she treated. She implemented research using those tests so that she could evaluate her clinical assumptions and hypotheses. And she developed a theory that could be used to plan and guide effective interventions. Throughout the development of sensory integration theory, Ayres attempted to validate her assessment methods and treatment procedures through research. Ayres conducted a number of studies designed to identify typologies of sensory integration dysfunction, first using the Southern California Sensory Integration Tests, the Southern California Postrotary Nystagmus Test, and other related assessments; and later, using the SIPT. These studies are commonly referred to as Ayres' "factor-analytic studies." Additionally, Ayres implemented two controversial intervention studies in an attempt to document the effectiveness of sensory integration treatment procedures (Ayres, 1972a, 1976, 1978). Findings from this research were used to revise and modify Ayres' original hypotheses, and thus played an important part in the evolution of sensory integration theory.

## Treatment Efficacy Studies

In an effort to validate the postulate that intervention can enhance sensory integration, Ayres implemented two intervention studies of children with learning disabilities. In the first study, Ayres (1972a) assessed the effects of sensory integration treatment programs on children with sensory integrative disorders and on children with auditory-language problems. Both experimental groups made significant gains in reading and in auditory-language skills. Ayres' (1976, 1978) goal in implementing her second treatment study was to determine which subtypes of learning-disabled children were most likely to benefit from therapy using sensory integration treatment procedures. Ayres found that children in the experimental group who had depressed durations of postrotary nystagmus made greater gains academically than did similar children in the control group.

Ayres believed that the results of these studies provided initial support for her hypothesis that improving sensory integration results in enhanced learning. The latter study also led her to conclude that *central* vestibular processing disorders were a common basis of learning problems, and that children with central vestibular processing disorders (including depressed durations of postrotary nystagmus) may respond more readily to programs that include the use of sensory integration treatment techniques than will children with prolonged durations of postrotary nystagmus.

In a subsequent critique of sensory integration intervention research, Densem, Nuthall, Bushnell, and Horn (1989) noted, however, that

> [c]omparative effectiveness studies are premature in areas of inquiry in which the significant variables and models of the process of change have not been clearly identified. . . . The research focus, therefore, needs to shift toward relating specific treatment variables to the process of development and learning during treatment, as well as to outcome measures. The question then becomes, not "How effective was the program?" but rather, "How does it work and for whom?" (p. 228).

Many of those who attended her lectures and other public presentations are aware that Ayres clearly recognized the need for further research designed to determine which children with sensory integration disorders responded best to specific treatment programs. She believed that the first steps in this process were (a) the development of a theoretical model of change, and (b) the identification of patterns or typologies of dysfunction.

## Factor-Analytic and Related Studies

In order to analyze patterns of dysfunction among learning-disabled children, Ayres used the statistical procedures of principal components, factor, and cluster analyses. The earliest studies that served as a basis for sensory integration theory were based on principal components and factor analyses. Principal components and factor analyses are conceptually similar in that both are empirical methods which can be used to determine whether some small number of underlying constructs can account for the variability in a set of test scores for a large group of people (Stevens, 1986). For example, we might administer two motor-free tests of visual perception (Space Visualization and Figure-Ground Perception), and three tests of motor proficiency (Postural Praxis, Bilateral Motor Coordination, and Sequencing Praxis) to a group of 200 children. We expect that some children will be better than other children in tasks that involve visual perception. Similarly, we expect that some children will be better coordinated than are other children. Finally, we expect that some children who are well coordinated will have poor visual-perceptual abilities, and some children who are clumsy will have very good visual-perceptual skills.

Knowing that this is the case, we expect children who are more skilled at visual-perceptual tasks to obtain higher scores on both tests of visual perception, and children who are not as skilled to obtain lower scores on both tests. Similarly, we expect very coordinated children to obtain high scores on all three motor tests, and children who are clumsy to obtain low scores on all three motor tests. Finally, we expect that children who obtain high scores on the tests of visual perception will not necessarily obtain high scores on the motor tests, and vice versa. In other words, we expect the two tests of visual perception statistically to correlate or to covary, and we expect the three tests of motor behavior to correlate or covary. However, we do not expect the tests of visual perception to correlate with the tests of motor proficiency (or, at least, we do not expect the strength of the correlation to be as strong). Principal components and factor analyses are statistical techniques that enable the researcher to examine the data in order to identify such sources of variability (patterns of correlations) among test scores. In our example, we expect two factors to be identified, one that includes the visual-perceptual tests and another that includes the motor tests. It is then up to the researcher to provide labels for, or to name, the factors. In this case, we might name a visual-perceptual factor and a motor factor.

Between 1965 and 1977, Ayres completed six factor-analytic studies of the Southern California Sensory Integration Tests and related measures, using data both from normal children and from children with perceptual-motor or learning disabilities (Ayres, 1965, 1966a, 1966b, 1969, 1972d, 1977). The theory of sensory integration evolved based on Ayres' interpretations of these data. Although the factors emerging in the studies were not identical, and the labels that Ayres attached to them varied over time, careful analysis reveals certain similarities that suggest the presence of several different, but relatively consistent, patterns of dysfunction. The patterns of dysfunction that appeared most consistently included:

1. *Dyspraxia*, or difficulty with motor planning, associated with *poor tactile discrimination*; commonly referred to as *somatosensory-based dyspraxia*
2. *Poor bilateral integration* associated with *vestibular-proprioceptive dysfunction* and poor postural-ocular mechanisms; commonly referred to as *vestibular bilateral integration disorder*
3. *Tactile defensiveness*, or an aversive reaction to being touched, sometimes associated with increased activity level and distractibility
4. *Poor form and space perception* (visual and tactile)
5. *Auditory-language dysfunction*
6. *Poor eye-hand coordination*

Ayres' goal was the identification of discrete patterns (typologies) of dysfunction. While these factor analyses indicated that domains of dysfunction could be differentiated, Ayres pointed out that they were not discrete typologies (Ayres, 1972d). A child could demonstrate more than one pattern, and some children were more correctly described as having *generalized sensory integrative dysfunction.*

In 1987, Ayres and her colleagues published the results of a seventh factor-analytic study based on the results of the Southern California Sensory Integration Tests (Ayres, Mailloux, & Wendler, 1987). However, this study also included preliminary versions of tests that were to become the praxis tests of the SIPT. The most consistent factors (represented primarily by the Southern California Sensory Integration Tests, the precursors of the SIPT praxis tests, and related clinical observations) that emerged were a factor that they named *visuo- and somatodyspraxia* and a factor represented by *poor bilateral motor and sequencing abilities.* Other, more unstable factors, appeared to reflect sensory processing deficits. The relationship between the results of this factor analysis and the more recent of the earlier factor analyses is shown in Figure 1–2.

More recently, in analyzing data from the SIPT, Ayres (1989) used cluster analysis in addition to principal components and factor analyses. Cluster analysis is conceptually similar to principal components or factor analysis, except that in the case of cluster analysis, the researcher is interested in using an objective technique to identify clusters or groups of subjects such that subjects within a particular cluster

| 1972 | 1976 | 1977 | 1987 | 1989 |
|------|------|------|------|------|
| Apraxia | Praxis-somatosensory | Praxis | Somatodyspraxia | Somatodyspraxia |
| Form and space | (Form and space) | (Form and space) | Visuopraxis | Visuomotor, form and space, visual construction |
| Hyperactivity, distractibility, tactile disorder | | Tactile defensiveness | | |
| Postural-ocular, bilateral integration | Postural-ocular, integration of two body sides | Postural-ocular, integration of two body sides | Bilateral motor and sequencing abilities | Bilateral integration and sequencing |
| Auditory-language | Auditory-language | Auditory-language | Auditory-memory | Praxis on verbal command |
| | Duration of post-rotary nystagmus | Duration of post-rotary nystagmus | Prolonged nystagmus | Postrotary nystagmus |
| | Eye-hand coordination | Eye-hand coordination | | Visuomotor Coordination |

FIGURE 1–2. Summary of factor analytic studies 1972–1989.

are similar to the other members of that cluster, but that members of any one cluster are different from members of any other cluster. In the example we described above, we expect an exploratory cluster analysis to identify four clusters, or groups, of children. We expect one group to be comprised of children who obtain high scores on both motor and visual-perceptual tests (high ability group), and another group to be comprised of children who obtain low scores on both groups of tests (low ability group). Finally, we expect the other two groups to be the high visual-perceptual–low motor group and the low visual-perceptual–high motor group. Cluster groups, like factors, are named by the researcher. In this case, we might name the clusters (a) normal ability, (b) general dysfunction, (c) motor dysfunction, and (d) visual-perceptual dysfunction.

Those patterns that emerged from the factor and cluster analyses of the SIPT data include:

1 Somatosensory processing deficits
2 Poor bilateral integration and sequencing
3 Impaired somatopraxis
4 Poor praxis on verbal command
5 Visuopraxis factor, more appropriately considered poor visual perception and visuomotor coordination
   a Poor form and space perception
   b Visual construction deficits
   c Visuomotor coordination deficits
6 Generalized sensory integrative dysfunction

These factor-analytic and related studies can be criticized appropriately for limitations in design. Because Ayres was constantly exploring new ideas, she used a different battery of assessments in each study. The result was that none of the studies was ever a true replication of a preceding one. Further, her sample sizes were consistently small relative to the number of test scores that were analyzed. Whenever this condition exists, the results are often unstable and cannot be generalized. That is, when sample sizes are small, there is great risk that individual tests will "load" on (correlate with) a given factor purely by chance. Had she replicated any of these studies, it is very likely that the patterns of factor loadings would have varied considerably. Therefore, in retrospect, a preferable approach might have been to use confirmatory factor-analytic techniques to "confirm" the existence of hypothesized constructs (factors) rather than to use exploratory factor-analytic techniques to "explore" her data for unknown underlying constructs. However, these limitations did not lessen the impact the studies had on the development of sensory integration theory; conservative interpretation of the results revealed reasonably consistent patterns of dysfunction that were represented by somewhat different individual test scores over time (see Fig. 1–2).

## AN EMERGING VIEW OF SENSORY INTEGRATION THEORY

These initial factor and cluster analyses of the SIPT marked a major step in the evolution of sensory integration theory. While many of the pattern labels appeared to differ from those that emerged from the earlier factor-analytic studies, we believe that this initial SIPT data generally expanded upon, and further clarified, the patterns identified through earlier research. For example, the earlier studies identified a vestibular bilateral integration disorder. The SIPT data indicate that the ability to plan and execute sequenced movements also is associated with bilateral integration. While the term "vestibular" was dropped from the pattern label, central vestibular-proprioceptive processing deficits continue to be hypothesized as the basis for some disorders in bilateral integration. However, by separating vestibular-proprioceptive disorders from bilateral integration and sequencing disorders, it is clearer that each can occur in isolation from the other. Thus, it is important that we recognize that these SIPT analyses add to, and build on, previous knowledge, rather than negate earlier findings.

Table 1–1 is a summary of the most recently hypothesized patterns of sensory integrative dysfunction that will be discussed in subsequent chapters. Included in Table 1–1 are not only the patterns of dysfunction, but also the components of the patterns, the hypothesized nature of the dysfunction, and the methods of evaluating for the presence of each pattern. We recognize that many readers may not yet be familiar with the SIPT or with the clinical evaluation procedures that are used in combination with the SIPT to identify disorders of sensory integration. We introduce the test names in order to begin to familiarize the reader with them. Where it is important that the reader understand the behavior or skill being assessed, we have described that behavior. Individuals interested in more information about these assessments are referred to the respective chapter (Table 1–1).

Some of the patterns in Table 1–1 (e.g., vestibular-proprioceptive, and especially sensory defensiveness) did not emerge from the SIPT data as the SIPT either do not provide a basis for evaluating the pattern, or do not include an adequate

**TABLE 1–1. HYPOTHESIZED PATTERNS OF DYSFUNCTION IDENTIFIED BY THE SENSORY INTEGRATION AND PRAXIS TESTS AND RELATED CLINICAL OBSERVATIONS**

| Pattern (Chapter) | Hypothesized Dysfunction | Components | Evaluations |
|---|---|---|---|
| Postural-ocular movements (Chapter 4) | Central processing of vestibular and proprioceptive inputs | Vestibular-ocular Vestibular-spinal | Postrotary Nystagmus Standing and Walking Balance Clinical observation of postural responses (e.g., balance, prone extension, muscle tone) Interview (balance, awareness of body movement and position in space) |
| | | Proprioception | Kinesthesia Standing and Walking Balance Clinical observation of postural responses (see above) Interview (see above) |
| Somatosensory (Chapter 5) | Central processing of tactile (and possibly proprioceptive) inputs | Tactile discrimination | Localization of Tactile Stimuli Graphesthesia Finger Identification Manual Form Perception |
| | | Proprioception | Kinesthesia Standing and Walking Balance (*Note*: The somatosensory pattern requires that tactile test scores be low with or without low scores on Kinesthesia and Standing and Walking Balance. When several postural responses are low, the vestibular-proprioceptive pattern is considered.) |
| Sensory modulation (Chapters 4 and 5) | Central processing of vestibular and proprioceptive inputs | Gravitational insecurity Aversive response to movement | Interview (fear or aversive response to movement) Clinical observation of fear or aversive response to movement |
| | Central processing of tactile inputs | Tactile defensiveness | Interview (aversive response to touch) Clinical observation of aversive response to touch |
| | Limbic system and/or reticular formation | Sensory defensiveness | Clinical observation of aversive or fearful response to touch, sound, movement, etc. Interview (aversive or fearful responses to sensory stimuli) |
| Bilateral integration and sequencing (Chapter 4) | Vestibular-proprioceptive inputs to higher level structures, including the supplementary motor area | Bilateral integration | Bilateral Motor Coordination Space Visualization Contralateral and Preferred Hand Use Clinical observation of bilateral coordination, midline crossing, right-left confusion |
| | (*Note*: When concurrent evidence of a vestibular-proprioceptive disorder is *not present*, cortical dysfunction should considered.) | Sequencing and projected or anticipatory movements | Sequencing Praxis Standing and Walking Balance Graphesthesia Oral Praxis Possibly, Postural Praxis Clinical observation of sequencing and projected movements |

(continued)

TABLE 1–1. HYPOTHESIZED PATTERNS OF DYSFUNCTION IDENTIFIED BY THE
SENSORY INTEGRATION AND PRAXIS TESTS AND RELATED CLINICAL OBSERVATIONS
(continued)

| Pattern (Chapter) | Hypothesized Dysfunction | Components | Evaluations |
|---|---|---|---|
| Somatopraxis (Chapter 6) | Tactile (and sometimes vestibular-proprioceptive) inputs to higher level structures, including the premotor areas (*Note*: When concurrent evidence of a somatosensory or vestibular-proprioceptive disorder is *not present*, cortical dysfunction should be considered.) | General motor planning, including sequencing and projected or anticipatory movements | Postural Praxis Bilateral Motor Coordination Sequencing Praxis Standing and Walking Balance Graphesthesia Oral Praxis Possible, Praxis on Verbal Command Clinical observation of supine flexion, and motor skill |
| Praxis on verbal command (Chapter 7) | Left hemisphere (*Note*: This is not considered a sensory integrative disorder.) | Auditory or language processing Motor planning bilateral and projected movements | Praxis on Verbal Command Postrotary Nystagmus (prolonged) Bilateral Motor Coordination Sequencing Praxis Standing and Walking Balance Oral Praxis |
| Visuopraxis (Chapter 7) (*Note*: This pattern is composed of three overlapping subpatterns. It is *not* a disorder of praxis.) | End product (*Note*: When concurrent evidence of a somatosensory or vestibular-proprioceptive disorder is *not present*, right, and sometimes left, hemisphere dysfunction is considered.) | Form and space perception Visuomotor coordination Visual construction | Space Visualization Figure-Ground Perception Constructional Praxis Design Copying Manual Form Perception Related visual perception test scores Motor Accuracy Design Copying Clinical observation of visuomotor skills Design Copying Constructional Praxis Clinical observation of two- and three-dimension construction |

number of assessments to determine definitively whether the pattern is present.
Also, we did not include generalized sensory integrative dysfunction in Table 1–1.
Upon careful analysis of the test scores of children in the generalized sensory
integrative dysfunction group, Ayres (1989) found that most have patterns that are
not clearly delineated as a distinct pattern of dysfunction. Rather, their test scores
vary and commonly reflect some combination of the other, more distinct, patterns
(Ayres, 1989).

## Theoretical Constructs

These patterns of dysfunction represent theoretical constructs that are operationally defined by groups of test scores that tend to correlate (factors). They are referred to as "meaningful clusters" of test scores when the emerging pattern is supported by the neurobiological and behavioral literature. (These meaningful clusters of test scores should not be confused with the SIPT cluster groups that represent groups of individuals rather than test scores.) *Constructs* are theoretical concepts that are indirectly observed or inferred from test performance and clinical observations. Examples of sensory integration constructs that only are indirectly observable include somatosensory perception, bilateral integration, and tactile defensiveness. At an even higher level on the continuum are the highly abstract constructs that can only be inferred. For example, we are unable to directly or indirectly observe sensory integration, inner drive, or learning (see Fig. 1–3).

When research suggests a correlation between two or more constructs, a relationship between those constructs may be hypothesized. However, a correlation does not determine or prove that one construct is the basis or cause of the other construct; *theoretical causal relationships are hypothesized* based on existing knowledge. Ayres reviewed the neurobiological and psychological research that provides the basis for theories of human behavior. When her review of the literature supported the probability of a causal relationship, Ayres postulated a cause-effect relationship between constructs. An example of a postulated relationship is: somatosensory processing contributes to motor planning. Another postulated relationship is: vestibular-proprioceptive functioning is a prerequisite for the development of bilateral integration and sequencing.

The patterns and hypothesized bases of dysfunction summarized in Table 1–1 are based only in part on the empirical evidence of a relationship. These hypothe-

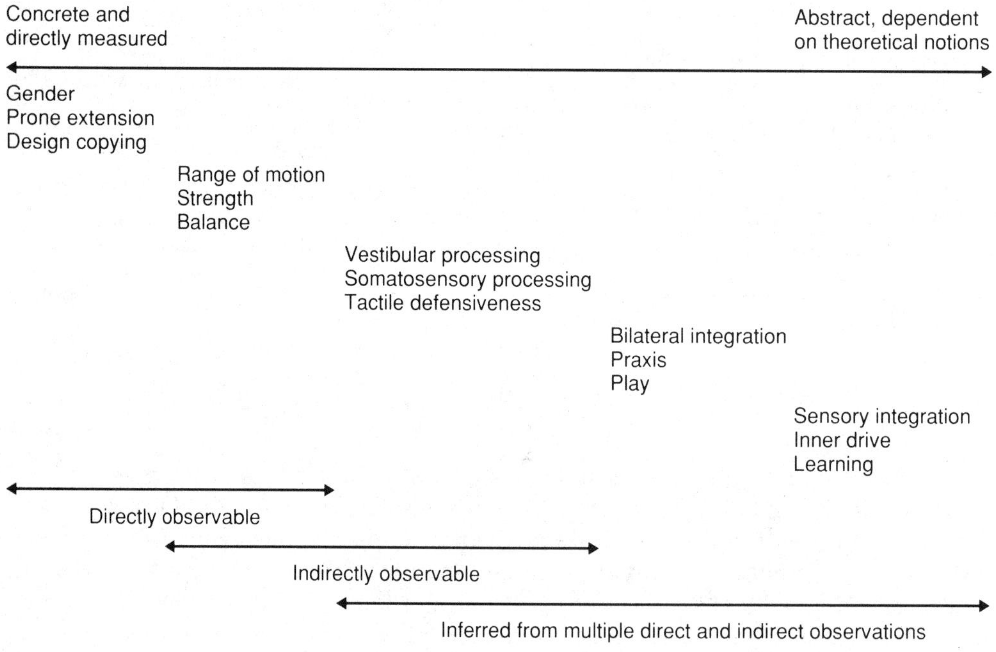

FIGURE 1–3. Continuum of complexity of theoretical concepts in sensory integration.

sized relationships between constructs are also derived from the basic assumptions of sensory integration theory.

## Assumptions of Sensory Integration Theory

As indicated above, sensory integration theory has three major, overarching postulates. The first major postulate specifies that normal individuals take in sensory information derived from the environment and from movement of their bodies, process and integrate these sensory inputs within the central nervous system, and use this sensory information to plan and organize behavior. The second postulate specifies that deficits in integrating sensory inputs result in deficits in conceptual and motor learning. The third major postulate guides intervention and specifies that provision of enhanced sensory experiences, provided within the context of a meaningful activity and the planning and production of an adaptive behavior, results in enhanced sensory integration, and in turn, enhanced learning.

A number of assumptions underlie each of these three major postulates of sensory integration theory. Some of these assumptions relate to the neural basis of sensory integration; others relate to the behavioral aspects of sensory integration.

*Assumption 1: Neural Plasticity.* Intervention procedures derived from sensory integration theory are hypothesized to effect changes in the brain. This is based on the assumption of sensory integration theory that there is *plasticity within the central nervous system.* Plasticity refers to the ability of brain structure to change or to be modified. This assumption, which is central to the theoretical basis of sensory integration intervention programs, makes it feasible to speculate that enhancement of the function of the nervous system is possible through the provision of controlled tactile, vestibular, and proprioceptive sensory inputs and the circular process shown in Figure 1–1.

According to Ayres (1989), the extent to which organism-environment interaction promotes development through intervention is dependent, in part, on the inherent plasticity of the brain.

> The brain, especially the young brain, is naturally malleable; structure and function become more firm and set with age. The formative capacity allows person-environment interaction to promote and enhance neurointegrative efficiency. A deficiency in the individual's ability to engage effectively in this transaction at critical periods interferes with optimal brain development and consequent overall ability. Identifying the deficient areas at a young age and addressing them therapeutically can enhance the individual's opportunity for normal development. (Ayres, 1989, p. 12)

Ayres consistently stressed the structural and behavioral aspects of plasticity of the young brain. In earlier writings, she assumed that a critical period for normal development of sensory integration is between 3 to 7 years of age (Ayres, 1979). Unfortunately, this has been incorrectly interpreted by some to mean that individuals older than 8 years of age can no longer benefit from sensory integration treatment procedures. Our experience in treating older children and adult clients with sensory integration dysfunction clearly indicates that these individuals have the potential for significant change, and experimental brain research indicates that plasticity persists into adulthood and possibly throughout life. Further, there is, as yet, no evidence that younger children with sensory integration disorders benefit more or change faster than do older children or adults who participate in sensory integration treatment programs.

In their critique of sensory integration theory, Ottenbacher and Short (1985) note that "recent environmental enrichment studies now indicate that brain alterations do occur in mature organisms and even in geriatric organisms" (p. 302). However, they also differentiate between plasticity (i.e., structural or morphological change), and learning (functional or "adaptive change in behavior as a result of experience") (p. 300). Behavioral change does not necessarily indicate a specific change in neural structure, and future research may lead to modification of the theory.

*Assumption 2: Developmental Sequence.* A second major assumption is that *the sensory integrative process occurs in a developmental sequence.* In normal development, increasingly complex behaviors develop as a result of the circular process, and behaviors present at each stage in the sequence provide, in turn, the basis for the development of more complex behaviors. When sensory integration dysfunction occurs, the circular process that leads to the normal development of sensory integration function is disrupted.

> Sensory integration theory assumes that the brain is immature at birth and also is immature [or dysfunctional] in some individuals with learning problems. Treatment for these individuals is aimed at recapitulating normal neuromotor development by providing therapeutic sensory and motor experiences. The goal of sensory integration therapy is to provide stimulation that will address certain brain levels (primarily subcortical), enabling them to mature [or function more normally], and thereby assisting the brain to work as an integrated whole. (Short-DeGraff, 1988, p. 200)

It should be noted that late in her career, Ayres rejected the earlier assumption of sensory integration theory that ontogeny recapitulates phylogeny, stating that placing so much emphasis on recapitulation has led to misunderstanding and to a narrow view of brain-behavior relationships (A. J. Ayres, personal communication, June 13, 1988).

*Assumption 3: Nervous System Hierarchy.* Closely related is the assumption that *the brain functions as an integrated whole, but is comprised of systems that are hierarchically organized.* Ayres consistently stressed the idea that the brain functions as a whole, but that "higher-level" integrative functions evolved from, and are dependent on, the integrity of "lower-level" structures and on sensorimotor experience. Higher (cortical) centers of the brain were viewed as those that are responsible for abstraction, perception, reasoning, language, and learning. Sensory intake, integration, and intersensory association, in contrast, were viewed as occurring mainly within lower (subcortical) centers. Further, lower parts of the brain were conceptualized as developing and maturing before higher-level structures; development and optimal functioning of higher-level structures were thought to be dependent, in part, on the development and optimal functioning of lower-level structures (Ayres, 1972b, 1974/1968a, 1974/1968b, 1975a, 1979, 1989).

Sensory integration theory has been criticized because of the inclusion of hierarchical concepts (Ottenbacher & Short, 1985; Short-DeGraff, 1988). However, as Short-DeGraff (1988) pointed out, Ayres incorporated both holistic and hierarchical concepts into her theory. Ayres used hierarchical concepts to facilitate communication of difficult ideas and as a guide for treatment; however, she never lost sight of the holistic, systems view of the brain. Unfortunately, the use of hierarchical concepts has led to an overemphasis on linear or reductionistic thinking when describing sensory integration theory and practice.

Thus, we propose that greater emphasis be placed on a *systems view* of the nervous system. In this view, Ayres' concept of an interactive, wholistic hierarchy is retained. According to Pribram (1986), "the essence of biological . . . hierarchies is that higher levels of organization take control over, as well as being controlled by, lower levels. Such reciprocal causation" (p. 507) exists throughout brain structures. This concept of simultaneous causation is expanded further in Chapter 2.

When children demonstrate evidence of inadequate central processing of sensory inputs, we suggest that it is most appropriate to think in terms of one or more systems not functioning optimally. This view includes the recognition that systems interact, and that both cortical and subcortical structures contribute to sensory integration. It also assumes that both *the person and the nervous system are open systems*. An open system is one that is composed of interrelated structures and functions that are organized into a coherent whole. An open system is also capable of self-regulating, self-organizing, and changing itself through the circular process shown in Figure 1–1. In this circular process, the action of the system (adaptive behavior, output, or interaction with the environment) becomes the cause (feedback and intake) of system change (cf. Kielhofner, 1985).

*Assumption 4: Adaptive Behavior.* Another assumption of sensory integration theory is that *evincing an adaptive behavior promotes sensory integration, and, in turn, the ability to produce an adaptive behavior reflects sensory integration.* While this assumption may appear to reflect circular logic, we propose that it represents a spiraling process of behavioral or sensorimotor change which occurs through the process of circularity, and which is characteristic of the open system. An adaptive behavior is one that is purposeful and goal-directed. It is a behavior that enables the individual to successfully meet the "just right" challenge and learn something new (Ayres, 1972b, 1979, 1985). Part of what is learned are new and more complex movements (Brooks, 1986). New movements, in turn, produce new forms of feedback.

More specifically, we learn movements from past experience only if we recognize that the prior movements were successful. Knowledge of success is presumed to be provided by the sensory feedback derived from the *production* and the *outcome* of the adaptive behavior. Active movement of one's own body produces vestibular-proprioceptive sensations (*production feedback*) that are organized within the brain and are believed to provide the basis for the development of neuronal models or memories of "how it feels" to move. Similarly, knowledge of the outcome of the adaptive behavior provides the basis for developing neuronal models or memories of "what is achieved" (*outcome feedback*) (Brooks, 1986). These neuronal models are then used as a basis for planning more complex movements. Active participation is a critical component. "Learning from previous experience thus depends on sensing and moving, not just on sensing" (Brooks, 1986, p. 14). Finally, we can speculate that the actual performance of increasingly complex movements indicates that new neuronal models have been developed.

*Assumption 5: Inner Drive.* The final assumption is that *people have an inner drive to develop sensory integration through participation in sensorimotor activities* (Ayres, 1979). While Ayres (1972b, 1975b, 1979, 1989) stressed the importance of inner drive to sensory integration and sensorimotor development, her discussion failed to clearly articulate the relationships among them. Ayres, however, did link inner drive and motivation to self-direction (self-guiding), and self-actualization (achieving). She indicated that children with sensory integrative dysfunction often show little motivation or inner drive to be active participants in their environment, to try new experiences, or to meet new challenges. Reciprocally, the improvement demonstrated by these children first appears in their improved belief in their own abilities, and in the satisfaction that they begin to find with mastery of the environment. According to Ayres, inner drive can be seen in the excitement, confidence, and effort that a child brings to an activity. Again, she implied that the circular process leads to a stronger inner drive to seek out self-actualizing or growth-promoting activities that in turn provide feedback that will enhance sensory intake and integration (Ayres, 1972b).

## THE SPIRAL PROCESS OF SELF-ACTUALIZATION: A NEW CONCEPTUAL MODEL OF SENSORY INTEGRATION

While Ayres' definition of sensory integration may seem deceptively simple, the theory of sensory integration is quite complex. Ayres also has been criticized for circularity and lack of clarity in some of her writings (Ottenbacher & Short, 1985). The following is an example of such circularity.

> An adaptive response is a purposeful, goal-directed response to a sensory experience. . . . In an adaptive response, we master a challenge and learn something new. At the same time, the formation of an adaptive response helps the brain to develop and organize itself. Most adults see this as merely play. However, play consists of the adaptive responses that make sensory integration happen. . . .
> When the sensory integrative capacity of the brain is sufficient to meet the demands of the environment, the child's response is efficient, creative, and satisfying. When the child experiences challenges to which he can respond effectively, he "has fun." To some extent, "fun" is the child's word for sensory integration. (Ayres, 1979, pp. 6–7)

We believe that, in part, the apparent circularity or lack of clarity in Ayres' writings reflects her early use of linear models to depict an open-system circular process (Ayres, 1976, 1979). To our knowledge, Ayres never actually used the term *open system* to refer to either the human organism or the nervous system. However, as we discussed earlier, her underlying assumptions regarding the sensory integration process not only are consistent with such a view, they require the adoption of such a view.

Based on our review and synthesis of Ayres' writings, we propose a new conceptual model of sensory integration that we call the *spiral process of self-actualization*. Consistent with the complexity of the theory, subspirals or feedback loops are embedded within the greater spiral process of self-actualization (Fig. 1–4). These feedback loops allow the open system to regulate and organize itself through the circular process. In proposing this model, we believe that we are reflecting Ayres' most recent thinking. However, we recognize that this model represents our interpretation of her work in light of current theory and research related to human behavior. It also incorporates contemporary systems theories that were not readily available when she was developing her theory. Undoubtedly, our interpretation also is influenced by our own clinical experience and professional knowledge.

An important component of this model is the inclusion of behavioral as well as neurobiological components. Although Ayres emphasized the neurobiological basis of sensory integration, she was clearly concerned about occupational behavior and the "well-being" of the children she treated. As early as 1972, Ayres talked about a self-actualizing process in which the ability to interact effectively with the environment is a necessary prerequisite for the successful and satisfying participation in daily life activities and, in turn, is dependent on the ability of the brain to process and effectively integrate sensory information. Play, self-esteem, and a sense of mas-

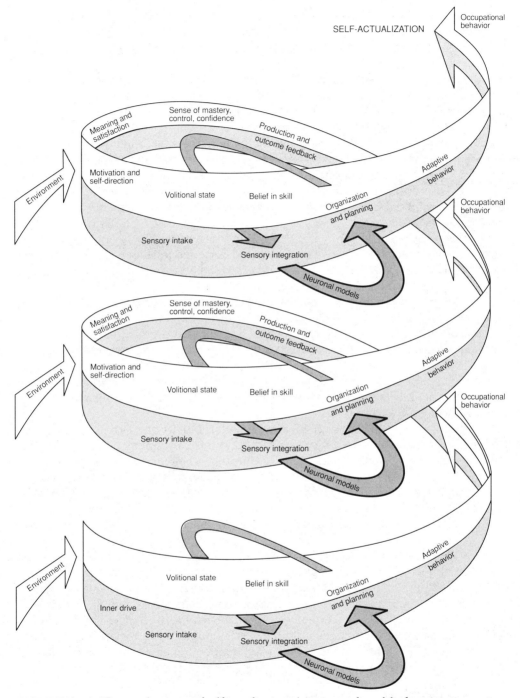

FIGURE 1–4. The spiral process of self-actualization: A conceptual model of sensory integration.

tery are among the behavioral components of the self-actualization process that she discussed in her writings (Ayres, 1972b, 1975a, 1979, 1985, 1989).

Because we recognize that some of the lack of clarity in Ayres' writings may have been due to her tendency to discuss assumptions pertaining to the three postulates (i.e., normal development, dysfunction, and intervention) within the same discussion, we have chosen to confine our presentation to the normal sensory integrative process. However, in so doing, we stress that there are parallel models that reflect the hypothesized *spiral process of dysfunction* and the hypothesized *spiral process of intervention.*

Because the spiral process of self-actualization is continuous, we must enter and begin to describe the process at some relatively arbitrary point. Therefore, we begin with *inner drive* and a subspiral that reflects the circular process shown in Figure 1–1 and that is represented by a medium-shaded line in Figure 1–4. Inner drive provides the impetus to actively seek out, and participate in, the sensorimotor activities that provide the opportunities for *sensory intake.* We have used the term *intake* rather than the more traditional term *input* because the taking in of sensory information, whether that information is derived from the environment or from the body, is an active process. In fact, the availability of sensory information does not ensure that the individual takes in the sensory information that is available. Further, *sensory integration* must occur. That is, the central nervous system must actively process, organize, and modulate sensory inputs from the body and the environment. A normal sensory integrative process implies an *organized and appropriate response* to sensory intake (i.e., an absence of hypo- or hyperresponsiveness).

There are many sources of sensory intake. Already discussed are (a) *production feedback*, which arises from the body and informs us about how it feels to move, and (b) *outcome feedback*, which arises when our actions produce a change in the external environment. Another source of sensory intake is the sensory stimuli derived from the physical and social environment. When we implement treatment programs that provide new opportunities for controlled sensory intake, we are intervening at this level. This important source of intake is represented by the arrows labeled *Environment.*

Further, active participation in a meaningful activity, and the planning and production of an adaptive behavior, are central to this conceptual model. *Meaningful* is defined as having significance, value, or purpose, when viewed from the perspective of the client; the term connotes the requirement of active interpretation of sensory information. In order for an activity to be meaningful, the client must be in control of, and be able to make sense of or interpret, the sensory experience. Therefore, whether or not an activity is meaningful depends on what the client experiences.

*Adaptive* implies that change has occurred in order for the individual to meet the demands of new or changing conditions in the environment so as to function more effectively within it. Finally, *behavior* is the output of the human open system and is an action or change in relation to the environmental change or stimuli. Behavior is what we can observe, what we evaluate, and what we hope to change. The commonly used term "adaptive response" is limited as it implies an automatic response to sensory intake. The term *adaptive behavior* is broader and allows for an individual to choose freely from among several effective strategies. An adaptive behavior

> is not an automatic or passive response to the environment. Before the system
> intakes information it must have a reason for doing so. Thus, the built-in, or
> acquired, purposes or goals of the system are critical. (Kielhofner, 1985, p. 7)

Adaptive behaviors, which may include both component postural and motor skills as well as complex conceptual or cognitive skills, must be organized and planned. Underlying both is the ability to conceptualize. The adaptive behaviors that we are most often interested in require motor planning. *Motor planning* or praxis involves

> conceptualization, planning, and execution of skilled adaptive interaction with the physical world. Praxis is the ability by which an individual figures out how to use his or her hands and body in skilled tasks like playing with toys, using tools (including a pencil or fork), building a structure (whether a toy block tower or a house), straightening up a room, or engaging in many occupations. Practicability includes knowing what to do as well as how to do it. (Ayres, 1989, p. 11)

Knowing "what to do" and organize "how to do it" refers to the *neuronal models* or memories that are used to plan new and more complex adaptive behaviors. Since these neuronal models of the body (body scheme) are hypothesized to develop as a result of the sensory feedback derived from the planning, the active performance (production), and the outcome of an adaptive behavior, production and outcome feedback are important for learning new skills. We cannot plan actions that are not yet learned. However, once a neuronal model of an action is developed, it can be used to plan new, more complex behaviors. Thus, we add a second loop (Figure 1–4, dark line) to our conceptual model. Production and outcome feedback provide a source of sensory intake that, once integrated, is used to develop these important neuronal models used in motor planning.

The final subspiral (Figure 1–4, white line), which parallels the first (medium-shaded) subspiral, reflects the core assumption of occupational therapy that humans have an occupational nature, and places sensory integration within the greater context of occupational science. The development of adaptive behavior is thought to be basic to *occupational behavior*. A core assumption of occupational science is that humans have an innate inner drive or need to participate in occupation. Further, the human occupations of play or leisure, school or work, and self-maintenance are intrinsically motivating, and the need for occupation is manifested by our mastery and achievement motives. In turn, we achieve *meaning* and *satisfaction* through feedback from participation in occupation (Kielhofner, in press). Thus, stimuli for planning and organizing adaptive behaviors include not only sensory intake, but also such volitional factors as *motivation* and *self-direction* for improvement.

White (1959) also hypothesized that children have an inner drive to master their environments, and that this drive can be observed in their play. A major format in which the child elicits adaptive behaviors is through participation in the occupation of play. When the play experience results in successfully meeting the "just right challenge," the child develops a *sense of confidence, sense of self-control,* and a *sense of mastery* that, in turn, provide meaning and satisfaction.

Csikszentmihalyi (1979) developed a model to explain intrinsic motivation or reward associated with play which appears to explain the significance of the "just right challenge." He hypothesized, based on his study of adolescent and adult play, that individuals seek challenges that are matched to their abilities. When an activity is too easy, the individual becomes bored. When the challenge is too great, the individual becomes worried. When the mismatch between personal ability and activity challenge becomes extreme, boredom and worry are replaced by anxiety. However, when the challenge level of the activity matches the skill of the individual, "flow" occurs. "Any activity that produces flow reliably helps people to *focus attention . . .,* and to establish a *feeling of control*" (p. 261).

Adaptiveness implies mastery over the environment rather than mastery of the person by the environment. When the individual feels in control of the environment, the locus of control is internal, within the individual, rather than external. The person who develops this sense of mastery also develops belief in his or her own abilities; that is, *belief in skill.* The realization of having the ability to do something enables one to become self-directing, and the individual becomes motivated to explore his or her capacity through the planning and production of adaptive behaviors, and the participation in meaningful occupation.

In summary, we hypothesize that through the spiral process of self-actualization, sensory integration and the corresponding adaptive behaviors lead to organized and appropriate occupational behavior, including self-care and self-management, play, and academic skills. As a child develops control over the environment and belief in his or her own skills, interaction with the environment becomes more meaningful and satisfying. To Ayres (1979), meaning and satisfaction are derived from the experience of moving and interacting effectively with the environment; she did not address the meaningfulness of activity per se. Rather, she believed that the child who is able to explore his or her own capacity through effective interaction with the environment derives meaning and satisfaction from organizing sensations from the body and the environment, and responding to them with an adaptive behavior.

Finally, *volition* is an important prerequisite for evincing an adaptive behavior. Evincing an adaptive behavior "requires effort — the kind of effort that a child gladly summons when he is emotionally involved in the task and believes he can cope with it" (Ayres, 1972b, p. 127).

## BOUNDARIES OF SENSORY INTEGRATION THEORY AND PRACTICE

Sensory integrative dysfunction is a developmental disorder that is hypothesized to result in disruption of the spiral process of self-actualization. While many other disorders also may disrupt this spiral process, sensory integration theory is intended to explain mild-to-moderate problems in learning and behavior in children, especially those problems associated with motor incoordination and poor sensory processing that cannot be attributed to frank central nervous system damage or abnormalities. Ayres hypothesized, based on clinical evidence of poor tactile discrimination or vestibular-proprioceptive mediated postural responses, that the deficits were related to central processing of sensory inputs. The theory is not intended to explain the neuromotor deficits associated with such problems as cerebral palsy (e.g., spasticity), Down syndrome (e.g., hypotonicity), or stroke (e.g., decreased tactile perception). Furthermore, the diagnosis of sensory integrative dysfunction requires that evidence of the hypothesized underlying basis (deficits in the *central* processing of vestibular, proprioceptive, or tactile sensory inputs) be present, and similarly, not attributable to either peripheral or cortical central nervous system dysfunction.

While the major focus of sensory integration theory is on young children, the theory is also applicable to adults who continue to demonstrate the manifestations of sensory integrative dysfunction that were present during childhood. However, the theory is not meant to explain adult-onset dysfunction. In fact, it is unlikely that an older person with an adult-onset learning, behavior, or neurological problem (e.g., dementia, cerebral vascular accident, schizophrenia) would have sensory integrative dysfunction unless that individual had sensory integrative problems as a child.

Similarly, children with mental retardation, cerebral palsy, or other developmental disorders attributable to frank central nervous system pathology may have concomitant deficits in sensory integration. One must always consider the possibility, however, that both their impairments in sensory processing and their motor deficits, including dyspraxia, can be attributed to the frank brain pathology. For example, children with severe hearing loss or children with Down's syndrome often have depressed postrotary nystagmus, hypotonicity, poor proximal joint stability, poor equilibrium, and difficulty extending against gravity to assume the prone extension posture. As will be discussed in Chapter 4, this cluster of symptoms is suggestive of deficits in central processing of vestibular-proprioceptive inputs. However, in the case of children with severe hearing loss, the problem can be attributed to damage to the eighth cranial nerve (i.e., peripheral damage). In children with Down's syndrome, the problem can be attributed to abnormalities of the cerebellum. In both cases, the problem probably is not due to deficits in integrating the sensory inputs per se.

While the boundaries of sensory integration theory previously have been clearly articulated (Ayres, 1972b, 1975a, 1979), there are many instances in the literature where these boundaries may have been exceeded (cf. Arendt, MacLean, & Baumeister, 1988; Bonder & Fisher, 1989; Densem et al., 1989). A similar problem exists in the SIPT manual (Ayres, 1989). Ayres used data from groups of children with known central nervous system disorders (i.e., cerebral palsy, mental retardation, spina bifida, brain injury, and, possibly, autism) to demonstrate that the SIPT were valid assessments of sensorimotor behavior. She also implied, however, that some of the sensorimotor deficits seen in these children reflect poor sensory integrative functioning. For example, in referring to 10 tested children with cerebral palsy, Ayres stated that

> the scores on Standing and Walking Balance (SWB), Motor Accuracy (MAc), and possibly Design Copying (DC) must be considered depressed by the neuromotor incoordination typical of cerebral palsy. This group as a whole has trouble with both visuopraxis and somatopraxis. Poor tactile perception is associated with the dyspraxia. (p. 210)

We feel that it is unfortunate that Ayres (1989) did not explicitly state that the praxis and tactile perception deficits were most likely attributed to the higher-level brain damage characteristic of children with cerebral palsy rather than indicative of impaired sensory integration (see also Chapter 8).

Boundaries also pertain to the treatment techniques and contexts (e.g., clinic, school) of clinical practice. *Sensory integration treatment techniques* involve the use of enhanced, controlled sensory stimulation in the context of a meaningful, self-directed activity in order to elicit an adaptive behavior. The emphasis is on the integration of vestibular-proprioceptive and tactile sensory input, and not just on the motor response. Thus, "an essential feature of sensory integrative procedures is the elaborate array of suspended equipment that can be used to provide potent and varied types of vestibular stimulation" (Clark, Mailloux, & Parham, 1989, p. 502).

Many of the treatment programs described in the occupational therapy literature and referred to as sensory integration probably are more appropriately referred to as sensorimotor, sensory stimulation, or perceptual motor approaches. *Sensorimotor* approaches emphasize the application of specific sensory stimulation through handling or direct stimulation with the purpose of eliciting a desired motor response (e.g., altered muscle tone, movement). In contrast, *sensory stimulation* involves the application of direct sensory stimulation (olfactory, touch pressure, vestibular, visual, and so forth) with the purpose of eliciting a more generalized behavioral response such as increased attention or arousal, calming or decreased heart rate, or minimized depression. Sensory stimulation is a component of both sensorimotor and sensory integration treatment, but in itself, it cannot be considered to be either. *Perceptual motor* activities are more cognitive than are the approaches described above, in that attention is focused on the coordinated execution of the task to be performed. Specific programs are designed so that the client can practice the skill to be learned (cf. Bonder & Fisher, 1989; Clark et al., 1989).

Moreover, some occupational therapists have found that specific sensory integration treatment procedures are beneficial for treating sensorimotor deficits in individuals whose problems cannot be attributed to deficits in sensory integration. For example, linear vestibular stimulation, provided by swinging on a suspended platform glider, might be used to affect the muscle tone in a child with cerebral palsy. In this instance, it is important to differentiate between a *sensory integration treatment program*, and a *sensorimotor treatment program into which sensory integration treatment procedures have been incorporated.* A major differentiating characteristic is the hypothesized goal of therapy: normalized muscle tone in a client with frank central nervous system pathology vs. improved ability to process and integrate sensory intake. Integrated approaches to treatment are discussed in more detail in Chapter 13.

We feel that it is important for occupational therapists to be explicit about the approach they used in treatment whenever reporting the results of their intervention programs. Moreover, when a theory, or its derived evaluation and intervention technology, are applied outside the circumstances of expected application, the therapist must recognize that the boundaries of the theory have been exceeded and that there is a need to apply the theory with caution.

## SUMMARY AND CONCLUSIONS

In this chapter we have presented an overview of the history of the development of sensory integration theory and practice, and our current perspectives of sensory integration theory. In this process, we have attempted to place sensory integration within the greater context of occupational therapy. Members of all helping professions share with us a common concern with functional independence. What makes occupational therapists unique is our emphasis on the process of "doing" occupational behavior. The term *praxis*, derived from the Greek, is more than motor planning; *praxis means doing.* Thus, it can serve to remind us that our primary concern is not sensory integration, but whether or not the clients we evaluate and treat are able to "do" what they need and want to "do."

The remaining chapters in Part I will expand on these important relationships between sensory integration, volition, and occupational behavior. The concept of volition as a model of mind in mind-brain-body relationships will be developed further in Chapter 2. Play, a major occupation of children, is both a context and an outcome of sensory integration treatment procedures. The relationship between play and sensory integration theory and practice will be the focus of Chapter 3.

We also initiated a process of critical analysis of sensory integration theory. Theory is provisional. As the results of additional research are disseminated and new perspectives or postulates formulated, each must be evaluated in relation to existing theory. Thus, critical analysis of sensory integration theory and practice should remain an ongoing process. The reader is encouraged to begin his or her own process of critical analysis of sensory integration theory as he or she reads the subsequent chapters of this book.

# REFERENCES

Arendt, R. E., MacLean, W. E., & Baumeister, A. A. (1988). Critique of sensory integration therapy and its application in mental retardation. *American Journal on Mental Retardation, 92,* 401–411.

Ayres, A. J. (1964). Tactile functions: Their relation to hyperactive and perceptual motor behavior. *American Journal of Occupational Therapy, 18,* 83–95.

Ayres, A. J. (1965). Patterns of perceptual-motor dysfunction in children: A factor analytic study. *Perceptual and Motor Skills, 20,* 335–368.

Ayres, A. J. (1966a). Interrelations among perceptual-motor abilities in a group of normal children. *American Journal of Occupational Therapy, 20,* 288–292.

Ayres, A. J. (1966b). Interrelationships among perceptual-motor functions in children. *American Journal of Occupational Therapy, 20,* 288–292.

Ayres, A. J. (1969). Deficits in sensory integration in educationally handicapped children. *Journal of Learning Disabilities, 2,* 160–168.

Ayres, A. J. (1972a). Improving academic scores through sensory integration. *Journal of Learning Disabilities, 5,* 338–343.

Ayres, A. J. (1972b). *Sensory integration and learning disorders.* Los Angeles: Western Psychological Services.

Ayres, A. J. (1972c). *Southern California Sensory Integration Tests manual.* Los Angeles: Western Psychological Services.

Ayres, A. J. (1972d). Types of sensory integrative dysfunction among disabled learners. *American Journal of Occupational Therapy, 26,* 13–18.

Ayres, A. J. (1974a). Reading—A product of sensory integrative processes. In A. Henderson, L. Llorens, E. Gilfoyle, C. Myers, & S. Prevel (Eds.), *The development of sensory integrative theory and practice: A collection of the work of A. Jean Ayres* (pp. 167–175). Dubuque, IA: Kendall/Hunt. (Original work published 1968).

Ayres, A. J. (1974b). Sensory integrative processes in neuropsychological learning disability. In A. Henderson, L. Llorens, E. Gilfoyle, C. Myers, & S. Prevel (Eds.), *The development of sensory integrative theory and practice: A collection of the work of A. Jean Ayres* (pp. 96–113). Dubuque, IA: Kendall/Hunt. (Original work published 1968)

Ayres, A. J. (1975a). Sensorimotor foundations of academic ability. In W. M. Cruickshank & D. P. Hallahan, *Perceptual and Learning Disabilities in Children: Vol. 2* (pp. 301–358). Syracuse, NY: Syracuse University Press.

Ayres, A. J. (1975b). *Southern California Postrotary Nystagmus Test manual.* Los Angeles: Western Psychological Services.

Ayres, A. J. (1976). *The effect of sensory integrative therapy on learning disabled children: The final report of a research project.* Los Angeles: University of Southern California.

Ayres, A. J. (1977). Cluster analyses of measures of sensory integration. *American Journal of Occupational Therapy, 31,* 362–366.

Ayres, A. J. (1978). Learning disabilities and the vestibular system. *Journal of Learning Disabilities, 11,* 18–29.

Ayres, A. J. (1979). *Sensory integration and the child.* Los Angeles: Western Psychological Services.

Ayres, A. J. (1980). *Southern California Tests of Sensory Integration Tests manual: Revised 1980.* Los Angeles: Western Psychological Services.

Ayres, A. J. (1985). *Developmental dyspraxia and adult-onset apraxia.* Torrance, CA: Sensory Integration International.

Ayres, A. J. (1989). *Sensory Integration and Praxis Tests.* Los Angeles: Western Psychological Services.

Ayres, A. J., Mailloux, Z. K., & Wendler, C. L. W. (1987). Developmental dyspraxia: Is it a unitary function? *Occupational Therapy Journal of Research, 7,* 93–110.

Bonder, B. R., & Fisher, A. G. (1989). Sensory integration and treatment of the elderly. *Gerontology Special Interest Section News, 12*(1), 2–4.

Brooks, V. B. (1986). *The neural basis of motor control.* New York: Oxford University Press.

Chinn, P. L., & Jacobs, M. K. (1987). *Theory and nursing.* St. Louis: C. V. Mosby.

Clark, F. A., Mailloux, Z., & Parham, D. (1989). Sensory integration and children with learning disabilities. In P. N. Pratt & A. S. Allen (Eds.), *Occupational therapy for children* (2nd ed., pp. 457–507). St. Louis: C. V. Mosby.

Csikszentmihalyi, M. (1979). The concept of flow. In B. Sutton-Smith (Ed.), *Play and learning* (pp. 257–274). New York: Gardner.

Densem, J. F., Nuthall, G. A., Bushnell, J. & Horn, J. (1989). Effectiveness of a sensory integrative therapy program for children with perceptual-motor deficits. *Journal of Learning Disabilities, 22,* 221–229.

Kielhofner, G. (1985). *A model of human occupation: Theory and application.* Baltimore: Williams & Wilkins.

Kielhofner, G. (in press). *Theoretical basis of occupational therapy.* Philadelphia: F. A. Davis.

Ottenbacher, K., & Short M. A. (1985). Sensory integrative dysfunction in children: A review of theory and treatment. In D. Routh & M. Wolrich (Eds.), *Advances in developmental and behavioral pediatrics* (Vol. 6, pp. 287–329). Greenwich, CT: JAI.

Pribram, K. H. (1986). The cognitive revolution and mind/brain issues. *American Psychologist, 41,* 507–520.

Sensory Integration International (1990). *Interpreting the Sensory Integration and Praxis Tests.* Torrance, CA: Author.

Short-DeGraff, M. A. (1988). *Human development for occupational and physical therapists.* Baltimore: Williams & Wilkins.

Sieg, K. W. (1988). A. Jean Ayres. In B. R. J. Miller, K. W. Sieg, F. M. Ludwig, S. D. Shortridge, & J. Van Deusen, *Six perspectives on theory for practice of occupational therapy* (pp. 95–142). Rockville, MD: Aspen.

Stevens, J. (1986). *Applied multivariate statistics for the social sciences.* Hillsdale, NJ: Lawrence Erlbaum.

White, R. (1959). Motivation reconsidered: The concept of competence. *Psychological Review, 66,* 297–333.

# CHAPTER 2

# Mind-Brain-Body Relationships

**Gary Kielhofner, DrPH, OTR**
**Anne G. Fisher, ScD, OTR**

*It takes no deep philosophical insight to recognize the connection between what a person does and what a person thinks he is, between what others expect of us and what they think of us.*

*Eccles & Robinson, 1985, p. 1*

Sensory integration is a complex phenomenon involving interrelationships among nervous system processes, sensorimotor behavior, and mental experience. These complex interrelationships can be observed in a normal child, Allison, when she goes to the neighborhood park, climbs onto a big swing, and begins to try to propel herself by pumping the swing. She has gotten the general idea of "how to do it" from observing older children, and she has attempted it several times before with variable results. This time Allison, as before, tries the movements she has seen other children make, extending her hips and leaning back while pulling against the chains of the swing. With each successive swing she begins slowly to feel something she had not quite felt before. The feeling is a synchrony between her movements, the force of gravity, and the trajectory of the swing. Soon she is one with the swing, with gravity, and with the movement of the swing in its pendular arc.

Underlying this feat is a complex integration of vestibular-proprioceptive, tactile, and visual information rushing to Allison's central nervous system, being integrated into meaningful patterns and emerging in her consciousness as an awareness of "how it feels" to propel oneself on this big swing and of "what is achieved" in the process (Brooks, 1986). What she feels are not only the sensations of acceleration through space and the wind on her face, but also a deep, *embodied feeling* of how the swinging is done. She experiences herself doing it, and what she feels is how it is to do it.

Allison also experiences a variety of emotions, including excitement, anxiety, and pleasure. She feels, precariously at first, in control of her body and the swing. She knows this through a self-reflective awareness of her capacity to do it. Moreover, she knows that she is doing something that her peers and parents perceive as a significant performance and she calls their attention to it. "Watch me, watch me!"

Thus, her swinging is simultaneously a richly integrated sensorimotor and psycho-social experience.

When her father asks her about the experience, she responds by saying "It was fun. I did it, I made the swing go." By this she means that it was physically pleasur-able to feel the acceleration of her body through space, and to finally achieve the sense of mastery over the swing. She also means that it was exciting to be on "the brink of danger" and yet to be in control of her body. And, finally, she means that it was fulfilling and affirming to do something "big kids" do. To Allison, these are all elements of a rich unitary experience she calls "fun."

This example illustrates the complex, but beautifully integrated experience of mind and body, mediated by the central nervous system. Human beings are both bodies with brains (the brain-body) and minds; we experience ourselves as such (Pribram, 1986). Allison is able to separate the *objects* of her experience (the big swing, gravity, leaning back while pulling against the chains of the swing, her father watching her) from the *phenomenological experience* of swinging (feelings of excite-ment and having fun, being competent and in control of her body, experiencing how it feels to swing). Beyond the conceptual separation of the objects and the experi-ence, only our theoretical and scientific systems have managed to separate mind and brain-body phenomena (Pribram, 1986).

Clearly we could describe Allison's experience in neurobehavioral terms, by carefully analyzing the rich array of sensory information available for intake, the sequence of motor actions she must plan and produce, and the need for her to monitor her adaptive motor behavior through sensory feedback. But no matter how detailed our analysis of this dimension of Allison's experience, it would still be obviously incomplete. Moreover, the same type of critique can be made of any attempt to describe Allison's experience from a purely psychological point of view.

This problem becomes even more acute when we focus on brain-behavior relationships as we attempt to explain what is involved when a child experiences sensory integrative dysfunction. Consider Joe, 9 years old, who is up to bat in a little-league practice session. Joe's brain lacks the ability to process and integrate sensory information from his body or the environment. Joe's inability to integrate sensory information seems to be related to the difficulty he experiences in planning and producing motor action sequences. As a result, his motor behavior is clumsy and his timing is off. But what does this tell us about *how or what Joe feels?*

Joe deeply wants to be able to play baseball well, but he feels extremely fright-ened as the pitcher gets ready to throw the ball. Joe knows the object of the challenge is to meet the pitched ball with the swing of his bat, but he does not know how to do it. He has little awareness of how it should feel to swing the bat and hit the ball. What he *can* feel are the eyes of his peers bearing down on him as the ball races in his direction. Joe becomes increasingly aware of an aching feeling in the pit of his stomach; his anxiety is acute and physically distressing. Joe has a deep and perva-sive feeling that he is "no good."

This emotional state manifests itself in Joe's brain as overarousal. As the ball approaches, Joe is unable to really watch it. The ball seems to disappear from his visual consciousness and he does not have an awareness of his relationship to it in time and space. He swings the bat almost in self-defense and in the vain hope that somehow it will connect with the ball. But he misses widely and the whole perform-ance has a tragicomic appearance. A chorus of jeers and laughter from his peers painfully drives home his error. And this is not a new experience for Joe. His discomfort with using his body for many of the coordinated actions required in sports is familiar to him. The harder he tries, the more difficult it seems to be to get things right. For Joe, not being able to physically execute the motor actions he wishes, and feeling uncomfortable around peers as his performance misses the mark, is a familiar and uncomfortable experience.

In Joe's case, we may speculate that inefficient brain processing is responsible for the quality of his motor performance. But, we can hardly argue that the inability of Joe's brain to process sensory information, and nothing else, caused the performance. Clearly, Joe's psychological state had something to do with how he performed. It is patently apparent that what went on as Joe performed badly was much more than just a case of poor sensory integration and uncoordinated motor behavior. Neither Joe's behavior nor his experience can be adequately captured by explanations grounded only in neuroscience. Rather, the important dimension of mental experience was also a critical part of what Joe did and felt.

Ayres (1972, 1979, 1989) clearly recognized the importance of mental factors in (a) the conceptualization, planning, and execution of adaptive behavior; (b) the *experience* of sensory integrative dysfunction; and (c) the creation of a positive therapeutic process. Her main reference to the mental aspects of the sensory integrative experience has been incorporated into the spiral process of self-actualization (Fig. 1–4) presented in Chapter 1. Ayres discussed the relationship between adequate sensory integration and the development of self-control, self-confidence, and a sense of mastery. She recognized that meaning and satisfaction are derived from effective interaction with the environment. Ayres also alluded to the *embodied sense of how it feels and what is achieved* when she discussed the importance of neuronal models of the mechanical self or body scheme in the planning and production of skilled motor behavior.

However, to Ayres, the development of a sense of mastery, meaning, satisfaction, and self-direction were the *end products* of sensory integration. Ayres only discussed the consequences of clumsiness and poor motor planning as *leading to* feelings of inadequacy and loss of control over the environment. "As young children [with sensory integrative dysfunction] they discovered that they couldn't do what their friends did, and they compared themselves unfavorably. They began to feel inferior and impotent, controlled by external forces, and bound to failure" (Ayres, 1979, p. 150). Treatment to increase motor competence was based on the principle that learning about what kind of motor actions effect intended changes in the environment provides the basis for the development of a sense of mastery. This sense of mastery was viewed as desirable because it "serves as a motivation for further efforts" (Ayres, 1972, p. 126). Thus, in the context of treatment, Ayres was concerned about the mind as secondary to the brain-processing deficit and the goals of therapy.

In fact, Ayres' strongest reference to mind was in what she referred to as the *art* of therapy, which stressed a sensitivity on the part of the therapist to what the child was experiencing and the need to let the child lead the therapy by selecting motor activities that were meaningful. The focus of this sensitivity was on obtaining a balance between providing structure and allowing the child freedom. Even here, the focus of treatment was on improving neural organization and promoting adaptive behavior.

> Watching the child as he performs, seeing his mood, his emotional state, and his motor action guides the therapist in providing the optimum amount of freedom or gentle manipulation to foster the constructive involvement of the child in a task with the gusto as well as intent to achieve that leads him to a more advanced level of neural organization. . . .

The kind of involvement necessary to achieve the state wherein the child becomes effectively self-directing within the structure set by the therapist cannot be commanded; it must be elicited. Therein lies the art of therapy. The opportunity can be offered, encouragement given, suggestions proffered. Physical assistance may help, but *unless the child wills to act upon the environment, he will not do so* [italics added]. Furthermore, he will not do so in a manner that can be called adaptive and growth-promoting and therefore therapeutic unless he finds it fulfilling to do so. Fulfillment comes with the right combination of challenge and success. (Ayres, 1972, pp. 258–259)

It is not surprising that no formal conceptualization of how mental and neurobehavioral phenomena are related has been developed and applied to the theory of sensory integration. Ayres' original work in developing the theory of sensory integration was based on a literature that did not grapple significantly with the problem of mind-brain-body relationships, or, worse, considered it to be an insignificant problem. The reductionist strategies that were dominant throughout neuroscience literature and practice separated and isolated phenomena for study (cf. Churchland, 1986). This resulted in a fragmentation within modern biological and behavioral sciences that pursued phenomena largely in isolation of each other (Boulding, 1956; Churchland, 1986). Consequently, until quite recently, there has been relatively little concern for how mental experience, neurophysiology, and behavior might be related (Churchland, 1986; Trevarthen, 1979).

This fragmentation in the knowledge base concerning mind-brain-body relationships has more than intellectual consequences. When therapists focus on one component of the dysfunctional complex (e.g., the state of the nervous system or neurobehavior), with relative inattention to mental phenomena—or vice versa—therapy becomes disjointed or incomplete (DiJoseph, 1982). A therapeutic approach that is able to consider both the brain-body and the mind, and appreciates how they are interrelated, has obvious advantages over a more narrow or fragmented approach. Thus, while sensory integration as a theory may not require a stronger conceptualization of the relationship between the brain-body and the mind, it is necessary to understand the complexity of this relationship as it pertains to the practice of occupational therapy based on sensory integration theory.

## PURPOSE AND SCOPE

The purpose of this chapter is to propose a model that will demonstrate the relationship of sensory integrative phenomena (i.e., neurological structures and neurobehavioral functions) to mental phenomena (i.e., emotional and conceptual processes) that influence the sensory integrative process. We first will propose our perspective on how the mind and the brain-body are interrelated, illustrating how mental phenomena influence and are influenced by the sensory integrative process. We will then argue that occupational therapy based on sensory integration theory requires the therapist to enable the child to achieve better brain organization through influencing both the mental experiences of the child and his or her capacity to choose adequately challenging sensorimotor activities. Finally, a conceptualization of mental processes involved in choices for action from another model of practice, the model of human occupation, will be integrated with sensory integration theory to demonstrate a more holistic approach to occupational therapy based in sensory integrative theory. The application of this integrated approach in clinical practice will be demonstrated using a case example.

When we refer to the integration of the model of human occupation with sensory integration theory, we are referring to the linkage of two compatible theories of practice. We do not mean to suggest the need for the development of a new, more global theory. Both sensory integration and the model of human occupation are practice theories in their own right. Each seeks to explain a specific domain of behavior and each maintains its integrity by retaining its identity as a distinct theory. Rather, what we are proposing is that the practice of occupational therapy can be enhanced by linking compatible theories when the needs of the client extend beyond the specific domain addressed by the primary theory that guides practice. We also believe that it is important to differentiate between an *integrated approach* that links compatible theories, and a more *eclectic approach* that combines elements of various theories, often without regard for their compatibility or for the relationship among their respective constructs. The integration of different approaches to practice with the theory and practice of sensory integration is addressed in more detail in Chapter 13.

## A PROPOSED VIEW OF MIND-BRAIN-BODY RELATIONSHIPS

### The Problem of Separating Mind from Brain-Body

A growing interdisciplinary movement has sought to overcome the conceptual fragmentation of the mind and the brain-body by developing more integrated theories that recognize the connections between diverse phenomena (Churchland, 1986). Over and over again, the point is being made that while chemical, biological, psychological, and sociological structures and processes may be of distinctly different orders, they are, at the same time, clearly interrelated and interdependent (von Bertalanffy, 1962). Moreover, it has been powerfully argued that no complete understanding of any phenomenon can be achieved while ignoring other interrelated phenomena. Thus, even a theory such as sensory integration, which seeks to explain the relationships among brain organization, sensorimotor component skills, and adaptive behavior, must recognize that the neurological phenomena under question are linked to, and profoundly influenced by, mental phenomena. With the increasing body of literature on the problem of separating the mind from the brain-body, we are now able to consider their interdependence seriously and explicitly in our discussion of the theory and practice of sensory integration.

Our proposed view of mind-brain-body relationships echoes several recurrent themes from the literature. As with any theory, our view is both preliminary and tentative. It will need further refinement and development as new knowledge emerges. However, it represents an important first step in understanding how mind-brain-body relationships can be understood in relation to sensory integration theory and practice. In taking this step, we have sought to formulate a perspective that (a) is consistent with available scientific evidence and occupational therapy models of practice, and (b) is logically coherent.

### Mind-Brain-Body Unity

Our perspective recognizes the mind, brain, and body as distinct aspects of a single system; they are functionally inseparable and interdependent. That the brain-body is governed by chemical and biological laws and the mind is governed by psychological laws indicates that they are not synonymous (Popper & Eccles, 1977). "Analysis by the methods of neurophysiology determines how neurons excite one another and generate patterned forces of behaviour. But neurophysiology is not intended to be a science of the mind" (Trevarthen, 1979, p. 188). Just as neurophysiologists are not able to fully explain mental experience, so psychologists and philosophers cannot explain all neurobiological processes. However, neither mental experience nor neurophysiological events can be explained fully without recognizing their interdependence. While the interdependence of mind-brain-body is central to this perspective, the implications — especially the clinical implications — cannot be fully appreciated without a closer examination of the nature of this relationship.

When we speak of the mind and the brain-body, we have to recognize that an important part of each is a set of ongoing processes: mental processes, brain processes, and body processes. That is, while the brain-body has clearly definable physical or anatomical structures, and while we can talk about such "mental structures" as personality, we must also recognize the ongoing, dynamic nature of the mind and the brain-body. Thus, the "stream of mental events" and the ongoing "stream of neurophysiological and neuromuscular events" are a fundamental part of what we mean by mind and brain-body. Moreover, mind and brain-body are linked by an interface between these processes, rather than by some mechanical or structural bond such as the neuromuscular junction that links the motoneuron to the muscle. At the point of their interface, mental and brain-body processes communicate with each other and exert a reciprocal causal influence on each other.

In fact, mental processes are fundamentally dependent on brain processes. As Trevarthen (1979) noted, "all the evidence from brain research indicates that any act or state of consciousness will involve most of the brain in excitation patterns of fantastic complexity" (p. 188). This means that all mental phenomena are produced by brain processes. When mental events proceed from neuronal events, they are being produced by large-scale brain "conditions" and "relationships." *Specific* mental experiences, however, are not stored in *specific* neuronal cells (Pribram, 1986). Rather, mental phenomena emerge from the gestalt functions of brain circuitry interacting with an ongoing stream of sensory information taken in from the environment. That is, the spatial-temporal patterning of electrical potentials in the brain are interpreted and given meaning, and provide the basis for conceptualization (Pribram, 1986).

While mental phenomena depend on the brain for their existence, they are not determined absolutely by the brain. Rather, we propose that brain processes create parameters that determine the potential for how the mind can operate, and that the brain has an influence on the content of the mind (e.g., how a person feels about a performance) by creating conditions in which the mental experience becomes probable. But, what actually is experienced is a function of an ongoing personal stream of awareness and of accumulated experiences within the human and nonhuman environment. For example, the brain makes it possible for Allison to learn how to move her body in order to propel herself on the big swing, to evaluate her own performance, and to become aware of how others view her newfound ability. But what she has learned to do, the particular content of her memories, and her self-reflections, are a product of her unique experience in interacting within a given physical environment and culture. Moreover, what she experiences each time she swings is influenced by multiple variables, including the ongoing state of the brain during the activity, memories of prior experiences (both long-term and immediately preceding the current experience), and who or what else is present in the environment.

When we speak of causation between the mind and the brain-body, we are not referring to the simple, linear form of causation with which we all are familiar. In simple causation, there is a clearly delineated temporal sequence (one event happens before a second event), and there is linearity (the first event clearly produces the second event). In the case of the mind and the brain-body, we are referring to other, more complex, forms of causation. Complex causation is more properly understood as a given set of events (e.g., the simultaneous and sequential firings of multiple neurons in the brain) that create possibilities and potentialities for a person to mentally experience something. These events do not directly make the experience happen. Moreover, causation may not involve, or be limited to, a temporal sequence. Rather, when Allison reflects on her experience, her brain-body is viewed as simultaneously creating conditions that allow her to think and feel about her experience. In this case, the events are *synchronous*; the mind and the brain-body have a causative influence on each other and that influence is exerted simultaneously.

While the causal role of the brain in creating the conditions for mental events to occur is more or less widely accepted, a less well-understood aspect of their interdependence is the causal influence of the mind on the brain-body. There is a persuasive argument, however, that the mind serves to integrate, and give order to, sensory information from the body and the environment that is being processed in the brain (Popper & Eccles, 1977). That is, the mind represents the interpretation of neurophysiological processes as meaningful experiences (Pribram, 1986). It thereby is the "integrating agent, building the unity of conscious experience from all the diversity of the brain events" (Eccles, 1977, p. 373).

In addition to this interpretive and integrative function, the mind also directly influences processes in the brain (Sperry, 1969, 1970). Sperry (1970) described this causal role as one in which mental processes *supervene* in neurophysiological events. That is, "subjective mental phenomena are conceived to influence and to govern the flow of nerve impulse traffic" (Sperry, 1969, p. 534).

Thus, the model of mind-brain-body interdependence argues that mental phenomena are both caused by, and emerge from, neurophysiological processes and that mental phenomena, in turn, act back on, and influence, ongoing large-scale neurophysiological processes (Fig. 2–1). The mind and the brain-body interface at the level of macro events. That is, it is not the excitation of specific neurons that

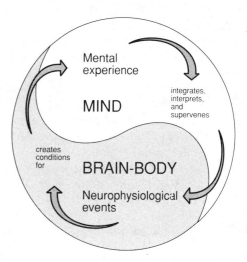

FIGURE 2–1. Synchronous interdependence of mind and brain-body.

produce specific mental experiences (e.g., memories) nor is it mental events influencing neurophysiology at the neuronal level. Rather, the mind and the brain-body articulate at holistic levels. The stream of awareness and the gestalt pattern of neuronal excitation throughout the brain are the level of interface between the mind and the brain-body. Moreover, mutual causation between the mind and the brain-body are assumed to be simultaneous. The mind and the brain-body coeffect one another in a synchronous fashion.

The ongoing stream of mental experience includes feelings, intentions, memories, and anticipations. Mental experience also includes the conceptual components of cognitive-perceptual-motor phenomena that are involved in the interpretation and orchestration of large-scale brain events. Thus, when Joe is up to bat, he feels anxious and dreads failure, and these mental events interfere with the cognitive-perceptual-motor interpretive capacities of his mind that might otherwise orchestrate the integration of sensory information for use in *more efficient* adaptive behavior. Additionally, his highly anxious emotional state, which translates into heightened arousal, also negatively influences his brain organization so that it is not in an optimal state to receive and organize the vestibular-proprioceptive, tactile, and visual information he needs to plan an appropriate action sequence to swing the bat effectively and hit the ball. Thus, to a significant degree, Joe's sensory integrative dysfunction is simultaneously influenced by mental events and interferes with mental events.

In summary, we recognize the mind and the brain-body as unique aspects of a single unitary system, and that each aspect has its own special properties and laws. The mind and the brain-body are mutually dependent on, and intimately interrelated with, neurophysiological events. Importantly, the complex causal relationship between the mind and the brain-body is *synchronous*. It is simultaneous and nonlinear. Neurophysiological events produce mental processes, and mental processes simultaneously shape neurophysiological events and behavior (see Fig. 2-1).

## Coordinated Change in Mind and Brain-Body

Thus far we have proposed how the mind and the brain-body operate in a synchronized fashion to mutually influence one another. The mind and the brain-body also influence each other through the process of *sequential causation*. Sequential causation enables the mind and the brain-body to codevelop and change over time. In this process, newly maturing capacities in the brain-body create new potentials for mental experience. Experiences lead to awareness of the possibility for new actions and, thus, stimulate new intentions. These intentions, formed in the mind, are realized in new motor behaviors that, in turn, expose the brain-body to a whole new array of sensory information (feedback). This sensory information facilitates brain development. This sequential intention-action-feedback process involves formation of conscious intentions (decisions to act) that are translated through brain processes into adaptive motor behavior. Adaptive motor behaviors, in turn, create new forms of production and response feedback that (a) are processed in the brain, (b) are interpreted in the mind, and (c) facilitate the development of neural organization. Viewed over time, the intention-action-feedback process results in an adaptive spiral that is superimposed on the spiral process of self-actualization we discussed in Chapter 1 (see Fig. 1-4). Importantly, this spiral is dependent on the synchronous cooperative action of the mind and brain we discussed earlier. Thus, *synchronous causation is superimposed on sequential causation.*

# DEVELOPING THE MIND-BRAIN-BODY LINK IN SENSORY INTEGRATION THEORY AND PRACTICE

Recognition that sensory integration and sensory integrative dysfunction involve a mind-brain-body process requires that we "couple" sensory integration theory with other theoretical frameworks that elaborate what is meant by mind. It is not enough to have a general, or vague, reference to the nature of the mind. That is, while recognition of a relationship between sensory integrative dysfunction, clumsiness, and self-esteem is an important beginning, it does not conceptually elaborate on how the child's view of self emerges, nor does it explain how that self-perception influences choices for behavior. If we consider that mental events are *at least as* complex as is the process of sensory integration, then we can readily see the requirement for a comparably sophisticated view of the mind. As we discussed earlier, this is not to argue that sensory integration theory should be expanded to provide an explanation of mental phenomena. Rather, it argues for a linkage or coupling, in practice, of sensory integration theory with another theoretical model that provides a more adequate conceptualization of the mind, in this case, the model of human occupation. We will propose that volition, a construct of the model of human occupation, provides a conceptual model of the mind that can be linked with the theory of sensory integration. To repeat Ayres' (1972) own words regarding the art of therapy, "unless the child *wills* [italics added] to act upon the environment, he will not do so" (p. 259); the term *volition* comes from the Latin word meaning to will or wish.

As we proceed, we will clarify further how linking these two models of practice can help us to understand more fully how synchronous causation is superimposed on sequential causation. To aid us in this process, we will refer to Figure 2–2, which the reader should recognize as an elaboration of one level (loop) of the spiral process of self-actualization shown in Figure 1–4. As we will see, *simultaneous* causation can be viewed as the ongoing, yet simultaneous, flow of interactions that occur *within* one level. That is, one level (or the single loop shown in Fig. 2–2) can be viewed as "simultaneous time." *Sequential* causation is that which occurs *between* levels and which enables the individual to move up to a higher level on the spiral. That is, movement to progressively higher levels is viewed as "sequential time."

## Volition as a Model of the Mind

The mind is a complex collection of conscious, preconscious, and unconscious feelings, beliefs, thoughts, and memories. Moreover, mental experience can be recognized as consisting of *three identifiable levels of conscious experience*: (a) immediate awareness of one's doing, (b) self-reflection in the midst of an experience, and (c) reflective self-awareness that builds on accumulated experiences. Schön (1983, 1987), in a related discussion, acknowledged the latter two levels, which he referred to as *reflection-in-action* and *reflection-on-action*, respectively. While Schön used these terms to refer to the professional reasoning process of the experienced practitioner, we believe that the concepts can be generalized to include the self-reflective processes associated with the performance of adaptive motor behavior.

Thus, to return to our example of Allison, we can recognize (a) that she has an immediate awareness of the physical actions and sensations of swinging (i.e., "how it feels" and "what was achieved"); (b) that she may reflect briefly, as she is swinging, on how much fun she is having or how she is doing; and (c) that she will leave the

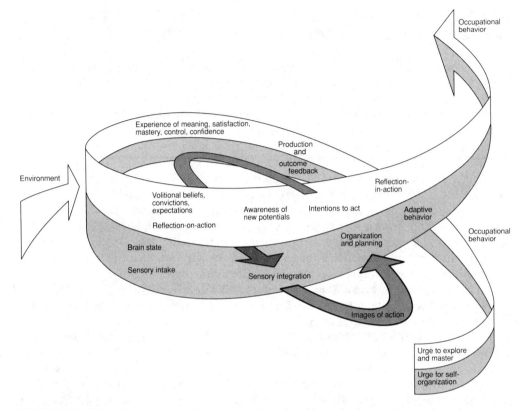

**FIGURE 2 – 2.** Synchronous interdependence of mind and brain-body superimposed on the sequential spiral process of self-actualization.

experience with an awareness of her capacity for swinging, of how enjoyable it was, and of the importance or meaning of the activity. The first level of awareness of "how it feels" and "what was achieved" relates to body scheme or neuronal models; we can also refer to these neuronal models as *images of action*. They represent an important *mental component* of the motor planning process. This level of the mind, represented in the spiral process of self-actualization (Fig. 1 – 4) and in Figure 2 – 2 by a dark line, will be discussed in more detail in Chapter 4.

In this chapter, we will focus on the latter two levels, reflection-in-action and reflection-on-action. The reason for this is straightforward. The latter two levels are least well developed in sensory integration theory, and they are the levels of the mind that are most fully elucidated by the model of human occupation. That is, the model of human occupation focuses on how persons *reflect while in* the midst of an experience (i.e., the states they experience *in action*) and on what persons come to believe about themselves and their actions as they later *reflect on* their experience (i.e., the states they experience *after action*).

The model of human occupation conceptualizes high-level intentional consciousness as a *volition subsystem* that organizes the conscious formation of intentions for action (Kielhofner, 1985). Volition is conceptualized as an organizational complex of both psychic energy and mental images. The energy is a *neurologically based urge* for self-organization. Because of a need for the brain to self-organize through action, there is hypothesized a corresponding *mental urge* for action. This mental urge for action provides the impetus for formulating an intention to have an effect on the environment and to experience control over personal behaviors and their outcomes. Thus, the brain's biological need to process sensory information translates into a psychological need to explore and achieve mastery. This concept of volitional energy parallels Ayres' concept of an inner drive to develop sensory integration through participation in sensorimotor activities (see Figs. 1–4 and 2–2).

In addition to psychic energy, volition contains images (beliefs, convictions, and expectations) that comprise a complex self-awareness concerning oneself as an actor in the world. These volitional images are of three types: (a) *personal causation*, or images concerning one's personal control, abilities, and likelihood of success in undertakings; (b) *values*, or images concerning what is important or significant in performance; and (c) *interests*, or images concerning what kinds of occupations are satisfying and enjoyable. Volitional images are *traits*. That is, these images are relatively stable and change only through accumulated experience. Further, because they are traits, we can expect them to endure unless experience sufficiently challenges them and brings about change to conform to the new experiences of reality. These volitional images influence choices that an individual makes for participation in various work, play, and daily living activities, that is, what adaptive behaviors an individual chooses to plan, organize, and produce.

More specifically, the underlying desire for exploration and mastery provides the energy for choosing behavior; behavior is chosen in accordance with subjective volitional images. Volitional energy and images—and, often, external stimuli— combine, producing a dynamic *state* we refer to as motivation; this state is one in which a person is disposed to initiate and sustain action (i.e., volitional traits and sensory information combine to create the potential and probability of a volitional decision). The motivational state is experienced as a willful state in which an individual feels attracted to and energized for performance, and obligated to perform.

While an urge to explore and master is necessary for providing the desire for action, volitional images (traits) are most critical for shaping the kind of action that will be chosen. For example, all other things being equal, persons will choose to engage in performances of which they feel capable, wherein they expect to experience pleasure, and to which they assign value. Thus, in the future we can expect Allison to choose swinging on the big swing as an activity because she feels competent at it, enjoys it, and sees it as an important accomplishment.

However, volitional images also converge with motivational states and an ongoing stream of experiences to collectively influence choices for action. For example, if we had observed Allison earlier, during the period of practice in which she learned to pump the swing, we would have found an admixture of (a) anxiety about her performance and possible negative outcomes, (b) positive expectations for mastering the skill of swinging, and (c) pleasure in experiencing control as she effected the swinging motion. These motivational states (feeling, memories, expectations) converged with her ongoing experiences (e.g., encouragement from her father, information gathered from her observations of "big kids" swinging) to create the mental conditions that properly oriented her toward learning the new skill of swinging. Together, these motivational states and environmental conditions provide the meaningful context in which sensory integration takes place. They create the mental conditions that supervene in neurological events and lend the organizing influence that assures proper sensory integration within the brain.

Moreover, ongoing decisions for action reflect an admixture of motives in which one or more volitional images may dominate, and the way in which various volitional images interact is often very complex. For example, some actions are chosen for their perceived value, despite uncertainty either about one's ability to do them or about how much fun they might be. Recall Joe, who persists at attempting to play baseball despite his difficulties in performance and the fact that he really doesn't enjoy playing baseball. Joe seems to be driven by a culturally assigned value associated with sports activities and his knowledge that peer approval can be gained by competence in sports. Eventually, Joe's feelings of incompetence and his lack of enjoyment may lead him to avoid baseball.

## Volitional Factors in the Genesis of Sensory Integrative Dysfunction

If volitional factors are considered in light of the conceptualization of mind-brain-body relationships offered earlier, we can see how they might contribute to the sequelae of sensory integrative dysfunction, that is, the spiral process of dysfunction that parallels the second postulate of sensory integration theory discussed in Chapter 1. It is hypothesized that sensory integrative dysfunction has its roots in some nonspecific form of brain deficiency. This means that the child encounters the world, and experiences it mentally, through a brain that is disorganized or limited in its ability to process and integrate sensory information taken in from the internal and external environment.

But this is only the beginning of the unfolding of the sensory integrative dysfunction. As the child engages in sensorimotor behaviors and experiences difficulty, a volitional image is formed. This volitional image may be affected in the following ways. First, the child may develop an awareness of personal inefficacy, lack of control, and expectation of failure. Second, the child may develop different expectations for pleasure in sensorimotor behavior (e.g., the child with tactile defensiveness who does not enjoy being touched by his or her parents, the child with gravitational insecurity who becomes inordinately fearful when his or her parents attempt to roughhouse). Third, the child may either (a) accept conventional valuation of activities and possibly devalue him- or herself when valued activities are found to be too difficult to perform; or (b) devalue those activities he or she has difficulty performing and, consequently, deviate from the normative values of peers.

These collective images, which appear in early childhood as rudimentary preferences and as a sense of self, become elaborated over time. They influence the formation of intentions to act. The child with sensory integrative dysfunction may choose to avoid sensorimotor activities that could provide his or her much-needed experiences. Thus, superimposed on the spiral process of dysfunction is a breakdown in the sequential intention-action-feedback loop.

Volition may also influence brain processes through the synchronous mode. Joe, who knows he has difficulty hitting a ball with a bat, enters the activity in an anxious state. His anxiety interferes with his ability to plan the projected motor action sequence of batting, and thus impairs not only his performance, but also the feedback he receives and the learning that could take place if Joe's brain was not overaroused. We can also imagine that Joe has a long history of failure to experience pleasure during most sensorimotor behavior. Coupled with a history of feelings of inadequacy, his performance is compromised even further, thereby also negatively impacting on the development of brain organization.

Volitional images not only influence the propensity to spontaneously develop intentions, they also shape how a child will react to the various stimuli in his or her environment. A child who has memories of positive experiences on the swing at the neighborhood park (i.e., mastery of the challenges and pleasure in the activity) will perceive the swing as providing distinctly different opportunities for action than will the child who fell off or who was unable to master the skill of pumping the swing. Thus, it is clear that environmental opportunities are not enough to ensure that children will seek out the sensorimotor experiences they need. This means that effective sensory integrative intervention programs must involve more than just the provision of sensorimotor activities designed to enhance sensory integration.

## VOLITIONAL FACTORS IN SENSORY INTEGRATION THERAPY

When we intervene, we generally set goals that the child will more spontaneously participate in skilled motor tasks (i.e., that he or she will spontaneously choose to engage in developmentally appropriate and adequately challenging sensorimotor behavior). Thus, *we also must incorporate goals of changing any volitional images that are a deterrent to spontaneous choice of motor behavior.*

The notion of changing volitional images raises a further problem of understanding *how* these images actually change. Volitional change is conceptualized as an open-system process (that parallels sensory integrative change) in which the action of the system (person) translates into structural changes via the open-system cycle. That is, the child behaves, generates feedback (reflection-in-action and reflection-on-action), and incorporates that feedback into his or her system, thereby altering brain functions or structures to accommodate the new information. The child then proceeds to behave on the basis of the new brain functions or structure. Over time, this cycle becomes a spiral — one that is either adaptive (self-actualizing) or maladaptive (dysfunctional) for the child.

### Trait and State

How the cycle of actions and experiences results in structural change in volitional images is a complex matter. The cycle may be more clearly understood when we clarify the distinction between states and traits. Volitional images are personal *traits*; that is, they are more or less stable images that an individual holds about him- or herself. In contrast, motivational *states* are the subjective experiences that persons have when they are engaging in action.

States and traits are mutually influential. For example, the person who lacks belief in his or her ability to perform a motor behavior is likely to be in an anxious state when engaging in a behavior that he or she perceives as having value or as being expected. On the other hand, if the person is skillfully led by a therapist to feel in control and to achieve mastery, the anxiety may give way to a sense of pleasure. These experiences (states), as they accumulate, begin to challenge the volitional images (traits) held by the child. Eventually these successful experiences lead the child to develop new images to replace the old ones. That is, where the child previously lacked belief in abilities and expectations for pleasure, he or she may come to have confidence to perform, and a pleasurable attraction to, certain sensorimotor activities.

## Mental States and Brain States

Our model of mind-brain-body relationships argues that the mind and brain-body simultaneously influence one another. That is, the child cannot experience control and pleasure in an action unless the brain is appropriately aroused and giving proper commands to the body (musculoskeletal system). Conversely, we may assert that the brain cannot be properly oriented to commanding intended actions and processing sensory information that these actions generate unless "proper" mental intentions are formulated. To bring this to a more practical level, we hypothesize that a child who is not experiencing something volitionally relevant does not, at that moment, have a brain properly oriented to organize sensory information for use in adaptive behavior.

By volitionally relevant, we mean that the action must be intended and experienced in terms of some desire to explore or master. Volitional relevance is personally defined by the individual's images of competency, pleasure, and value as they relate to the particular behavior. A child who is experiencing "intentional irrelevance" (i.e., someone who does not have a purpose for his actions as defined by the value, interest, and sense of competence he or she assigns to it) will not have a brain-organizing experience.

Figure 2–2 illustrates the proposed relationship between volition and the brain as they codevelop. This model of volition-brain-body interactions can be understood not only as a normal developmental sequence, but also as a model of successful therapeutic intervention. Furthermore, it can be used as a comparative model to more fully understand the nature of sensory integrative dysfunction.

## Consideration of Mind in the Course of Intervention

To demonstrate how we might link concepts from the theory of sensory integration and the model of human occupation into an integrated occupational therapy intervention program, we will return to Joe. When Joe was evaluated by his occupational therapist, he was found to have a pattern of low test scores which suggested problems with processing tactile as well as vestibular-proprioceptive information. As we might have expected, these sensory processing deficits were associated with problems in planning and producing bilateral and projected action sequences, motor planning, and visuomotor coordination.

Superimposed on this is Joe's poor sense of self. Joe is interested in, and values, baseball, probably because he perceives that other people who are important to him (i.e., his parents and his peers) are interested in, and value, baseball. He correctly perceives, however, that he is not good at baseball. Joe also correctly perceives that other people know that he is not good at baseball. When Joe comes up to bat, he expects to fail. When he *does* fail, his belief that he is "no good" (at baseball, but perhaps also "no good" at all) is fueled. Thus, the cycle perpetuates itself.

We can plan Joe's intervention along one of two lines — or we can combine both lines of reasoning. We can either capitalize on the fact that Joe values baseball and has the motivation to play it, and we can control and adapt the game of baseball in such a way that he can succeed. Or we can guide Joe through a process of becoming interested in a different activity that he values and that he also feels competent to perform. Because we know that Joe's skills at baseball are very poor, but that his interest and values for baseball are very high, we will probably choose both to improve his skills *and* to alter his interests. We will try to help him to improve his ability at baseball so that the probability increases that he will actually hit the ball when it is thrown toward him during a game with his friends. We will do that by (a) improving his sensory integration ability and his motor planning and visuomotor skills, and (b) creating opportunities for him to practice batting in a controlled situation where the ball is thrown directly at his bat (so that he learns what it feels like to swing the bat successfully). When attempting to improve his underlying sensory integrative dysfunction, we will intentionally create activities that provide opportunities for Joe to intake controlled tactile and vestibular-proprioceptive stimuli, while at the same time demanding from him adaptive responses that are clearly related to batting the ball (e.g., hitting a ball with a stick held at either end while swinging to and fro in a net hammock suspended from the ceiling) (Fig. 2–3). We will be certain to point out to Joe the similarities between the treatment activities and the demands of baseball (e.g., the need to watch the ball carefully) in order to enhance his motivational state.

With regard to changing his interests and values, we may also embrace two strategies. First, with Joe's help, we will create activities that are fun and highly motivating to Joe, in the context of direct intervention based on the principles of sensory integration. However, many of those activities will not be so obviously related to improving his skills at baseball (e.g., riding on a bolster suspended at both ends from the ceiling, pretending the bolster is a horse). The key to utilizing this

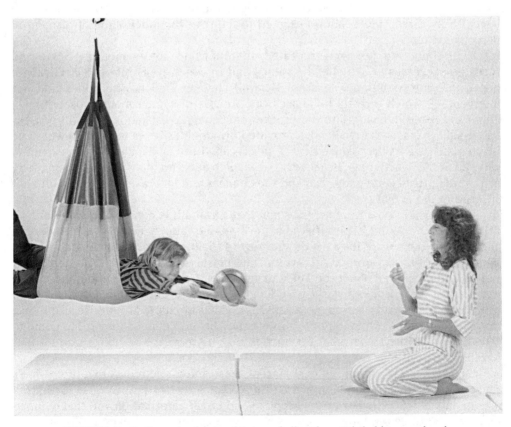

FIGURE 2–3. Prone in the net, hitting a ball with a stick held in two hands.

strategy successfully will be to create activities that (a) Joe is interested in doing, (b) he values and believes his friends and parents would value, (c) he can succeed at performing, and (d) address his needs with regard to sensory integration. If Joe is able repeatedly to succeed at activities that meet these criteria, he may begin to alter his beliefs about his skills and about himself. A second strategy that the therapist might find useful would be to sit down with Joe and talk about his interests, suggesting some new activities that he had not thought of before and facilitating his participation in activities that he identifies as interests.

When Joe enters treatment with Elizabeth, an experienced occupational therapist, Elizabeth has access to all this information about Joe. Her primary goal in intervention is to interrupt the abnormal process of sequential causation that Joe has developed. That is, she wants to change both his ability to process and use available sensory information *and* his beliefs about his ability to act. Joe has experienced problems in both of these areas for a long time and they have mutually influenced his development.

Elizabeth knows that no single interaction with Joe will result in resolution of the conflict between Joe's volitional traits and what Joe is experiencing. Rather, in any single treatment session, Elizabeth hopes to be able to influence the process of synchronous causation by simultaneously influencing Joe's sensory integration abilities and his emotional state. That is, she believes that by developing activities that are (a) highly motivating (and fun) for Joe and (b) challenging, but within his capabilities, she can help to engender a state of optimum arousal in Joe. In that state, Joe will be able to produce appropriate adaptive behaviors and reap the maximum benefit from direct intervention designed to improve the functioning of his central nervous system.

Over time, and following repeated alterations to Joe's emotional state and repeated successes at activities he values and in which he is interested, Elizabeth hopes that Joe's volitional sense of self will change. That is, she hopes that her intervention, which directly influences the process of synchronous causation, will ultimately result in changes to the process of sequential causation. Joe will possess better skills to meet the challenges provided by activities he values and in which he is interested; he will recognize that he possesses those skills; and he will expect to succeed at those activities. Because he expects to succeed, he will enter the activity in a more optimal state of arousal and the chances will increase that he actually *will* succeed at the activity.

Let us look in on a treatment session that Elizabeth is conducting with Joe. We will "observe" how one expert therapist develops a treatment activity so that she can address simultaneously Joe's needs with regard to both emotional state and sensory integration. This session occurred within the first 6 weeks of Joe's treatment, after Elizabeth had learned about the kinds of activities that motivate Joe, but before Joe had learned that Elizabeth was a good judge of his skills and abilities. Joe has been successful at doing all the treatment activities he has attempted so far. He also thinks that the swings and other equipment are "really neat." He looks forward to going to therapy but, at the same time, he worries that he may not be able to do all that Elizabeth asks of him.

Elizabeth believes that the best kind of sensorimotor activities to address Joe's sensory integrative dysfunction will be those that provide opportunities for him to take in enhanced vestibular-proprioceptive and tactile information and that demand bilateral coordination, motor planning, and visuomotor coordination. She also believes that Joe must be given as much control as possible over the activities in which he engages. She encourages him to design and select equipment to create those challenges. She guides him in his choices and sometimes creates new activities that reflect the choices that he has made previously.

Elizabeth has learned that Joe especially likes working on the trapeze, but that he is still a little concerned that he won't be able to succeed at certain treatment activities. She also knows that Joe really likes concrete evidence of his achievements; at Joe's request and no matter what the activity, Elizabeth puts a mark on the blackboard each time Joe succeeds at hitting the target with a ball, catching the ball, kicking over the blocks, or whatever the activity demands. The "score" that Joe receives in this manner is cumulative; he continues to add to it every week. At this point, Joe has 436 points; he is looking forward to the time when he will "break 1000."

When Joe first suggested that they keep score in this manner, Elizabeth was curious about his request. She queried Joe about what he would do with the points. "Nothin'," he said, "just collect 'em." He also told her that he didn't want to play *against* anyone; he just wanted to keep counting his points.

When we enter the clinic, Elizabeth and Joe have been working for about 20 minutes. Elizabeth has noticed that Joe has mastered the activity and seems to be getting a little bored. Wanting to increase the challenge, but to continue to work on a task requiring a similar kind of motor planning, Elizabeth has just arranged two stacks of mats about 3 feet apart on the floor. She has suspended the trapeze so that it hangs from the ceiling between the two stacks of mats. On the floor between the mats, Elizabeth has piled a short stack of cardboard blocks. The task for Joe is to swing from one set of mats to the other without knocking over the blocks (Fig. 2–4). Each time Joe succeeds, Elizabeth counts the blocks that he successfully jumped over and adds that number of points to his score; she also adds one more block to the pile so that the challenge gradually becomes greater and greater. When Joe knocks over the blocks, the game begins again.

Joe can reliably jump over six or seven blocks before knocking the pile over. However, in this particular "round," Joe has managed to clear nine blocks, an all-time record. As Elizabeth begins to record his nine points, Joe interrupts her. "I think I should only get six points," he says.

"Why?" asks Elizabeth. "That's the best you've ever done."

"Because," Joe answered, "those first three blocks are lower than the mats I'm jumping off of. That's not fair. I shouldn't get points for those. Besides, I don't need easy points anymore."

Elizabeth added six points to Joe's score, as requested. After that, she began to ask him whether or not he *wanted* particular points, rather than just deciding for him. Sometimes he took the points and sometimes he did not, but he always thought about it carefully.

That seems to be a turning point in Joe's intervention. While he continued to require concrete and externally provided evidence of his success, he also was beginning to examine critically the criteria by which success was judged. That is, he seemed to want his accumulating points to represent the mastery of self-determined challenges. Further, Joe was requesting an active role in the process. He seemed increasingly to believe that his skills were adequate to meet important challenges and that he, rather than Elizabeth, was the best judge of his performance. Further, his beliefs about his skills accurately reflected the gains that he was making in his

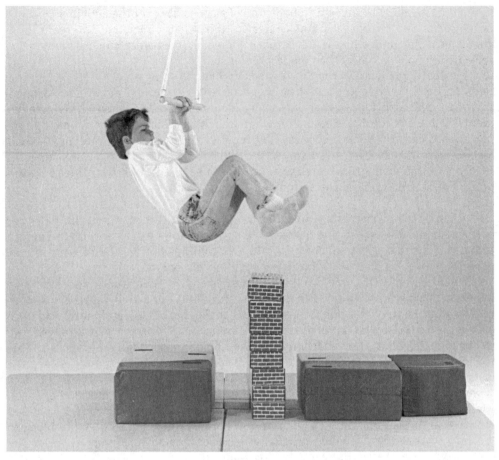

**FIGURE 2–4.** Holding onto the trapeze, swinging from mat to mat.

ability to process and use sensory intake. In carefully addressing the synchronous nature of Joe's problems, Elizabeth has begun to help him to alter the sequential development of his abilities and his beliefs.

## SUMMARY

We have presented a model of the mind-brain-body relationships that is derived from linkages between the theory of sensory integration, the volition construct of the model of human occupation, and existing theories of mind-brain-body relationships. When we apply this model, we learn that intervention aimed at changing the brain and its capacity for sensory integration and motor behavior cannot be achieved unless we *simultaneously* change those volitional traits that influence the ways in which the brain takes in and processes information prior to, during, and following motor performance. More specifically, we have argued that a client cannot *sequentially*, over time, improve his or her abilities to integrate sensory information and use that information in the planning and production of new, more complex, adaptive behavior unless that client also increases the (a) belief in his or her ability and (b) capacity to value and experience pleasure from motor performance. A corollary, of course, is that interventions designed to *sequentially* improve volitional traits in a client with sensory integrative dysfunction cannot succeed fully unless the intervention *simultaneously* focuses on improving the client's sensory integrative functioning. But that is another story, to be told elsewhere.

We also have learned that we intervene by guiding the client to choose to participate in sensorimotor activities that the client *wants* to do and thinks he or she *can* do. That is, the choices must be activities that are intrinsically motivating and that the client values. We also want to be sure that, in direct intervention, we remove all possible negative consequences of performance that the client may have suffered in real life (i.e., injury, embarrassment, failure). As we will discuss more directly in the next chapter, we want to create a playful environment for treatment and help the client to play in a way that requires the use of his or her emerging skills.

# REFERENCES

Ayres, A. J. (1972). *Sensory integration and learning disorders.* Los Angeles: Western Psychological Services.

Ayres, A. J. (1979). *Sensory integration and the child.* Los Angeles: Western Psychological Services.

Ayres, A. J. (1989). *Sensory Integration and Praxis Tests.* Los Angeles: Western Psychological Services.

Boulding, K. (1956). General systems theory: The skeleton of science. *Management Science, 2,* 197–208.

Brooks, V. B. (1986). *The neural basis of motor control.* New York: Oxford University Press.

Churchland, P. S. (1986). *Neurophilosophy: Toward a unified science of the mind-brain.* Cambridge, MA: MIT Press.

DiJoseph, L. M. (1982). Independence through activity: Mind, body, and environment interaction in therapy. *American Journal of Occupational Therapy, 36,* 740–744.

Eccles, J., & Robinson, D. N. (1985). *The wonder of being human: Our brain and our mind.* Boston: New Science Library.

Kielhofner, G. (1985). *The model of human occupation: Theory and application.* Baltimore: Williams and Wilkins.

Popper, K. R., & Eccles, J. C. (1977). *The self and the brain.* New York: Springer-Verlag.

Pribram, K. H. (1986). The cognitive revolution and mind/brain issues. *American Psychologist, 41,* 507–520.

Schön, D. A. (1983). *The reflective practitioner: How professionals think in action.* New York: Basic Books.

Schön, D. A. (1987). *Educating the reflective practitioner.* San Francisco: Jossey-Bass.

Sperry, R. W. (1969). A modified concept of consciousness. *Psychological Review, 76,* 532–536.

Sperry, R. W. (1970). An objective approach to subjective experience: Further explanation of a hypothesis. *Psychological Review, 77,* 585–590.

Trevarthen, C. (1979). The tasks of consciousness: How could the brain do them? *Brain and Mind* (CIBA Foundation Symposium No. 69, new series, pp. 187–215). New York: Excerpta Medica.

von Bertalanffy, L. (1962). General systems theory: A critical review. *General Systems, 7,* 1–20.

CHAPTER **3**

# Play Theory and Sensory Integration

**Anita C. Bundy, ScD, OTR**

*Doing things for the fun of it constitutes play.*
*But what is the use of doing things just for fun? What is the use of play? Rather, has it any use? If it had no use we do not believe a desire for it would have been so firmly implanted in our natures, and in the nature of every living thing. . . . The first few years of a child's life . . . seem spent almost wholly in play. Nothing gives us more uneasiness than to see a child who does not play. We consider it a sure sign of sickness, either of body or mind. . . . [As a result of playing], the child grows. Growth is the primary use of play, and this is as true of intellectual growth as of physical.*

*West, 1888, p. 469*

Imagine this scenario. A small group of us are preparing to observe an occupational therapy treatment session. The session is to be based on the principles of sensory integration theory. We're standing off in a corner of the clinic, near the back door that leads to a hallway and other offices in the building. The clinic is a large room; thick mats cover the floors, and swings and other equipment line the walls.

Ricky, an 11-year-old boy with sensory integrative dysfunction, bounds through the front door into the clinic, eager to begin his therapy session. "What do you want to start with today, Ricky?" asks Sally, Ricky's occupational therapist. Without a moment's hesitation, Ricky responds, "The bull! I want to ride the bull!"

The "bull" is a large, padded, cylindrically shaped swing (sometimes called a bolster swing). It is suspended by two ropes, attached at either end, to a single hook mounted in the ceiling. Before mounting the bull, Ricky queries Sally as to what the record is for the longest ride on the wild, bucking beast, and who holds it. Sally responds that she thinks the record is about 1 minute and that he, Ricky Ranchero, is the current champion.

Ricky rides the bull by lying on his stomach on top of it and "hugging it for dear life." Sally grabs the ropes and, making wild whooping noises, shakes the swing as hard as she thinks Ricky can tolerate. Ricky maintains his hold on the bull for a full 30 seconds. All the while, he yells out "Ricky Ranchero, winner and still champion," and other cheers of accomplishment.

Gradually, Ricky begins to lose his grasp on "the beast" and slides around the bull until he is riding underneath, still holding on valiantly (Fig. 3–1). Sally shakes

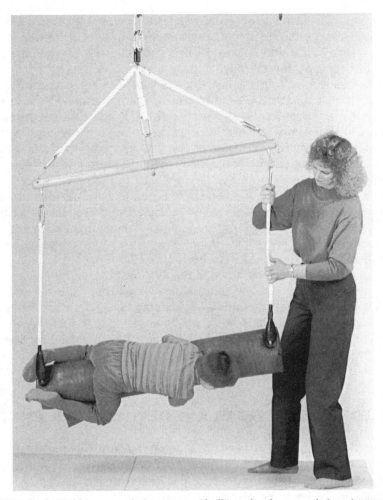

**FIGURE 3–1.** Holding on to bolster swing "bull" as the therapist shakes the swing.

the ropes somewhat less vigorously. She cheers Ricky on, trying to coach him to extend his ride for as long as possible. After several more seconds, Ricky begins to yell that he's "losing it," and drops softly onto the padded surface beneath him. "That was about the hardest ride you ever gave me, I think," Ricky says, and the two begin developing a strategy for Ricky's next ride.

This was truly an excellent treatment session. As silent, unobtrusive observers to this treatment session, we were enthralled. The interaction between Ricky and Sally was exquisite, like a finely tuned dance. They seemed oblivious to our presence. And, having not seen Ricky for many months, we were very impressed by the gains he obviously had made as a result of the treatment Sally had carefully planned and conducted with him. We were proud to be a part of a profession that clearly had made such a difference in the life of this young man.

Our reverie was interrupted by the arrival of another observer, one who was totally unaware of what she was watching. "No wonder kids like to come here," she remarked. "She's *just playing* with him."

As occupational therapists, our "hackles were raised" by this comment. We have been called "play ladies" for too many years. Didn't this woman realize that it was Sally's skill that made the treatment session appear to be so effortless and playful? Didn't she realize that it was, in part, Ricky's difficulty with playing that had led to his referral to occupational therapy?

The obvious answer to these questions is "no." Clearly, she did *not* recognize what an accomplishment this playful treatment session really was. And she is not alone. Some major theoreticians (cf. Montessori, 1973) also have suggested that play is secondary to the serious business of learning. In her original book, Ayres (1972) wrote a brilliant description of the use of play and the creation of a playful environment. However, she entitled it "The Art of Therapy" and the word "play" does not appear anywhere in the chapter. Nor is play listed in the index of her book.

Ayres was aware that she was "ahead of her time." She avoided discussing the contribution that play made to therapy because she feared being criticized for lacking a "scientific basis" (A. J. Ayres, personal communication, March 13, 1988). Had Ayres attempted to justify play in her early work, quite possibly the theory of sensory integration never would have been created.

Today play *is* a respectable topic, a respectable goal, and a laudable achievement. The benefits of play are becoming widely recognized (Rubin, Fein, & Vandenberg, 1983). As occupational therapists, we list play as an important lifelong occupation (Kielhofner, 1985). Therefore, we have an important responsibility to understand play, to evaluate it, to promote it, and to validate the effectiveness of its use as treatment. To do this, we must begin by defining play in a way that will enable us to facilitate it and, thereby, realize all the benefits that are associated with it.

## THE PROBLEM WITH PLAY: DEFINING AN ENIGMA

Why bother defining play in a book about sensory integrative theory? Isn't defining play like defining "red" or "blue"? All of us know what red and blue are when we see them. Yet most of us are unable to define them meaningfully; that is, in a way that enables others to recognize them.

Ask people on the street if they know what play is. Certainly, most will say they do. Ask them to define it. They will probably say things like "fun," "opposite of work," or "what kids do." Ask them if they would recognize play if they saw it, and of course they'd say yes, but they may think you are crazy even to ask such an "obvious" question.

Defining play *is* like defining a color. While the distinction between red-orange and orange-red is of little concern to most people, it may be of great concern to the artist whose livelihood may require using the precise colors needed to recreate a sunset.

Play is to occupational therapists what red is to the artist — a tool. Occupational therapists make a living (and often enable others to do so), by creating therapeutic situations in which the risks and consequences are minimized, thereby allowing our clients to try out things they could not, or would not, try in their normal lives (Vandenberg & Kielhofner, 1982). That is, occupational therapists make a living by creating "play" and by enabling others to play. Thus, it is crucial that we be able to distinguish play from nonplay. This distinction is as important for occupational therapists using sensory integrative theory as a tool of treatment as it is for occupational therapists using any practice theory, regardless of the age of the clients.

Further, we have a responsibility to our emerging profession to develop the constructs of our practice and to validate these constructs with research. Without a working definition of constructs such as play, neither theory nor clinical practice can be fully validated through research.

The problem of defining play has plagued theorists and researchers from many professions for years (Rubin et al., 1983). In contrast, occupational therapists who have written about play frequently have assumed that their audience knows what play is and that a definition is not necessary. Those few occupational therapists who have offered a definition have stated only that play is an intrinsically motivated and pleasurable behavior (cf. Daub, 1983; Florey, 1971), or have attempted to define it by citing various developmental taxonomies of play (Clark, 1985; Michelman, 1969; Takata, 1974). Still others (cf. Reilly, 1974) believed that defining play is impossible. In the one text written by occupational therapists devoted entirely to play, Reilly (1974) stated that "only the naive could believe from reviewing the evidence of the literature, that play is a behavior having an identifiable nature" (p. 113). She preferred, instead, to discuss play in a theoretical fashion, as an "appreciative learning system." However, as Pratt (1989) indicated, "practice in occupational therapy demands more than a theoretical explanation of play" (p. 295).

The body of knowledge in occupational therapy has been drawn from several sciences, including biology, psychology, sociology, and anthropology (Hopkins, 1988). Each of these "parent fields" contains a body of literature on play. Much of our knowledge of pediatric play is based on the literature of developmental psychology. In addition, the literature of education (another practice profession that, like occupational therapy, views play as an important means to promote development) also contains a significant body of literature on play. It seems appropriate, therefore, that we begin the process of defining play by examining concepts from developmental psychology and educational literature.

According to Rubin et al. (1983), definitions of play reported in developmental psychology literature are of three types: (a) descriptions of the characteristics that mark the occurrence of play and separate it from other behaviors; (b) taxonomies describing play behaviors in the context of children's social and cognitive development; and (c) descriptions of the environmental contexts likely to evoke playful behaviors. We will discuss each and relate them to occupational therapy and sensory integration in the following sections.

## The Characteristics of Play

Probably the most common method of defining play is by listing traits thought to characterize it or to separate it from other occupations (usually work). A number of terms traditionally have been used, including "pleasurable," "voluntary," and "spontaneous." Following a thorough review of the literature defining play, Rubin et al. (1983) identified six traits that most authors agree are the hallmarks of play: (a) intrinsic motivation; (b) attention to means rather than ends; (c) organism rather than stimulus dominated (what can *I* do with this object rather than what does this object do?); (d) nonliteral, simulative behavior; (e) freedom from externally imposed rules; and (f) requiring the *active* participation of the player.

Because each of these traits provides the occupational therapist with important guidelines for assessing whether or not play occurred during a given treatment session, each requires some additional discussion. As we will show, these traits become intertwined and difficult to separate during any play transaction (Neumann, 1971).

## INTRINSIC MOTIVATION

Rubin et al. (1983) indicated that, of these six traits, intrinsic motivation alone is almost universally acknowledged as the essential element of play. By their definition, intrinsic motivation refers to the concept that the individual engages in the activity because something about the activity itself is appealing rather than because someone else told the individual that he or she should, or must, do it. For instance, in the above example, it might be that the idea of riding an animal such as a bull is intrinsically motivating to Ricky and that any activity that incorporated riding bulls might motivate him.

While intrinsic motivation frequently is defined as motivation derived from the appeal of the activity itself, some authors (e.g., Berlyne, 1966; Neumann, 1971; Piaget, 1962; White, 1959) relate intrinsic motivation to the "inner drive of the individual." However, these authors seem to have varying opinions as to why play is intrinsically motivating. For example, White associated intrinsic motivation with mastery; Piaget associated it with practice of skills; and Berlyne linked it with maintaining optimum levels of arousal.

Intrinsic motivation often is considered to be the most important trait of play; however, it is difficult to observe and to measure (Smith, Takhvar, Gore, & Vollstedt 1985). Often intrinsic motivation is assumed to be present because the individual has chosen the activity or appears to be enjoying it. In the above example, it is quite clear that Ricky finds riding the bull to be an intrinsically motivating activity. Mastery, practice, arousal, and motivation intrinsic to the activity all may contribute to Ricky's obvious motivation to engage in the activity.

## ATTENTION TO MEANS RATHER THAN ENDS

When an individual is playing, he or she is *more concerned* with the process (means) of play than with its outcome (ends). For Ricky, it was primarily the thrill of riding the bull that led him to request that game, repeatedly, over the course of a number of treatment sessions.

However, Ricky also was interested in the outcome of the game. He kept track of the amount of time he was able to ride the bull and engaged in a sort of long-distance competition with a friend of his, "Bronco Billy," who also happened to be treated by Sally on a different day. Had Ricky been more interested in beating Billy (ends) than in the thrill of the ride (means), the activity would have become more like work (albeit enjoyable work) than like play.

It also is interesting to note that Sally, who was very involved in the whole play episode, *was* more interested in the ends than the means of the activity. Sally wanted Ricky to gain better proximal stability. She helped to facilitate the creation of an activity that provided Ricky with opportunities to take in enhanced vestibular stimulation while resisting the pull of gravity and the movement of the swing. Sally was definitely enjoying the treatment activity, just as Ricky was enjoying it, but Sally was working, while Ricky was playing. Only the most skilled occupational therapists can make their work look like play.

## ORGANISM RATHER THAN STIMULUS DOMINATED

In order for an individual to play with an object or toy, he or she must be familiar with the object. He or she must know what the object is, what it does, and something about what to expect from interacting with the object. Information about an object or toy comes from *exploring* the object; exploration is stimulus-dominated behavior.

Exploration may occur in stages with the individual gradually interacting more and more with the object. The individual may first merely look at the object from a distance or watch someone else playing with it. If the object appears sufficiently safe, the individual may proceed closer to gather more information. He or she may poke, prod, mouth, or touch the object. The individual who is exploring appears to be asking "What does this object *do*?"

Play, on the other hand, is characterized by activity that suggests the individual believes that he or she can do anything he or she wants to with the object (organism-dominated behavior). That is, the individual knows how to interact with the object and finds the feelings or sensations generated by play with the object to be intrinsically motivating.

Generally, an individual does not have to go through the whole exploration process with each new object he or she encounters. Most individuals can extend, or generalize, their knowledge and actions to toys and objects that are similar to those with which they are familiar. They can move immediately into playing with the moderately novel object and can adjust to any differences encountered when playing with the *new* object.

Sometimes a child's difficulty playing appears to be related to difficulty with exploration and with generalizing what he or she knows about using one toy to the use of a similar toy. Consider the following account of Katrina, a 5-year-old child of normal intelligence who was raised in a middle-class family. Katrina was being evaluated for possible sensory integrative dysfunction. When all the standardized testing had been completed, the therapist suspended a large rectangular swing, actually a glider, from two hooks in the ceiling. She then asked Katrina whether she could think of something to do with the swing. Katrina looked puzzled and answered that she couldn't think of anything. After some time passed, Katrina said that she could push the swing, and proceeded to do so. She pushed it a number of different directions and at different speeds, but she never attempted to get on it, even though she played almost daily on the swings in her backyard and in the park.

Finally, the therapist suggested that Katrina climb onto the swing and she did. However, she neither tried to figure out how to make the swing go, nor asked for a push. After a short period of time, Katrina got off the swing and sought out the Sit 'n' Spin that was identical to the one she had at home. Apparently, Katrina's neuronal model for "swing" did not include the glider. Further, although she clearly enjoyed equipment that provided movement, her exploratory skills were not adequate to enable her to derive similar pleasure from the swing.

Katrina's behavior with the glider stands in stark contrast to Ricky's behavior with the bolster swing. Ricky's behavior suggested that he knew very well what to attempt with the bolster swing. In fact, observations of Ricky, later in his treatment session, suggested that he knew *many* things to do with the bolster swing.

Katrina only explored the swing from a distance. She seemed to lack any idea of what to do with it. She appeared to be trying to figure out what it could do, but in a manner more like that of very young children. By 5 years of age, most children we have observed know immediately that the glider is a swing, even if they have some difficulty "making it go."

When the therapist, hoping to facilitate Katrina's play, suggested that Katrina continue her exploration from *on top of* the swing, she again appeared bewildered. She ceased exploring and eventually returned to a toy with which she was familiar enough to play, a toy that her parents had painstakingly taught her to use. Had the therapist gotten on the glider with Katrina and both showed her and "talked her through" how to propel it, Katrina probably would have gotten the idea. However, the need of a 5-year-old to have someone else help her explore a swing is highly unusual.

Exploration is quite normal as a precursor to play, especially in very young children, or with very novel toys. However, Katrina's exploration was impaired as it did not lead to her becoming familiar enough with a moderately novel toy to be able to use it in play. Further, Katrina appeared to have extraordinary difficulty generalizing her ideas for using the playground swing to her use of the glider swing. This was confirmed by her mother, who indicated that each time Katrina got a new toy, someone had to teach her to use it. Otherwise, she simply took it apart or used it as a prop in fantasy play. Katrina not only lacked skills in exploration and play, she lacked the ability to generate ideas of what to do in play.

Although individuals like Katrina are not commonly encountered on the caseloads of occupational therapists, we do see them. Often they are individuals who have severe sensory integrative deficits or who have other more pervasive developmental disabilities, such as autism. Helping them to play, or to take an active role in directing their own therapy, presents a special challenge to the therapist.

## NONLITERAL, SIMULATIVE BEHAVIOR

When Rubin et al. (1983) described play as nonliteral behavior, they were referring only to an individual's ability to pretend or to engage in fantasy play. While we believe that pretending is very important, we think that it is only one aspect of a larger construct of play, the suspension of reality (Neumann, 1971). Another, equally important, facet of the suspension of reality is represented in the need for the therapist to minimize or eliminate the consequences that might normally be associated with the client's performing the same activity in "real life" (Vandenberg & Kielhofner, 1982).

We will now discuss both aspects of the suspension of reality, pretending and reducing the consequences of reality. Most important is that the individual should be free to transform him- or herself, and the treatment activity, into anything he or she desires (Neumann, 1971); and that a primary role of the occupational therapist is to make sure that the constraints of objective reality do not prevent the individual from playing (Ellis, 1973; Vandenberg & Kielhofner, 1982).

Clearly, pretending is an important part of Ricky's treatment session. Only imagination could allow Ricky to transform the therapeutic equipment he was riding into a "bull" and himself into its victorious rider. One of the "paradoxes of play" (Bateson, 1972b) is represented in Ricky's transformation of the swing into the bull. In making the swing into something that it is not (a bull), the therapeutic activity takes on "real" meaning for Ricky. This increased level of meaningfulness of the activity probably would not have been present if the activity consisted only of Ricky, himself, trying to stay on the swing as long as possible while Sally shook it.

Again, the contrast between Ricky and Sally becomes evident. Both Sally and Ricky are actively involved in creating an imaginative game. However, while Ricky is absorbed in pretending, Sally has a dual role. She must help to sustain the playful frame (Bateson, 1971, 1972b) for Ricky and, at the same time, she must be equally active in adjusting the activity so that her "literal" goal of improving Ricky's proximal stability can be met.

For individuals with sensory integrative dysfunction, objective reality commonly presents many constraints that interfere with play. Not the least among those constraints may be fear of moving or fear of being touched. Gravity also presents an inordinate constraint to many individuals whose muscle tone or postural responses may not be adequate to enable them to resist it fully. Complex toys may inhibit the individual whose motor planning skills are poor. It is the responsibility of the therapist to orchestrate the treatment session, and the treatment environment, so that these constraints are minimized or eliminated. In creating a safe environment that is free of the consequences that prevent the individual from succeeding at certain activities in "real life," reality is temporarily suspended and both play and therapeutic gain are facilitated.

The freedom to suspend reality is an important trait of play and a powerful facilitator in the therapeutic process. However, we must offer two important cautions to the occupational therapist providing treatment based on sensory integrative principles.

First, there are some individuals who apparently are "fearless"; they seem to be unaware of *any* constraints imposed by reality. Commonly, these individuals bolt into the treatment area and "fly" headfirst over pieces of equipment left in their paths. They also may perform other dangerous feats such as letting go while hanging upside down from the trapeze. We must be particularly vigilant when treating these individuals. Further, we may need to be particularly careful about encouraging them to overuse pretending in their treatment sessions. If apparently fearless behaviors also occur at home and at school, these children may need our help to distinguish real from pretend.

Second, we need to be aware that not all good occupational therapy involves either play or the alteration of reality. Many individuals may not automatically generalize skills they gain in therapy to their everyday lives. While play is a powerful tool for *gaining* skills in treatment, the therapist also may have to engage the individual in certain "real life" tasks to be sure that, once skills have been attained, they are being used. At the very least, we need to follow up on the outcomes of our therapy by checking with the client and his or her family or by observing the client using newly acquired skills in the context of activities performed in everyday life. The following scenario illustrates this point.

Linda, an occupational therapy student, had been working for a short time with Max, an 8-year-old child who had sensory integrative dysfunction. She asked him how he felt about his treatment, to which he responded, "It's fine; it's fun, but I still can't play dodgeball. I cover my eyes when someone throws the ball at me and then it hits me. And I can never hit anybody else with the ball. I aim it, but it just flies off and then the other kids laugh." For some time, Linda and Jill (the supervising therapist), aware that Max wanted to get better at dodgeball, had incorporated catching and throwing a Nerf ball into Max's sensory integration treatment activities. His skills seemed to have become much better. Thus, they were a little dismayed by his complaint.

Then Linda decided to take Max outside and engage him in some skills-training with a ball like the one he used in gym class. She had him throw the ball repeatedly and practice dodging when she threw it at him. She offered two bits of advice repeatedly, "Keep your eyes on the ball, and throw low."

When Max returned to therapy the next week, Jill asked him how it went with the dodgeball. "It went a little better," he replied. "I did what Linda told me and it helped."

"What *did* Linda tell you?" asked Jill.

"Keep my eyes on the ball, and throw low," came the reply.

While the primary treatment approach used with Max had been based on sensory integration principles, Linda and Jill responded to Max's needs to generalize his developing skills to the "real world" by breaking their typical treatment routine to work on what was bothering Max most at that moment, dodgeball. For Max, dodgeball was not play; it truly was work (and, at the moment, not very enjoyable work). "Playing" dodgeball, to Max, however motivating it was, meant anxiety and embarrassment, not the typical feelings associated with play. Thus, the session between Linda and Max could not be described as play in any sense. In fact, Max insisted that they search for the appropriate ball so that their "game" would be as close to reality as possible.

Max had already made many improvements in treatment and, in fact, had many of the skills he needed to be able to succeed at dodgeball. However, *he* didn't recognize that the skills he used in treatment were the same skills he needed for dodgeball. Further, he didn't seem to understand that he needed to throw low to be successful and when confronted with a *real* dodgeball sailing toward him, he continued to close his eyes, even though he had long since learned to watch the Nerf ball he caught during treatment activities.

Linda and Jill were implementing good occupational therapy. They left behind both play and sensory integration when they needed to do so. They were not bound by the belief that when Max gained skills in treatment, he would automatically use them in "real life." They asked for *his* assessment of the results of treatment. Further, they felt free to conduct a session in which reality was *not* suspended. And they made a real difference in the life of their young client.

In summary, the freedom to suspend aspects of reality by pretending and by minimizing the constraints of reality are powerful tools for use in therapy. We must be aware, however, that there are times when the demands of real life *must* be dealt with in therapy, and there are times when allowing an individual to suspend too many aspects of reality might, in the end, be more harmful than helpful to the client.

## FREEDOM FROM EXTERNALLY IMPOSED RULES

Play is an activity that is controlled by the player. It is not imposed by an adult or even another child. It cannot be controlled by too many rules, or it will not occur. But play is a paradox (Bateson, 1971). Knowing the "rules" (i.e., understanding the process and the expected outcomes) enables the player to be safe, to plan his or her actions, and to be free to play. For example, a person playing dodgeball behaves entirely differently than a person playing soccer or volleyball. The individual playing dodgeball by volleyball "rules" probably would not be allowed by the team to play for very long.

Therapy, like cooperative play, can never be totally controlled by the client. In therapy, the therapist has objectives that must be met (Rast, 1986); play can be used to facilitate those objectives, but it cannot replace them. However, for any treatment objective, there is a considerable amount of latitude in how the objective will be achieved. As we will discuss in more detail in Chapters 10 and 12, therapy activities are most successful when they are selected and directed by the client. There are no "rules" for achieving particular goals by using particular activities or pieces of equipment. The use of specific equipment to meet specific objectives is bounded only by the creativity of the therapist and the client.

Once the rules that insure the client's safety have been established, there is little need for other external rules to be applied. The client should be as free as possible to select from an array of activities that have been carefully chosen for their therapeutic potential. He or she should be free to transform the equipment and him- or herself into whatever is desired. In selecting and transforming the activity, the client has a part in establishing the "rules" of the activity. The client should be free to negotiate changes in the activity and in the rules, as he or she sees fit (Bateson, 1972a).

Control of a treatment session is always shared between the client and the therapist. In addition to providing the client with freedom to select and transform activities, there are many ways for a therapist to be sure that a treatment session meets the therapeutic objectives that have been set without removing intrinsic motivation, or the freedom of the client to suspend reality or establish his or her own rules. The skilled therapist adjusts the level of the challenge by altering the activity to make it just a little harder or a little easier or by changing the activity altogether. The therapist can easily carry over a pretend theme or be certain that the new activity is even more motivating than the original activity was. In so doing, the client is enabled to retain both an adequate degree of internal control and the feelings of control as the therapist moves toward meeting her objectives. The play frame is retained and therapeutic gain is facilitated.

It is a mistake to believe that activities result in only one outcome at a time. Children and adults gain many skills and other benefits from their play, but we have never known an individual to state (or even think) before he or she goes to play, "I guess I'll go improve my skills today." People play because it is pleasurable, but they gain more than just pleasure from their play (White, 1989). The same should be true for therapeutic intervention. Ricky initially decided to enroll in therapy because he wanted to be "better at playing sports" with his friends. What motivated him to come each week, however, was that therapy was fun.

## REQUIRING THE ACTIVE PARTICIPATION OF THE PLAYER

When an individual truly is playing, he or she is totally absorbed in the activity. The activity is neither so difficult as to cause worry or anxiety nor so easy as to result in boredom. That activity represents the "just right challenge" (Berlyne, 1969; Csikszentimihayli, 1975, 1979). These words are the same words typically used to describe successful treatment activities. Riding the bull represented such an activity for Ricky. Sally's altering the force with which she shook the swing when Ricky began to lose his grasp represents the therapist's adaptation to the activity to maintain the "just right challenge."

Unless the individual is actively involved, the activity is neither therapeutic nor play. Further, unless the activity results in an adaptive behavior from the individual, it is not therapeutic. As it is defined in Chapter 1, an adaptive behavior is one that is done just a little better than it has ever been done before. However, we must caution therapists that "just a little better" also may be interpreted as *being just a little easier to do or being just a little more spontaneous*. In Max's case, it meant being skilled enough to *play* dodgeball with the other kids, rather than just "suffering" through it.

When activities represent the "just right challenge," clients may repeat the activity over and over again in the course of the treatment session until they have "mastered" the challenge. Once an activity has been mastered, it no longer represents a challenge to the client and is, therefore, less useful in therapy. However, much practice is required before an activity truly is mastered. In each case, a new neuronal model of how it feels to do it is formed through practice. Altering the activity ever so slightly often presents a new challenge and a need to modify the neuronal model. We must take care that, in an attempt to elicit adaptive behaviors from our clients or, *out of our own boredom*, we do not change activities too rapidly. We must take our cues from our clients. An individual who is engrossed in an activity is playing. If the activity has been carefully chosen, that individual also is producing adaptive behaviors and realizing therapeutic gains.

There are no "rules" about how many activities should be done in a treatment session or how long each activity should last. Activities should be allowed to continue until they are no longer motivating for the client or until the client has mastered the challenge.

Therapists frequently ask whether or not comparing successful treatment activities to play means that the activities necessarily must be "fun" to be good treatment. Having observed many individuals, both in play and in therapy, we prefer to examine whether or not he or she is absorbed by the activity rather than looking for signs of obvious fun or delight (although these certainly may be present). Often, individuals are too engrossed in the activity (whether play or therapy) to be aware even that they are having fun. After the activity is over, they may remark that it was fun or pleasurable, but laughing or smiling or other signs commonly associated with "fun" were notably absent when the activity was in progress.

Further, many of the clients we treat rarely associate fun with activities involving movement or touch. We believe that it is a sure sign of progress made in therapy when an individual begins to remark afterward than an activity was fun. Several clients have queried us about whether or not a particular activity was "fun" in ways that have made us think that they have made new associations between fun and activities involving movement and touch.

## SUMMARY

Several characteristics commonly used to define play have been described, and their relationship to therapy discussed, as they apply both to the client and the therapist. We believe that it is important for therapists to remember these traits since they provide important guidelines for evaluating treatment to insure that play *is* being used when such is the intent. Further, we hope that therapists will recognize when play is not necessary or even should be avoided.

## Play as Developmental Hierarchies (Taxonomies)

Rather than defining play by its characteristics, a number of authors have offered taxonomies that define developmental hierarchies associated with various types of play. Among the best-known of these taxonomies was that developed by Piaget (1962), who described a developmental sequence of play reflecting children's acquisition of cognitive skills (i.e., practice, symbolic, games with rules). Similarly, Parten (1932) formulated a taxonomy of behaviors that described the development of social play (i.e., onlooker, solitary, parallel, associative, and cooperative play). Both Parten's and Piaget's taxonomies are widely used by occupational therapists. In addition, Knox (1974), an occupational therapist, developed a taxonomy describing preschoolers' play skills; the Knox play scale later was revised by Bledsoe and Shepherd (1982) and renamed the Preschool Play Scale. This taxonomy, which measures play in four different domains (Space Management, Material Management, Imitation, and Participation) is commonly used by therapists both in clinical practice and in occupational therapy research (Bledsoe & Shepherd, 1982; Bundy, 1987, 1989; Clifford & Bundy, 1989; Harrison & Kielhofner, 1986; Howard, 1986; Knox, 1974).

According to Rubin and colleagues (1983), there are two primary areas in which defining play by using a taxonomy is particularly beneficial: in the evaluation of individual children's play development, and in research. By narrowing play into categories, it becomes more readily observable; thus, the play of individuals with various disabling conditions can be compared with that of normal individuals. This comparison can be done individually, as therapists do when evaluating a client with suspected play deficits, or when determining the effectiveness of treatment on the improvement of play skills. This comparison also can be done with groups, as researchers do when investigating the effect of a particular disorder on play.

The problem with using a taxonomy to define normal play lies with the implications this has for defining play deficits. Taxonomies of play are generally based on social or cognitive behaviors associated with chronological or mental age. However, when using taxonomies as the only definition of play, it is virtually impossible for therapists to simultaneously consider an individual's *preferences* for play. When one considers both the traits that define play, and the use of a taxonomy as a definition of normal play, the problem becomes apparent.

For example, does a preschool-aged child who has a motor planning disorder and who does not like to play on the playground (as do most children his or her age), but who *really likes* to play indoors, have a play deficit? Is that deficit comparable to that of the preschooler who really wants to join his or her peers on the top of the jungle gym but cannot figure out how to get there? Both seem to have a deficit in play, but the two deficits are very different. In the first case, the child prefers activities at which he or she is successful, and avoids other play activities that his or her peers really like. However, in the second case, the child is unable to do the types of activities he or she most wants to do.

Defining play by the use of a taxonomy alone does not allow the therapist to distinguish between these two types of deficits. Thus, the therapist may be unable to develop the optimal treatment plan for these two individuals.

## The Environment of Play

According to Rubin et al. (1983), the third method for defining play comes from descriptions of the context in which play behaviors occur. While these definitions usually appear in the procedures sections of research reports of play, they also can help us to think about the most desirable characteristics of our treatment environments. They are indirect definitions of play, characterized by those things that the investigators (and therapists) believe will evoke play behaviors. Rubin and his colleagues (1983) have summarized a number of environmental components that are commonly used by researchers to elicit play. These include:

> (1) an array of familiar peers, toys, or other materials likely to engage children's interest; (2) an agreement between adults and children, expressed in word, gesture, or established by convention, that the children are free to choose from the array whatever they wish to do within whatever limits are required by the setting or the study; (3) adult behavior that is minimally intrusive or directive; (4) a friendly atmosphere designed to make children feel comfortable and safe; and (5) scheduling that reduces the likelihood of the children being tired, hungry, ill, or experiencing other types of bodily stress. (p. 701)

Clearly, the rationale for defining play as behaviors that occur in contexts such as those described above is that when a child is in a safe environment, surrounded by interesting toys and nondirective adults, the chances increase that the child will be intrinsically motivated and free of external rules. Thus, the chance for play to occur is maximized.

The difficulty with defining play by its context lies with the assumption that the adults responsible for creating the playful environment view play in the same way that children view it. Further, this definition assumes that the behaviors elicited are actually play behaviors. Clearly, therapists must be vigilant observers of the individuals they treat to be certain that play is occurring, when such is their intent. Merely setting up a theoretically playful situation does not ensure that play can, or will, occur.

## An Educational Perspective on Play

Rubin and his colleagues (1983) have provided us with a structure for examining and facilitating play, and with important considerations for differentiating play from nonplay. In another theoretical treatment of play literature, Neumann (1971), an educator, developed a definition of play that includes many of the same elements Rubin and his colleagues discussed. However, Neumann's criteria for play make the definition somewhat simpler, and thus more easily applied when examining therapeutic sessions for the presence of play.

Neumann described three criteria for play. These included internal locus of control (freedom to choose); internal determination of reality; and intrinsic motivation. Neumann (1971) believed that internal locus of control, rather than intrinsic motivation (Rubin, Fein, & Vandenberg, 1983), was the most important criterion for play. Further, she stated that within any single play transaction the criteria become almost inextricably intertwined, but that all the criteria depend on the presence of a degree of internal control.

For example, Neumann (1971) indicated that if the individual is in control, then he or she is able to determine who and what to play with, and how and where to play. The individual who is in control is free to suspend reality in such a way as to transform a swing into a bull and him- or herself into a fearless rider. When internal reality is present, another child would be free to determine the "fate" of the "bean bag monsters" lurking in the "waters" of the mat. While the individual may choose to make the transaction similar to objective reality, the therapist must remember that a treatment session that successfully incorporates play will include a reality made to order for, and by, the individual.

Neumann (1971) believed that when the three criteria were present as a part of any transaction, that transaction could be considered to be play. However, Neumann also acknowledged that while these criteria describe the maximum optimal conditions under which play occurs,

> . . . rarely does one have total internal control, total intrinsic motivation, or total internal reality. Consequently, play and nonplay must be considered as opposing end-points of a continuum of transaction between the individual and the environment. The degree to which the criteria for play are fulfilled determines where on the continuum the transaction belongs. (p. 163)

The consideration of play as a continuum is perhaps the most significant contribution Neumann (1971) made to us. As occupational therapists we are interested in play, in part because play is a powerful medium for treatment. However, Neumann also cautioned us about being careful in our use of play as a tool.

> The consideration of play on a continuum is particularly important in implementation of play for educational or other purposes. Since implementation of play implies external motive, namely someone attempting to use play for a specific purpose other than play itself, care must be taken to provide opportunity for internal criteria so that play, as defined along a continuum, does occur. If the

transaction is not play, then play is not being implemented and any value or goals sought by using play specifically will not be attained. (p. 164)

In much the same way that therapists view a successful treatment session, Neumann (1971) believed that any act of play is a transaction between the child and the environment "during which specific aspects of the environment and of the child are manipulated by the child" (p. 137). According to Neumann (1971), the criteria help to determine what is, and what is not, play. She stated, however, that play transactions are more fully portrayed when the ways in which the play is carried out and the objects and other people involved in the transaction also are described. For example, the reader would have known very little about Ricky's play if we had not depicted the swing, the clinic, and Sally's role in the transaction.

Neumann's advice to describe play transactions in enough detail that others can visualize them is a particularly cogent suggestion to those of us who frequently describe a client's play abilities in reports to parents and others. The clients we treat often are able to play quite well under certain circumstances, but may be unable to play at all in other situations (Bundy, 1989). It is important that we provide parents and others with the information they need to be able to facilitate the play of our clients outside of therapy.

This does not mean that we want parents and others to conduct therapy with our clients. We will discuss that issue in Chapter 11. We *would* like them to be able to play with our clients in a way that each finds satisfying and rewarding. Many times, by describing key aspects of playful treatment sessions, we can facilitate play between our clients and other important people in their lives.

## TOWARD A WORKING DEFINITION OF PLAY FOR OCCUPATIONAL THERAPISTS

Based on Neumann's (1971) work, the following working definition of play is proposed for use by occupational therapists seeking to use play as a part of treatment. Play is a transaction between an individual and the environment that is intrinsically motivated, internally controlled, and free of many of the constraints of objective reality. Since it is not always possible (or desirable) for individuals to be in complete control of their environments, to fully determine their own reality, or to be in the presence of the objects or playmates that might be most intrinsically motivating at the time, play transactions are considered to represent a continuum of behaviors that are more or less playful, depending on the degree to which the criteria are present (Fig. 3–2).

When clients play during occupational therapy based on the principles of sensory integration theory, they play in certain predictable ways. That is, not all kinds of play lend themselves to use in this type of therapy. In treatment based on the principles of sensory integration, clients use their sensorimotor skills to interact with an environment specially designed to provide opportunities for enhanced sensory intake. They may repeat specific transactions, practicing until they master the challenge. They become absorbed in their play and demonstrate the acquisition of adaptive behaviors. They often transform themselves, the therapist, and elements of the environment into something that they are not.

Because the creation of playful treatment sessions is difficult, therapists must be prepared to evaluate each activity in each treatment session to determine where on

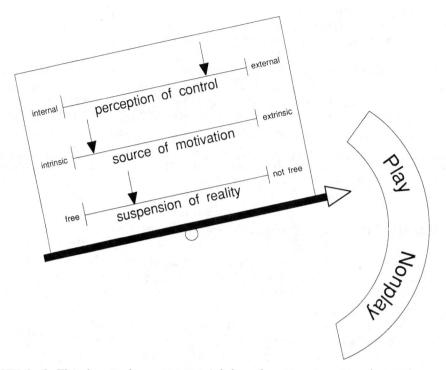

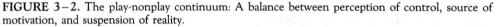

FIGURE 3–2. The play-nonplay continuum: A balance between perception of control, source of motivation, and suspension of reality.

the play-nonplay continuum each transaction falls with regard to each of the criteria for play. Ellis (1973, pp. 126–127) has offered a series of questions which the therapist may ask in order to determine how well the goal of play has been met. Listed by the criterion to which they apply, these questions include:

*Intrinsic Motivation*

    1a. Is the client undertaking the behavior in order to achieve a payoff?

OR  1b. Is the client behaving only for the experiential reward associated with the process?

    2a. Does the setting or situation (including the therapist) impose consequences that, by requiring given behaviors, prevent the client's concern for the process of his or her behavior?

OR  2b. Does the setting provide interactions that are freed from an externally applied final consequence?

*Internal Locus of Control*

    1a. Is the behavior controlled by somebody other than the client?

OR  1b. Is the client controlling the behavior?

    2a. Is something in the setting so constraining the behavior that the choices among responses available to the client are limited?

OR  2b. Does the setting permit choices at each point in a stream of behavior to rest with the client?

*Internal Reality*

    1a. Is the client forced by circumstances to recognize all the constraints of reality?

OR   1b. Is it possible for the client to bend some aspects of the real situation by suspending temporarily associations between events in favor of an imagined situation?

2a. Does the setting prevent a relaxation from concern with the real connection between events and consequences?

OR   2b. Does the setting allow the suspension of some aspects of reality?

## THE POTENTIAL OF PLAY IN THERAPY

When Ayres (1972) wrote about the "art of therapy," she described the skilled therapist as one who facilitates a child's mastery of the environment. Her terminology is similar to that used by White (1959), who compellingly argued that humans require a long and playful "apprenticeship" in order to become masters of their environments.

If play is the vehicle by which individuals become masters of their environments, then play should be among the most powerful of therapeutic tools. Further, if therapists are able to promote an individual's play, then they should announce that as an accomplishment, rather than feeling that they must couch their treatment goals in something "more meaningful" or "more reimbursable." "The child's play can thus be viewed as serious business, though to him it is merely something that is interesting and fun to do" (White, 1959, p. 321).

Therapy based on the principles of sensory integration is conducted by providing the individual with activities that incorporate opportunities for enhanced sensory intake, provide the "just right challenge," and demand from that individual an adaptive behavior. Treatment is thought to be most successful when the activities are intrinsically motivating and when the individual is actively involved, in control, and directing the flow, of the session. All discussions of sensory integration therapy inevitably contain mention of the need to be sure that the client is safe from both physical and psychological threat; in other words, that there are no adverse consequences to attempting difficult challenges and that the constraints of objective reality have been kept at bay (see Chapter 10).

The above description is about as close to a description of play as it is possible to imagine. Not all play is good therapy and not all good therapy is play. However, treatment based on sensory integration theory, when carried out in the fullest sense, describes a special subset of play transactions in which all activities include enhanced sensory stimulation.

Creating a playful environment and facilitating the play of individuals with disabling conditions is not an easy task (Anderson, Hinojosa, & Strauch, 1987; Rast, 1986). In fact, Rast cautioned that play and therapy almost appear to be mutually exclusive.

> A child's play is an intrinsically motivating activity done voluntarily and for its own sake; therapy proceeds according to the therapist's plan to achieve definite treatment objectives. Also, play is characterized by a combination of engagement and enjoyment, characteristics that may be desirable in therapy, but are not necessarily typical of it. (p. 30)

We believe that, while not all occupational therapy is play, play is what therapists using the principles of sensory integration strive to attain. Play and nonplay are a continuum of behaviors, not an either-or situation (Neumann, 1971). If it is necessary for the therapist to be relatively more directive in a session, then the therapist might want to compensate for that by emphasizing activities that are particularly motivating to the client or by supporting a lot of pretending in the session.

Therapists are aiming to meet therapeutic objectives within as playful a framework as it is possible for the child and the therapist to create together. In her concluding remarks, Rast (1986) summarized this beautifully.

> Therapy goals often fail to gain an impaired child's attention or cooperation because they tend to be too remote or abstract to be experienced as intrinsically motivating. Play, by contrast, offers just such intrinsic motivation. . . . Play activities, however, should neither be used primarily as a device to disguise therapy nor held as a reward until the completion of a session. When properly conceived and utilized, play activities have the power to translate the multifaceted aspects of environmental interaction into experiences that are directly meaningful to the child in the "here and now." Thus, rewarding engagement in play activities in the present can contribute to future achievements. (p. 40)

As therapists, we strive to provide the client with the sense that he or she is playing. We make available activities that the client will find intrinsically motivating and that provide challenges closely matching his or her skills. However, we also must orchestrate the session so that it is treatment. That is, we must have a plan. We must know exactly the type and the amount of sensory stimulation that will lead to the adaptive behaviors we seek from the client. We must be prepared to alter activities ever so slightly so that they meet the dual purposes of play and therapy. We must take our lead both from theory and from the responses of our client. While the client is playing, we are conducting treatment. The client has the benefit of both play and skilled therapeutic intervention.

Play and playfulness are powerful therapeutic tools. Play promotes competence. The playfulness of the therapist (and ideally of the child) helps to create an atmosphere in which play can occur. When play and playfulness are coupled with skilled therapeutic intervention, they often can make a real difference in the lives of the clients we treat. Therapists using sensory integrative principles in the most skillful manner with children who have disordered central nervous systems should strive to create play in their treatment sessions. Play promotes the spiraling process of self-actualization.

## THE CONTRIBUTION OF SENSORY INTEGRATION TO PLAY

### What Sensory Integration Theory Implies

The ability to process and integrate sensory information effectively and to use that information to plan and produce efficient interactions with the environment enables the individual to control his or her actions and provides the individual with a sense that he or she is in control. Transactions that truly are play are dependent on the player's ability to be in control (Kooij & Vrijhof, 1981; Neumann, 1971; Rubin et al., 1983). Further, individuals who believe that they are more internally than externally controlled may be better players (Morrison, Bundy, & Fisher (in press); Kooij & Vrijhof, 1981).

Thus, it is logical to conclude that some individuals who have sensory integrative dysfunction also may have difficulty playing. Certainly the individual who is at the mercy of gravity, or fear, cannot feel in control of many of the activities that characterize play. As Lindquist, Mack, and Parham (1982) have stated eloquently,

It is apparent that the relative adequacy of sensory integrative abilities will influence how the child plays. At the sensorimotor level, the child's ability to integrate and organize sensation is of paramount importance in using the body effectively in play. At the constructive level, such end products of sensory integration as praxis, eye-hand coordination, and visual perception will influence the quality of the child's interactions with objects. And at the social level, end products of sensory integration — self-esteem and self-confidence — may influence the child's willingness and ability to interact, cooperate, and compete with peers in social play. (p. 434)

To play optimally, individuals must feel that they are in control and are free to choose what to play with and how to play; they must be able to suspend reality; they must be able to interact with the people and objects that they find intrinsically motivating. Because sensory integration is one of the foundations for play, sensory integration theory provides therapists with an *indirect* means of evaluating some of the neurobehavioral antecedents to play. Deficits in sensory integration are most clearly related to individuals' abilities to interact with people and objects in their environments and to feel as though they are in control. Sensory integrative deficits also may affect the types of activities that the individual finds to be intrinsically motivating (Clifford & Bundy, 1989).

A deficit in the ability to integrate and organize vestibular-proprioceptive input manifests itself in impaired postural-ocular responses, gravitational insecurity, or aversive responses to movement. Similarly, a deficit in tactile processing may result in poor motor planning or tactile defensiveness. Although some of these manifestations may result in an individual's having a decreased ability to play, it is a "quantum leap" from poor tactile discrimination to impaired play skills. We must make that leap with care.

## What the Research on Play and Sensory Integration Theory Suggest

The premise that sensory integrative dysfunction results in impaired play skills in young children was investigated in a series of studies conducted by Bundy (1987, 1989) and Clifford & Bundy (1989). They observed 61 boys (30 normal and 31 diagnosed as having sensory integrative dysfunction) during 30 minutes of free play, both indoors and outdoors. They recorded play behaviors on the Preschool Play Scale (Bledsoe & Shepherd, 1982; Knox, 1974). The results demonstrated that the mean scores of the boys with sensory integrative dysfunction were significantly lower than those of the normal boys on the overall score of the Preschool Play Scale and on three of its four dimensions: Space Management, Material Management, and Participation. However, further analysis of the data revealed that approximately one third of the boys with sensory integrative dysfunction received scores on the Preschool Play Scale that were no more than 6 months below the norm for their chronological ages, and well within the range for the normal boys. Thus, sensory integrative dysfunction does not always result in play deficits.

Further, although Bundy (1987) found statistically significant correlations between scores on the Preschool Play Scale and scores on the Bruininks-Oseretsky Test of Motor Proficiency (Bruininks, 1978), none of the correlations exceeded $r = 0.40$; most were much lower. Thus, boys with the poorest motor coordination (and theoretically the worst sensory integrative dysfunction) were not necessarily those boys whose play skills were the most impaired and vice versa.

Finally, Clifford and Bundy (1989) demonstrated that both normal preschool-aged boys and preschool-aged boys with sensory integrative dysfunction more frequently expressed preference for toys that supported sensorimotor play (e.g., swings, slides) over toys that supported other types of play (construction, symbolic). However, when the boys' expressed preferences for various types of play (percentage of toys they selected from each category) were compared with their actual performance in those domains of play (scores on related Preschool Play Scale domains), many boys had apparently altered their play preferences to match their abilities. Fewer than one third of the boys with sensory integrative dysfunction expressed strong preference for any domain of play in which their play skills were not age appropriate.

## What Sensory Integration Theory and Play Research Do Not (or Cannot) Tell Us

The research conducted to date has indicated that sensory integrative dysfunction *does not always* result in disruption to play skills and behaviors. However, the research in this area has been limited to preschool-aged boys with heterogeneous types of sensory integrative dysfunction. Thus, the research is riddled with unknowns. For example, what consequences does sensory integrative dysfunction have to the play of older children and adults? Are individuals with sensory integrative dysfunction less playful than are normal individuals? Does sensory integrative dysfunction differentially affect the play of boys and girls? And, what are the consequences of altering play preferences (particularly in children) to reflect the individual's actual abilities?

Certainly, tactually defensive children who always avoid playing with other children for fear that they will be touched, deprive themselves of one of the most important arenas in which to develop the social skills they will need throughout their lives. Is the same true of motor skills? How much motor play is required for the individual to practice the motor behaviors he or she will need to function adequately in daily life (Clifford & Bundy, 1989)? Further, Vandenberg (1981) has suggested that social interaction is more apt to occur in the context of gross motor than fine motor play. If that is true, then the child who avoids gross motor play may inadvertently deprive him- or herself of the chance to develop and practice social skills. And these are only a few of the many questions that remain to be answered through future research.

While only Bundy and Clifford (Bundy, 1987, 1989; Clifford & Bundy, 1989) have systematically studied the play skills of individuals with sensory integrative dysfunction, a few related studies describing the play (or leisure) of children with learning disabilities (mainly school-aged children or adolescents) have been completed (Bryan, 1976, 1978; Levy & Gottlieb, 1984; Margalit, 1984). Although the results of these studies cannot answer fully the questions we have posed, they suggest that the questions are valid and have important implications for treatment.

Margalit (1984) reported that the leisure time of learning-disabled adolescents was apt to be comprised largely of passive, solitary activities such as television watching. Other researchers (cf. Bryan, 1976, 1978; Levy & Gottlieb, 1984) have concentrated on the sociometric status of learning-disabled children and on their ability to enter social situations appropriately. Not surprisingly, most of these researchers have found their subjects to be relatively isolated and to lack the skills to initiate and respond to social situations.

If the results of these studies can be extrapolated to the individuals who are referred to us for sensory integrative dysfunction (and any extrapolation of this nature certainly must be done with caution), then it is important that we do all we can to facilitate the play skills of these individuals. In some cases, this may mean working to improve the individual's sensory integration. In other cases, it may mean working directly on the play skills. Most times, it probably means both.

It is important to reiterate that the questions posed above have not been addressed in studies with individuals who have sensory integrative dysfunction. Therefore, we cannot answer those questions adequately. The few studies that have been done have not demonstrated that all children with sensory integrative dysfunction necessarily have deficits in play (Bundy, 1987, 1989; Clifford & Bundy, 1989).

Clearly, the ability to process and integrate incoming sensory input may influence, in some way, an individual's ability to play. Thus, sensory integration theory provides therapists with some information that may explain some of an individual's problems in play. Likewise, observations of an individual's play can provide therapists with valuable information about that individual's sensory integrative capacities. Finally, play is a critical component of sensory integration treatment programs. However, sensory integrative theory is not primarily about play. It is a theory about the neurobehavioral foundations for play and the spiral process of self-actualization that is influenced by sensory integration. Play is an extremely complex function. It is the end product of the interaction among a number of inborn traits and acquired skills; sensory integration is only one of the many foundations of play.

## PRINCIPLES FOR ASSESSING PLAY AND TREATING PLAY DEFICITS IN CHILDREN WITH SENSORY INTEGRATIVE DYSFUNCTION

The relationship between sensory integration and play is not simple, nor is it clear, either from the theory or the existing research. Following is a brief discussion of four points related to the play skills of individuals with sensory integrative dysfunction.

*If you want to know about how well an individual plays, watch that individual play.* Watch that individual for signs that sensory integrative dysfunction interferes with his or her ability, but watch for more than that. Watch to see how well he or she plays. Further, it is important to observe individuals playing in a number of different types of environments. A study by Vandenberg (1981) suggested that the playthings available to individuals in various settings had a marked effect on the types of play in which the children engaged. Vandenberg found that more social interaction occurred in settings that encouraged gross motor play than in settings that encouraged fine motor play. He believed that children in the latter settings had less need to interact with their peers and that the activity itself "pulled for" parallel play. This study has important implications for therapists who have limited time, but who may wish to assess the social play skills of their clients.

Occupational therapy evaluations, especially evaluations of sensory integrative function, are time consuming and costly. Many therapists feel that they cannot justify the expenditure of additional time to observe individuals playing. However, the importance of play to an individual's life cannot be overemphasized. Sensory integrative dysfunction, by itself, is not a problem to be addressed by occupational therapy. It becomes a problem for occupational therapists when it disrupts an individual's abilities to assume his or her expected life roles, including the role of player.

*If you want to know whether or not an individual is happy with his own play skills, ask that individual.* Ask the child's mother; ask the child's teacher. Find out who the child's best friend is and why he or she likes that friend. Ask who he or she would really like to play with if he or she could play with anyone; find out why. Even if the child is very young, find out what the child most likes to do and what the child least likes to do; find out why. Much information, both about the individual and about his or her sensory integrative dysfunction, can be gleaned in this way. There may well be important differences between the child who is happy with his or her time spent in play, even if that time is spent doing something very different from peers, and the child who really wants to do what everybody else does, but does not have the skills to be able to do those things. The latter individual is certainly at more risk for impaired self-esteem (Clifford & Bundy, 1989).

While asking questions of an individual is certainly the most direct way to get answers, there also are assessment tools that address individual preferences in play. Most of these tools are quite simplistic as well as quick and easy to administer; some involve only pointing to pictures of preferred toys (Wolfgang & Phelps, 1983). The advantage of using a tool to ascertain this information is that it gives individuals a chance to respond to a number of choices. Thus, the therapist has a more global picture of the child's preferences in play.

*Don't assume that improving an individual's sensory integrative functioning will automatically improve his or her play.* Play, like many of the more well recognized end products of sensory integration (e.g., improved motor skills and self-esteem), is a complex phenomenon. Over time, individuals learn what they can and cannot do in play. Often their beliefs about their skills do not change just because their skills or sensory integration improve. Many therapists have had the experience of suggesting an activity to a client who responds that he or she "can't do that." The therapist may be quite sure that the client could perform the activity. If the therapist is able to coax the individual into trying, the client may be quite delighted with his or her newfound skill. However, the very fact that many clients balk at trying activities in which they previously may have been unsuccessful suggests that self-perceptions are not necessarily automatically adjusted to reflect improvements in skill or in sensory integrative functioning.

Further, newly developed skills that may be accomplished in the therapy room under the vigilant eye and hand of the therapist may not be generalized automatically to the playground or to the home. In observing children, both on an adventure playground and in therapy, Levitt (1975) found that the level of the children's skills was higher in the structured therapy session than on the playground. It may well be that, before a child can use a skill spontaneously, that skill must be practiced many times in an environment free of the consequences that would be associated with performing that same skill in "real life." The example of Max learning to play dodgeball is only one of countless such examples we have seen.

*If the goal is to improve both an individual's play and his sensory integrative functioning, play with the individual.* The individual with deficits in both play and sensory integration needs the therapist as a model player, and the assistance of the therapist in learning how to play (Lyons, 1984). In fact, Sutton-Smith (1980) has suggested that the roles of the coach and of the spectator may be even more important than those of the player in establishing play transactions. The therapist working with the individual who has difficulty playing needs to take extra care to be certain that all the elements of play (intrinsic motivation, internal control, and freedom to suspend reality) are present in the therapeutic sessions.

If the child is older than 3 or 4 years of age, talk to the child about the differences between the way he or she perceives the world and the way other people perceive it. Encourage him or her to bring a friend to therapy. It is easy for the therapist to schedule a treatment session that meets the needs of the client, but also includes a friend. Parents can be very helpful in assisting their child to choose a friend who will comply with the therapeutic regimen. The chosen friend usually loves to come and, even with older children, the stigma of therapy is thereby easily eliminated. We are not suggesting that treatment based on sensory integrative theory can, or should, be conducted with two clients simultaneously. We will discuss that issue more fully in Chapter 10. Rather, we are suggesting that conducting treatment with one client and a normal friend has many advantages for the client, including the development of social skills.

## CONCLUSION

Play is a powerful tool for treatment. For many individuals, the most important byproduct of occupational therapy may be the improved ability to play. If it is carefully planned and conducted, therapy using the principles of sensory integration may be very helpful in facilitating the development of play. Likewise, play, as a part of a well-orchestrated treatment plan, can result in improvements in sensory integration. While sensory integrative dysfunction may result in disruptions to play, we should not assume that all individuals who have sensory integrative dysfunction also have deficits in play. Clearly, further research is needed in this area.

## REFERENCES

Anderson, J., Hinojosa, J., & Strauch, C. (1987). Integrating play in neurodevelopmental treatment. *American Journal of Occupational Therapy, 41*, 421–426.

Ayres, A. J. (1972). *Sensory integration and learning disorders.* Los Angeles: Western Psychological Services.

Bateson, G. (1971). The message "this is play". In R.E. Herron & B. Sutton-Smith (Eds.), *Child's Play.* New York: Wiley.

Bateson, G. (1972a). Metalogue: About games and being serious. In G. Bateson, *Steps to an ecology of the mind* (pp. 14–20). New York: Bantam.

Bateson, G. (1972b). Toward a theory of play and fantasy. In G. Bateson, *Steps to an ecology of the mind* (pp. 177–193). New York: Bantam.

Berlyne, D. E. (1966). Curiosity and exploration. *Science, 153*, 25–33.

Berlyne, D. E. (1969). Laughter, humor and play. In G. Lindzert & E. Aronson (Eds.), *The Handbook of Social Psychology* (Vol 3). Reading, MA: Addison-Wesley.

Bledsoe, N. P., & Shepherd, J. T. (1982). A study of reliability and validity of a preschool play scale. *American Journal of Occupational Therapy, 36*, 783–788.

Bryan, T. (1976). Peer popularity of learning disabled children: A replication. *Journal of Learning Disabilities, 7*, 34–43.

Bryan, T. (1978). Social relationships and verbal interactions of learning disabled children. *Journal of Learning Disabilities, 11*, 107–115.

Bruininks, R. H. (1978). *Bruininks-Oseretsky Test of Motor Proficiency examiner's manual.* Circle Pines, MN: American Guidance Service.

Bundy, A. C. (1987). *The play of preschoolers: Its relationship to balance and motor proficiency and the effect of sensory integrative dysfunction.* Unpublished doctoral dissertation, Boston University.

Bundy, A. C. (1989). A comparison of the play skills of normal boys and boys with sensory integrative dysfunction. *Occupational Therapy Journal of Research, 9*, 84–100.

Pratt, P. N. (1989). Play and recreational activities. In P. N. Pratt & A. S. Allen (Eds.), *Occupational Therapy for Children* (pp. 295–310). St. Louis: C. V. Mosby.

Clifford, J. M., & Bundy, A. C. (1989). Play preference and play performance in normal boys and boys with sensory integrative dysfunction. *Occupational Therapy Journal of Research, 9*, 202–217.

Csikszentmihayli, M. (1979). The concept of flow. In B. Sutton-Smith (Ed.), *Play and learning* (pp. 257–274). New York: Gardner.

Csikszentmihayli, M. (1975). Play and intrinsic rewards. *Humanistic Psychology, 15*(3), 41–63.

Daub, M. M. (1983). The human development process. In H. L. Hopkins & H. D. Smith (Eds.), *Willard and Spackman's Occupational Therapy* (6th ed., pp. 43–86). Philadelphia: J. B. Lippincott.

Ellis, M. J. (1973). *Why people play.* Englewood Cliffs, NJ: Prentice-Hall.

Florey, L. (1971). An approach to play and play development. *American Journal of Occupational Therapy, 25,* 275–280.

Harrison, H., & Kielhofner, G. (1986). Examining reliability and validity of the Preschool Play Scale with handicapped children. *American Journal of Occupational Therapy, 40,* 167–173.

Hopkins, H. L. (1988). Current basis for theory and philosophy of occupational therapy. In H. L. Hopkins & H. D. Smith (Eds.), *Willard and Spackman's Occupational Therapy* (7th ed., pp. 38–42). Philadelphia: J. B. Lippincott.

Howard, A. C. (1986). Developmental play ages of physically abused and non-abused children. *American Journal of Occupational Therapy, 40,* 691–695.

Kielhofner, G. (Ed.). (1985). *A model of human occupation: Theory and application.* Baltimore: Williams & Wilkins.

Kooij, R. V., & Vrijhof, H. J. (1981). Play and development. *Topics in Learning and Learning Disabilities, 1,* 57–67.

Knox, S. H. (1974). A play scale. In M. Reilly (Ed.), *Play as exploratory learning: Studies of curiosity behavior* (pp. 247–266). Beverly Hills: Sage.

Levitt, S. (1975). A study of the gross motor skills of cerebral palsied children in an adventure playground for handicapped children. *Child Care, Health and Development, 1,* 29–43.

Lieberman, J. (1977). *Playfulness: Its relationship to imagination and creativity.* New York: Academic Press.

Lindquist, J. E., Mack, W., & Parham, L. D. (1982). A synthesis of occupational behavior and sensory integration concepts in theory and practice, Part 2: Clinical applications. *American Journal of Occupational Therapy, 36,* 433–437.

Lyons, M. (1984). A taxonomy of playfulness for use in occupational therapy. *Australian Occupational Therapy Journal, 4,* 152–156.

Margalit, M. (1984). Leisure activities of learning disabled children as a reflection of their passive life style and prolonged dependency. *Child Psychiatry and Human Development, 15,* 133–141.

Michelman, S. M. (1969). Research in symbol formation and creative growth. In W. L. West (Ed.), *Occupational therapy functions in interdisciplinary programs for children.* Rockville, MD: Maternal and Child Health Service, US Department of Health, Education, and Welfare.

Montessori, M. (1973). *The Montessori method.* Cambridge, MA: Bentley.

Morrison, C. D., Bundy, A. C., & Fisher, A. G. (in press). *The contribution of motor skills and playfulness to play. American Journal of Occupational Therapy.*

Neumann, E. A. (1971). *The elements of play.* New York: MSS Information.

Parten, M. B. (1932). Social participation among preschool children. *Journal of Abnormal Psychology, 27,* 243–269.

Piaget, J. (1962). *Play, dreams and imitation in childhood.* New York: Norton.

Rast, M. (1986). Play and therapy, play or therapy? In C. Pehoski (Ed.), *Play: A skill for life* (pp. 29–42). Rockville, MD: American Occupational Therapy Association.

Reilly, M. (Ed.). (1974). *Play as exploratory learning: Studies in curiosity behavior.* Beverly Hills: Sage.

Rodriguez, B. K. (1989). *Play, locus of control and depressive symptomatology.* Unpublished master's thesis, University of Illinois at Chicago.

Rubin, K., Fein, G. G., & Vandenberg, B. (1983). Play. In P. H. Mussen (Ed.), *Handbook of child psychology (4th ed.): Vol. 4. Socialization, personality and social development* (pp. 693–774). New York: Wiley.

Smith, P. K., Takhvar, M., Gore, N. & Vollstedt R. (1985). Play in young children: Problems in definition, categorization and measurement. *Early Child Development & Care, 14,* 25–41.

Sutton-Smith, B. (1980). A "sportive" theory of play. In H. Schwartzman (Ed.), *Play and culture* (pp. 10–19). West Point, NY: Leisure.

Takata, N. (1974). Play as prescription. In M. Reilly (Ed.), *Play as exploratory learning: Studies of curiosity behavior* (pp. 209–246). Beverly Hills: Sage.

Vandenberg, B. (1981). Environmental and cognitive factors in social play. *Journal of Experimental Psychology, 31,* 169–175.

Vandenberg, B., & Kielhofner, G. (1982). Play in evolution, culture and individual adaptation: Implications for therapy. *American Journal of Occupational Therapy, 36,* 20–28.

West, M. A. (1888). *Childhood: Its care and culture.* New York: Law, King & Law.

White, R. W. (1959). Motivation reconsidered: The concept of competence. *Psychological Review, 66,* 297–323.

Wolfgang, C., & Phelps, P. (1983). Preschool play materials preference inventory. *Early Childhood Development and Care, 12,* 127–141.

# Part *II*

## DOMAINS OF FUNCTION

# CHAPTER 4

# Vestibular-Proprioceptive Processing and Bilateral Integration and Sequencing Deficits

**Anne G. Fisher, ScD, OTR**

*There is an "unpublished rumor" that children with sensory integrative dysfunction crave what they need. If this is true, we must ask ourselves: If children with sensory integrative dysfunction, specifically those with central vestibular-proprioceptive processing deficits, crave vestibular-proprioceptive stimulation, why aren't these children self-correcting?*

The title of this chapter refers to *vestibular-proprioceptive* processing deficits. The occupational therapist familiar with sensory integration theory or the related literature is acutely aware that, historically, the emphasis has been on vestibular and not proprioceptive functioning. We prefer to use the term vestibular-proprioceptive processing for two reasons. First, the vestibular system is a source of specialized proprioceptive inputs. (The term *proprioception* was derived by Sherrington (1906) from the Latin *proprius* to refer to perception of sensations that originate in receptors that are stimulated by an organism's *own* movement. Thus, Sherrington identified both vestibular and muscle-spindle receptors as the primary sources of proprioceptive inputs.) Second, many of the clinical assessments we use do not enable us to differentiate between vestibular and proprioceptive contributions to postural control and motor performance.

We therefore use the term *vestibular-proprioceptive* to refer to inputs derived from active movements of one's own body, and the terms *vestibular* and *proprioceptive* to refer to specific groups of vestibular-proprioceptive receptors. More specifically, the vestibular receptors are the semicircular canals, the utricle, and the saccule, which are stimulated by movement of the head and by gravity. Proprioceptors include the specialized receptors of the muscles, joints, and skin that are stimulated by *active* movement of muscles and joints.

The occupational therapist studying or clinically applying the theory of sensory integration needs to be aware that in the literature on sensory integration an inordi-

nate amount of attention has been placed on the evaluation and treatment of vestibular or vestibular-proprioceptive processing deficits. Vestibular processing disorders
have been associated with learning disabilities and motor coordination deficits
(Fisher, Mixon, & Herman, 1986; Frank & Levinson, 1975–1976, 1976–1977; Horak,
Shumway-Cook, Crowe, & Black, 1988), and treatment directed toward the vestibular
system has been advocated as a basis for remediating the underlying problem
(Ayres, 1978, 1979; deQuiros & Schrager, 1979; Frank & Levinson, 1975–1976, 1976–
1977). Finally, there has been a trend toward an increased emphasis on the use of
vestibular stimulation as a therapeutic modality (Fisher & Bundy, 1989). According
to Clark, Mailloux, and Parham (1989), the emphasis on the use of "potent vestibular
stimulation, the type that is provided by swinging in net hammocks" (p. 501) and
other forms of suspended equipment, is a unique characteristic of sensory integration treatment programs. As a result, vestibular stimulation often has been inappropriately equated with sensory integration treatment.

    This emphasis on the vestibular system has been compounded by confusion
regarding the appropriate use of terminology, misconceptions regarding the nature
of *central* vestibular-proprioceptive deficits as defined by the theory of sensory
integration, and disagreement regarding the existence of such deficits (cf. Bonder &
Fisher, 1989; Brown, Haegerstrom-Portnoy, Yingling, Herron, Galin, & Marcus, 1983;
Clark et al., 1989; Fisher et al., 1986; Horak et al., 1988, Polatajko, 1985; Shumway-
Cook, 1989). Moreover, the validity of clinical assessment of vestibular-proprioceptive processing deficits, and, in fact, the very existence of central vestibular-proprioceptive processing deficits in children with motor coordination deficits and learning
disabilities, remains controversial, in spite of recent evidence regarding their validity (Fisher et al., 1986; Horak et al., 1988). Therefore, the occupational therapist
employing sensory integration theory, assessment, or treatment techniques must be
able to differentiate among (a) beliefs that are logically drawn from underlying
assumptions or that are supported by empirical evidence, (b) beliefs that are illogi-
cally drawn from underlying assumptions or that are not supported by empirical
evidence, (c) misconceptions about the intent of the underlying assumptions or the
theoretical implications of empirical evidence, and (d) disagreements about the
interpretation of the assumptions and empirical evidence that have been published
in occupational-therapy, physical-therapy, medical, educational, psychological, and
neurobehavioral literature.

## PURPOSE AND SCOPE

    The purpose of this chapter is to provide the occupational therapist with the
background knowledge needed to appreciate these critical issues, which are central
to the understanding and appropriate application of sensory integration theory. An
important emphasis will be the attempt to link theoretical assumptions with empirical evidence and with clinical practice.

    We believe that any discussion of the relationship between theory, research,
evaluation, and treatment is most meaningful if it takes place within a relevant
context. We will therefore begin our discussion at the point in time where it begins
for the clinician; specifically, when the client is referred to occupational therapy for
evaluation. We will present two brief case descriptions of individuals with central
vestibular-proprioceptive processing deficits. Emphasis will be placed on the diversity of the presenting clinical manifestations of central vestibular-proprioceptive

process deficits seen in individuals who are subsequently identified as having sensory integrative dysfunction.

We will then review the neurobehavioral aspects of the vestibular and proprioceptive systems as they pertain to the basic assumptions or postulates of sensory integration theory, and to the evaluation and treatment of vestibular-proprioceptive processing deficits. Building on the case presentations and the theoretical basis for central vestibular-proprioceptive processing deficits, we will discuss hypothesized types of vestibular-proprioceptive dysfunction. These include *postural-ocular movement disorder, gravitational insecurity,* and *intolerance or aversive response to movement.* Because *disorders of bilateral integration and sequencing* are believed to be related to vestibular-proprioceptive processing deficits, they also will be discussed. Disorders of bilateral integration and sequencing are considered to be a specific *disorder of motor planning* characterized by problems with planning and producing bilateral and projected action sequences. Throughout this chapter, we will include a discussion of the theoretical and empirical evidence supporting the existence of vestibular-proprioceptive and related disorders.

Specific disorders are identified through the process of evaluation. Once we have an idea of the types of disorders we might expect to see, we can then discuss the specific evaluation methods used to identify vestibular-proprioceptive processing deficits. Because the Sensory Integration and Praxis Tests (SIPT) (Ayres, 1989) are discussed in more detail in Chapter 8, and because they are limited in their ability to identify vestibular-proprioceptive processing deficits, the emphasis here will be on information obtained through interview, other standardized tests, and nonstandardized or subjective clinical observations that are used to supplement the SIPT. As before, we will include discussion of the existing evidence supporting valid clinical assessment of vestibular-proprioceptive processing deficits.

We will conclude with a brief discussion of the theoretical issues that pertain to the treatment of deficits in vestibular-proprioceptive processing and in bilateral integration and sequencing. This section is intended to provide the theoretical background for applying the principles of sensory integration treatment discussed in later chapters.

# CLINICAL PICTURE OF VESTIBULAR-PROPRIOCEPTIVE DYSFUNCTION

Individuals who have central vestibular-proprioceptive processing deficits vary markedly in their presenting symptoms. The following two cases demonstrate the extent to which individuals can differ. Both of these cases are presented because they are typical of the individuals in whom the presence of central vestibular-proprioceptive deficits was confirmed through assessment of vestibulo-ocular and vestibulo-spinal responses in a visual-vestibular laboratory. These laboratory methods for assessing vestibular control of eye movements and balance are described in more detail by Fisher et al. (1986), Horak et al. (1988), and Shumway-Cook, Horak, & Black (1987).

## Todd

Todd is 8 years, 9 months of age. He was referred for an occupational therapy evaluation because his mother is concerned about the amount of time he needs to spend on his schoolwork. While he is functioning at grade level, Todd needs to spend several hours each night studying.

Todd's mother describes him as being a "very likeable kid." He is relatively easygoing, and it is fun to do things with him. He is also a perfectionist who "works hard to do his best." She feels that one of his strengths is perseverance. "When he makes up his mind that he wants to do something, he will practice and practice until he gets it." But, she is also aware that he is a bright child (his tested IQ is 129), and she is concerned that a "bright child has to work so hard to get it." She would like to see him spend more time "having fun with the other kids" and less time doing schoolwork.

Todd's mother is also concerned about his coordination. She describes Todd as being awkward. "He has to first watch the other kids and then he has to practice a lot before he catches on." Learning to tie his shoes was difficult for Todd, and he didn't accomplish shoe tying until he was 8 years of age. At age 7, he had a similar experience with learning to ride a two-wheeled bicycle, an activity he still does not enjoy.

When asked about himself, Todd indicated that he "does fine" in school, but acknowledged that he has to work hard to get As and Bs. He stated that his greatest skill is his ability to memorize things, and he thinks that this ability helps him when he takes tests. The thing that he would like to do most is to play competitive games with the other kids, but "I'm not good enough." Aware that they are easier for him, Todd prefers more unstructured activities such as swimming, boating, and art. He also loves to ride the roller coaster, but says that most other amusement park rides (e.g., Ferris wheel) are boring.

Todd's occupational therapy evaluation included assessment of his sensory integrative functioning. Compared with other boys his age, Todd had difficulty with balance reactions, extending his body against gravity into the prone extension posture, and stabilizing his trunk. His overall muscle tone appeared to be low (hypotonic) and his postural muscles, especially his extensor muscles, seemed to be weak. Todd tended to compensate by moving quickly from one position to another so that he did not have to maintain stable positions for any length of time.

Todd also had difficulty performing bilateral motor tasks, especially those involving *anticipatory or projected movement sequences.* For example, despite the fact that every weekend he and his father practice throwing and catching (because he wants to be able to play baseball with the other children), Todd had difficulty catching a bounced tennis ball when the occupational therapist varied the force or direction of the bounce.

Catching a ball requires Todd to anticipate where he will need to place his hands so that they will be where they need to be when the ball reaches him. He must project into the future, and plan his movements according to the conditions that will exist when he catches the ball. Todd, however, tended to place his hands at his midline without considering the direction of the bounce. This strategy worked well for Todd when the ball was predictably bounced directly to him, but it was not an effective strategy for catching a ball that was bounced to a different place each time.

Another task that was especially difficult for Todd was jumping in a series of six 8-inch squares that were drawn on the floor like a hopscotch. The task, as described to Todd, was to jump on both feet into each of the six squares, one at a time. He was told to begin by jumping into the first square, and then to go all the way to the end. He was asked to do this without stopping and without stepping on the lines. In spite of demonstration and several practice trials, Todd had difficulty performing the task as one continuous action sequence. He hesitated before starting, paused or momentarily stopped jumping in the middle of the sequence, and, when he got to the end, he had trouble stopping and standing stationary outside the last square in the manner in which he had been instructed. His performance suggests that Todd not only has difficulty jumping in a coordinated manner with both feet together, but that he also has difficulty initiating, sequencing, and terminating bilateral, projected motor action sequences.

Todd's scores on the SIPT were consistent with his clinical picture. His lowest scores were on Bilateral Motor Coordination and Sequencing Praxis, suggesting that Todd has difficulty in performing bilateral motor functions and reproducing sequences of movement, respectively. Todd also made a number of right-for-left reversal errors when he positioned the blocks on the three-dimensional Constructional Praxis test. His mother also has noted reversals in his written work. Finally, neither the interview of his mother nor his test results suggested evidence of problems with tactile discrimination, visuomotor coordination, form and space perception, or sensory defensiveness.

## Chris

Chris is 28 years old. She has a master's degree in special education and teaches children with developmental delays in an urban public school system. Chris referred herself for an occupational therapy evaluation, after attending a 3-day workshop on sensory integration theory, because of a history of "clumsiness and rotten balance." Due to the limited availability of relevant standardized assessments for adults, Chris' occupational therapy evaluation, including assessment of her sensory integrative functioning, relied heavily on interview and observation of her performance.

Chris describes herself as someone who has been clumsy all of her life. "I was the family 'klutz.' I was always falling, tripping over my own feet." At school, when everyone else was playing games, "I used to just sit at the side and watch. Sometimes I could find someone to talk to me, but most of the time, my classmates preferred to play with the other children."

An overriding component of Chris' descriptions of her childhood was a pervasive fear of movement. For example, riding on escalators was very scary for her. When Chris' mother would take her shopping, her mother would want to take the escalator to another floor. "I would refuse to get on. When my mother tried to insist, I would inevitably end up on the floor screaming. My mother would get very angry, but now I think that she just was embarrassed."

Sometimes, thinking that Chris just needed experience with movement, her father would take her to the playground or try to roughhouse with her. Her father would become very frustrated because she would get scared and refuse to participate. His response was to give up trying to help her. Chris has an older sister who is quite attractive and well-coordinated. He would ask Chris, "Why can't you be like her?"

Now that she is an adult, Chris continues to become easily nauseated when she rides in cars, even for very short distances. She has flown only once, and when she did so she became disoriented. "I felt as if I was upside down." Riding escalators or other moving equipment continues to be a problem, but she usually is able to avoid having to use them (e.g., using stairs instead of escalators).

Evaluating Chris in the clinic was difficult because she would become tense and her body would stiffen whenever she attempted any activity that required that her feet leave the floor. She could stand on one foot for about 10 seconds if she kept her eyes open and held her breath, but she was unable to stand on one foot with her eyes closed. She was able to extend her body against gravity into the prone extension position only if she held her breath, and she was unable to hold the position for more than 4 or 5 seconds. Flexing against gravity into the supine flexion position was somewhat easier. Chris could flex at the hips and knees, and she could lift her upper trunk, bringing her legs and shoulders up into the flexed position. However, she had difficulty flexing her neck, as was demonstrated when she led with her chin rather than her forehead while righting her head. Finally, Chris demonstrated marked winging of the medial border of her scapulae when she assumed a quadruped position.

Because of her history of difficulty tolerating movement, Chris was given the opportunity to try some of the suspended equipment used in sensory integration treatment programs. She was able to sit on a bolster suspended from the ceiling at both ends (bolster swing) and swing gently as one does on a suspended porch swing (Fig. 4–1). She also was able to get into a sitting position on a small rectangular platform (glider) suspended from the ceiling at both ends. As long as the movement of the glider was linear, and it moved no more than a few inches, she was able to tolerate it. If, however, it began to swing sideways or in a circle, she would become extremely tense and grab onto the suspension ropes.

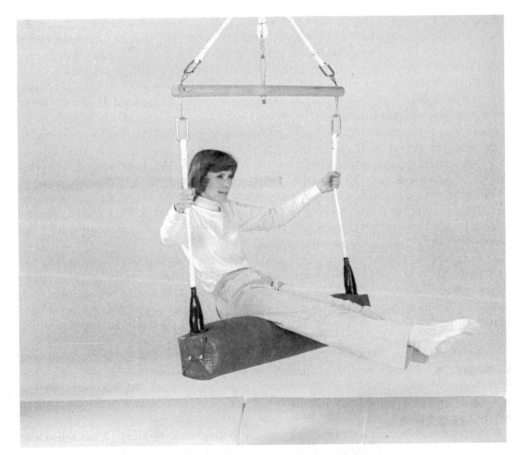

FIGURE 4–1. Using a bolster swing as a large swing.

Perhaps the most remarkable finding from the evaluation was that Chris had a poor sense of where her body was in space. During the interview, it became apparent that she had developed many compensatory strategies, but that her sense of where her body was in space was more conscious than internal. For example, when she was asked to cross her feet at the ankles prior to assuming the supine flexion posture, she had to look at her feet to determine whether she was doing the right thing. When she assumed the prone position on the floor, she could not identify where "up" was unless weights were placed on her back. "Up" was then identifiable, but only because "I can feel the floor pushing me." A similar situation occurred when she assumed a prone, head-down position over a therapy ball. In the course of her development, "up" had became known as "on top of my head"; and front had become known as "the way I am looking." While this worked for her when she was upright, when she assumed a prone or head-down position, these cognitive compensatory strategies for determining where "up" is were no longer adequate.

# NEUROBEHAVIORAL BASIS OF VESTIBULAR AND PROPRIOCEPTIVE DYSFUNCTION

The experienced occupational therapist is acutely aware that vestibular-proprioceptive functioning cannot be assessed directly. Rather, we must infer, based on the results of our clinical assessment, whether or not there is adequate evidence for concluding that vestibular-proprioceptive deficits are present. Do Todd and Chris have vestibular-proprioceptive processing deficits? What is the neurobehavioral and empirical evidence that provides the basis for the theoretical assumption that central vestibular-proprioceptive processing deficits contribute to the problems each of these individuals is experiencing?

Vestibular-proprioceptive processing is hypothesized to contribute to the perception of active movement of the body in space; the development of body scheme; and postural responses, especially those involving extensor muscles (e.g., extensor muscle tone, equilibrium). Recent research suggests that proprioceptive inputs are involved in the programming and planning of bilateral projected action sequences (Goldberg, 1985). In the following section, we will discuss the neurophysiological and behavioral evidence to support a relationship between vestibular-proprioceptive processing and the behavioral deficits manifested by Todd and Chris. We will assume a basic understanding of neuroanatomy and vestibular-proprioceptive neurophysiology, focusing instead on the less familiar and more applied aspects of vestibular-proprioceptive functioning. Where appropriate, we will introduce implications for intervention.

## Vestibular System

The vestibular system traditionally is viewed as having a role, along with the visual system and proprioception, in three major functions: subjective awareness of body position and movement in space; postural tone and equilibrium; and stabilization of the eyes in space during head movements (compensatory eye movements).

### VESTIBULAR RECEPTORS

The vestibular receptors are the hair cells (cristae) located within the semicircular canals, the utricle, and the saccule of the vestibular labyrinth. The semicircular canals are angular accelerometers that detect changes in the direction and rate of angular acceleration or deceleration of the head. Angular acceleration of the head results in rotary head movements; that is, head movements that, if continued long enough, result in the head turning in a circle (e.g., spinning, head nodding).

Within each vestibular apparatus are three semicircular canals, endolymph-filled ducts oriented at right angles to each other so that they represent all three planes in space. When the head is tilted forward 30°, the horizontal canal is oriented in the horizontal plane, and the two vertical canals are vertical and oriented at right angles to each other. The hairs of the cristae ampullaris of the semicircular canals project into the cupula, a gelatinous wedge that is free to move like a swinging door within the endolymph. When the head moves (accelerates), the inertia of the endolymph causes it to lag behind head movement. The result is displacement of the cupula and bending of the hairs in the direction opposite head movement. When head movement stops (decelerates), the inertia of the endolymph causes the cupula to "keep going." The result is displacement of the cupula and bending of the hairs in the same direction that the head had been moving. Several seconds after the head stops moving, or after it has rotated at a constant velocity for several seconds, the endolymph "catches up" and the cupula and the hairs return to their normal resting positions. Because the hair cells in each pair of canals are maximally stimulated by head rotation in the same plane, the hair cells are able to detect movement of the head in the three orthogonal (right-angle) planes of three-dimensional space. The most efficient stimuli to the semicircular canals are angular, transient (short-term), and fast (high-frequency) head movements of at least 2° per second; when the head moves at slower speeds, the endolymph, cupula, and hair cells all move at the same speed as the head (Fisher & Bundy, 1989; Roberts, 1978; Wilson & Melvill Jones, 1979).

The utricle is a linear accelerometer that detects linear head movement and head tilt. The utricle is located in the horizontal plane when the head is erect, and the hair cells in each quadrant of the utricle are systematically oriented in a different direction. Embedded in a gelatinous layer over the hair cells are calcium carbonate formations called otoliths, which are denser than the surrounding endolymph. As the head moves, the force of gravity and linear acceleration act on this otolithic membrane to displace the hairs of the hair cells. Those hair cells that are aligned in the direction of gravitational pull, head tilt, or linear acceleration are maximally stimulated. Thus, systematic variation in the orientation of the utricular hair cells results in the utricle also being able to detect head movement or head tilt (position) in the three orthogonal planes of three-dimensional space. Finally, the utricle responds to linear, sustained, and low-frequency stimuli (i.e., stationary head position or slow head movements less than 2° per second) (Fisher & Bundy, 1989; Roberts, 1978; Wilson & Melvill Jones, 1979).

Despite much speculation concerning the possible roles of the saccule (e.g., vertical accelerometer, vibratory receptor), its precise function remains unknown. The only confirmed function of the saccule, identified in animals, is in acoustico-neural transduction, and the significance of saccular acoustic reception remains unclear (Cazals & Aurousseau, 1987). Therefore, we will not discuss the saccule further.

The most effective stimuli for the semicircular canals and the utricle represent opposite ends of a continuum (Fig. 4–2). The functional implication of this continuum for treatment is that any head position or head movement will result in the stimulation of some combination of vestibular receptor hair cells. Reciprocally, the combination of hair cells that are stimulated tells us about head position and the

| SEMICURCULAR CANALS | | UTRICLE |
|---|---|---|

← ─────────────────────────────────────────────────────────── →

**Stimuli**

| Head movements that are at least 2° per second, angular, and transient (phasic) | Head movements that combine semicircular canal and utricular stimuli | Head movements that are slower than 2° per second, linear, and sustained |
|---|---|---|

**Response**

| Phasic extension of the downhill limbs, phasic flexion of the uphill limbs, and transient righting of the head and upper trunk | Response varies, depending on the most "salient" stimulus | Tonic extension of the downhill limbs, tonic flexion of the uphill limbs, and maintained righting of the head and upper trunk |
|---|---|---|

FIGURE 4–2. Continuum of effective stimuli for and response of the semicircular canals and the utricle.

speed and direction that we are moving in space. Therefore, *treatment planning should give consideration to activities that provide stimuli (a) in all body (head) positions, and in all planes of three-dimensional space; (b) that vary in speed from static (position) to fast; (c) that are linear and angular; and (d) that are transient and sustained.*

## VESTIBULAR SYSTEM–MEDIATED POSTURAL RESPONSES

The responses that are elicited as a result of utricular or semicircular canal stimulation "act on antigravity extensor muscles so as to elicit *compensatory* head, trunk, and limb movements, which serve to oppose head perturbations, postural sway, or tilt" (Fisher & Bundy, 1989, p. 240). However, as might be expected, there are differences between the kinds of postural responses ultimately elicited by stimulation to the different receptors. Utricular inputs, conveyed primarily via the lateral vestibular spinal pathway to limb and upper-trunk alpha and gamma motoneurons, result in ipsilateral facilitation of extensor muscles and inhibition of flexor muscles. Semicircular canal inputs are conveyed primarily via the medial vestibulospinal pathway to axial alpha and gamma motoneurons, and result in bilateral facilitation of neck and upper-trunk muscles. Utricular inputs elicit more sustained postural responses (i.e., tonic postural extension and support reactions, whereas semicircular canal inputs elicit more transient or phasic equilibrium responses (Fisher & Bundy, 1989; Roberts, 1978; Wilson & Melvill Jones, 1979).

More specifically, transient or angular head movements that stimulate the semicircular canals result in (a) phasic stabilization of the head and upper trunk in the upright position, (b) phasic (rapid, transient) extension of the weight-bearing limbs on the side toward which the individual is rotating or tilting (downhill side), (c) phasic flexion of the weight-bearing limbs on the contralateral (uphill) side, and (d) phasic compensatory abduction and extension of nonweight-bearing limbs. Sustained head tilt or linear head movements that stimulate the utricle result in (a) tonic (maintained) extension of the downhill weight-bearing limbs (support reactions), (b) maintained flexion of the uphill weight-bearing limbs, (c) maintained compensatory abduction and extension of the non–weight-bearing limbs, and (d) maintained stabilization of the head and upper trunk in the upright position (Fisher, 1989; Roberts, 1978; Wilson & Melvill Jones, 1979). The functional implication for treatment is that if the goal is to facilitate tonic postural or support reactions, activities that provide utricular stimulation may be more appropriate. If the goal is to encourage the use of more phasic or transient postural reactions, then activities that provide semicircular canal stimulation may be indicated (see Fig. 4–2).

An example of an activity that provides relatively pure semicircular canal stimulation is rotation (spinning) in a suspended net hammock. Movement of the head in space is fast and angular, and as long as the speed of rotation varies, transient accelerations and decelerations occur. An activity that provides a relatively pure utricular stimulus is lying prone over a stationary therapy ball or barrel. As long as head position remains constant, gravity provides a sustained, linear, constant-velocity stimulus. However, most head movements elicited by common sensory integrative treatment techniques fall between these two extremes, and head movements that we commonly think of as being "slow" (e.g., a child who is slowly rocked back and forth while lying prone on a ball) are actually too fast to be effective stimuli for the utricle. We therefore need to examine our treatment activities to determine the most "salient" stimulus-and-response characteristics of the activity.

For example, imagine a child positioned prone in a suspended net hammock that "slowly" swings forward and backward through an arc of about 30°. Swinging forward and backward in a net hammock is a relatively good activity for stimulating the utricular hair cells and promoting tonic postural extension. Although the head movement is technically angular, the radius of arc is great enough for the head movement to be thought of as linear. Finally, to the extent that the child maintains his or her head tilted out of the vertical position, the linear sustained force of gravity acts on the head to facilitate extension (righting) of the head and upper trunk. However, since one complete cycle is 60°, the net would have to swing slowly enough to take 30 seconds to complete one full cycle in order to be slow enough to be a *pure* utricular stimulus. Yet, even when the cycle is completed in less than the *ideal* 30 seconds, utricular-mediated tonic postural responses clearly predominate.

Now, imagine a child jumping up and down on a trampoline. The activity is more linear than angular, and gravity provides a relatively constant stimulus that promotes the tonic postural-support reactions of the legs (downhill limbs) needed to maintain the upright position when landing on the trampoline. As long as the child is able to continue jumping without losing his or her rhythm, we should see less extension in the legs when the child is jumping up, and more extension in the legs when the child is coming down. However, if the child lands slightly off balance, as often happens on a trampoline, there will be a transient change in velocity and direction of head movement, and a phasic equilibrium reaction should be elicited that prevents the child from falling.

## VESTIBULAR-MEDIATED OCULAR RESPONSES

In addition to its connections with postural muscles, the vestibular system also has connections with eye muscles. Like the postural responses elicited as a result of stimulation to the vestibular system, vestibulo-ocular responses are *compensatory* in nature. We will discuss two compensatory eye movements that are elicited as a result of stimulation to the vestibular system; these are (a) the vestibular-nystagmus or *vestibulo-ocular reflex* (VOR) and (b) *optokinetic afternystagmus* (OKAN). We will also discuss a related perceptual response, the sensation of *circularvection.* Other eye movements (e.g., smooth pursuit or tracking movements; saccadic eye movements used in reading or to quickly shift the eyes from the paper on the desk to the blackboard) are mediated primarily by the visual system (cf. Baloh & Honrubia, 1979; Leigh & Zee, 1983).

We will discuss these responses in some detail because a full understanding of how they are measured and interpreted is important to understand the literature that claims to refute the validity of vestibular-based sensory integrative deficits. More specifically, we will discuss three measures of the integrity of the vestibular system. These are *peak slow-phase eye velocity, duration* of vestibular nystagmus, and *time constant* of vestibular nystagmus. Slow-phase eye velocity is a measure of *peripheral* vestibular function. Duration and time constant are measures of *central* vestibular processing *as long as slow-phase eye velocity is normal.* In sensory integration theory, we hypothesize *normal peripheral* and *impaired central* vestibular processing. As we will see later in this chapter, research showing normal peripheral vestibular responses has been misinterpreted to mean normal central vestibular processing.

*Vestibular nystagmus* consists of compensatory slow-phase eye movements in one direction followed by saccadic fast-phase eye movements in the other direction. There are two types of vestibular nystagmus, (a) perrotary nystagmus, which occurs *during* rotation, and (b) postrotary nystagmus, which occurs *following* rotation. During perrotary nystagmus, when the head moves in one direction, the eyes move "slowly" in the opposite direction to compensate for the head movement. These compensatory slow-phase eye movements of vestibular nystagmus function to stabilize visual images on the retina when the head moves. Because these relatively slow compensatory eye movements in one direction are followed by quick saccadic eye movements (fast-phase) in the opposite direction, vestibular nystagmus is characterized by rhythmic, back-and-forth eye movements. Our discussion will focus on the compensatory slow-phase eye movements that reflect the vestibular-mediated component of nystagmus.

During angular acceleration (rotation) of the head, the speed of the slow-phase eye movements (slow-phase eye velocity) increases as the speed of head movement increases. However, when the speed of rotation remains constant, slow-phase eye velocity of perrotary nystagmus does not remain constant. Instead, after about 2 seconds, it gradually declines until the eyes stop moving. When the rotation is suddenly stopped, nystagmus is induced in the opposite direction; this is referred to as postrotary nystagmus. Like perrotary nystagmus, postrotary nystagmus slow-phase eye velocity continues at a fairly steady rate for about 2 seconds and then gradually declines to zero (Cohen, Henn, Raphan, & Dennett, 1981; Fisher et al., 1986; Leigh & Zee, 1983; Raphan, Matsuo, & Cohen, 1979). The initial 2-second plateau and subsequent gradual decline in slow-phase eye velocity of perrotary and postrotary vestibular nystagmus is depicted in Figure 4–3. Also shown are the time constants for the decay of nystagmus ($TC_D$) and for the vestibular afferents ($TC_C$). These are discussed in the next section.

The time course of perrotary and postrotary nystagmus is usually described in terms of the *duration* of nystagmus and the *time constant* of slow-phase eye velocity decay. The time constant is a measure of how fast the slow-phase eye velocity declines from peak velocity to about two-thirds of the initial peak slow-phase eye velocity (Fisher et al., 1986). Although the time constant can be measured only in laboratory settings, where nystagmus is recorded using electronystagmography, it sometimes is considered a better measure of the time course of nystagmus than is duration (Fisher et al., 1986).

As described earlier, when the head rapidly accelerates or decelerates, the cupula of the semicircular canals is displaced transiently; this displacement results in an increased rate of firing of the cupular afferents of the vestibular nerve. During *constant velocity rotation,* and after rotation is suddenly stopped, the cupula gradually returns to its normal resting position. As shown in Figure 4–3, the gradual decline in the rate of firing of the cupular afferents is much faster than, but otherwise follows a similar pattern to, the decline of slow-phase eye velocity of vestibular nystagmus. That is, the cupula returns to its normal resting position long *before* nystagmus stops. More specifically, the time constant and duration of firing of the *cupular afferents* is approximately 5 to 8 seconds and 20 seconds, respectively (Cohen et al., 1981; Heide, Schrader, Koenig, & Dichgans, 1988; Koenig & Dichgans, 1981). By contrast, the time constant and duration of *vestibular nystagmus* is much longer, and averages approximately 14 seconds and 40 seconds, respectively, when an adult is rotated at a constant velocity of 60° per second (Fisher et al., 1986). These relationships between the time constant and duration of the cupular afferents and the time constant and duration of nystagmus are shown in Figure 4–3.

The difference between the time course of vestibular nystagmus and the relatively shorter time course of the cupular afferent has been attributed to a brainstem mechanism that stores information related to slow-phase eye velocity. There is evidence that this storage mechanism is impaired in individuals with vestibular-based, sensory integrative dysfunction (Fisher et al., 1986). In normal individuals, the velocity storage mechanism is hypothesized to be responsible for the prolonged time constant and duration of perrotary and postrotary nystagmus, beyond that which could be accounted for by cupular displacement (Cohen et al., 1981; Magnusson, Pyykko, Schalen, & Enbom, 1988; Raphan et al., 1979). This velocity storage mechanism is also thought to be responsible for circularvection and optokinetic afternystagmus, two additional functions that have been shown to be impaired in individuals with vestibular-based sensory integrative dysfunction (Fisher et al., 1986). We will therefore turn our attention to these two vestibular-mediated responses.

Many individuals have had the experience of sitting in a parked car and perceiving the sensation that the car in which they were sitting was moving forward when

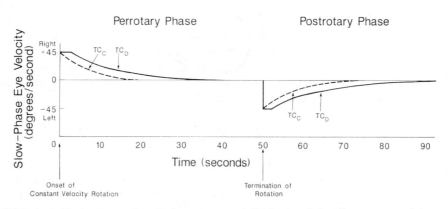

FIGURE 4–3. Time course of vestibular nystagmus (solid line) and the afferent nerve of the cupula (broken line). When an individual is rapidly accelerated and then rotated at a constant velocity of 60° per second to the left, the peak slow-phase eye movements (vestibulo-ocular reflex) are to the right (plus), but only about 45° per second (solid line). After about 2 seconds, the speed of the slow-phase eye movements begins to decline, and after about 40 seconds, the eyes stop beating (velocity = zero). Then, when rotation is suddenly stopped, postrotary nystagmus is generated to the left (minus); the postrotary response is in the opposite direction and is essentially a mirror image of the perrotary response. The time constants of the cupular afferents ($TC_C$) and nystagmus ($TC_D$) are indicated with arrows (see text for details).

the car that was parked next to them backed out. This illusion of self-movement in one direction, induced by movement of the visual surround (moving car) in the opposite direction, is called *circularvection*. We become particularly aware of circularvection when we "know" that we are stationary, but "perceive" that we are moving. Under normal circumstances, we don't expect our stationary environment to move; we expect to move within a stationary environment.

Although circularvection can be associated with illusion, in most situations circularvection *accurately* contributes to our conscious perception that *we are moving within a stationary environment or visual surround.* When the head moves in one direction, there is apparent relative "movement" of the visual surround in the opposite direction. When the visual surround appears to "move" (called *optokinetic stimulation*), as it does when we ride in a car or when we turn our heads in space, slow-phase eye movements are generated that attempt to track the "movement" of the visual surround. As with vestibular nystagmus, they are followed by saccadic fast-phase eye movements in the opposite direction. These eye movements are called *optokinetic nystagmus* (a phenomenon easily observed in an individual looking out the window of a moving vehicle.

Within seconds after initiation of optokinetic stimulation, one begins to feel, and appropriately so, as though he or she is moving (circularvection). Optokinetic nystagmus is initiated simultaneously with the onset of optokinetic stimulation, and continues as long as there is relative movement of the visual surround. However, optokinetic nystagmus also persists *after* the termination of optokinetic stimulation, that is, after the visual surround stops "moving" and there is no longer a moving visual surround for the eyes to track. This response is termed *optokinetic afternystagmus* (OKAN).

Let us now consider the relevance of the vestibular system to sensory integration theory and clinical investigation of sensory integration dysfunction.

## THEORETICAL IMPLICATIONS AND CLINICAL SIGNIFICANCE

Individuals who have been identified as having vestibular-based sensory integrative dysfunction also have been identified, through laboratory testing of circularvection, time course of vestibular nystagmus, and OKAN, as having impairments of velocity storage. Optokinetic afternystagmus, like circularvection and time course of nystagmus, is dependent on "sensory integrative centres in the brainstem which are responsible for velocity storage" (Jell, Phillips, Lafortune, & Ireland, 1988, p. 201).

Thus, in contrast to individuals who have peripheral vestibular lesions, individuals with central vestibular processing deficits will have normal peak slow-phase eye velocity (Horak et al., 1988), but shortened durations and time constants of vestibular nystagmus. Individuals with central vestibular processing deficits also will have diminished or abnormal circularvection and depressed durations of OKAN (cf. Fisher et al., 1986; Heide et al., 1988).

More specifically, Fisher et al. (1986) found that adult subjects with sensory integrative dysfunction and *clinical evidence* of impaired vestibular processing have depressed scores on the known valid laboratory measures of tonic central processing of vestibular inputs associated with velocity storage. However, their subjects demonstrated no indication of peripheral vestibular dysfunction; peak slow-phase velocity of perrotary or postrotary vestibular nystagmus was normal.

Horak et al. (1988) assessed the vestibulo-ocular reflex and postural responses under varying conditions of increasing sensory conflict in children with peripheral vestibular impairments (associated with hearing loss) and in children with learning disabilities and motor incoordination. Children with peripheral vestibular impairments demonstrated depressed peak slow-phase velocity of vestibular nystagmus and impaired postural reactions only when *both* visual and somatosensory (body contact and proprioception) inputs were eliminated or disrupted. The children with learning disabilities and motor incoordination had normal vestibulo-ocular peak slow-phase velocity, but impaired postural reactions under *all* conditions of sensory conflict (see also Shumway-Cook et al., 1987).

Considered together, the results of these investigations suggest that there is a group of individuals with learning disabilities and motor incoordination who have central, not peripheral, deficits in processing vestibular inputs. Furthermore, "despite intact peripheral vestibular information, [learning-disabled] children with sensorimotor impairments could not appropriately integrate vestibulospinal inputs with visual and somatosensory inputs for postural orientation" (Shumway-Cook, 1989, p. 241).

When reading the experimental literature on the relationship between vestibular system functioning and learning disabilities or sensory integrative dysfunction, it is important to differentiate between those studies in which indicators of *peripheral* vestibular function are measured (peak slow-phase eye velocity during vestibular nystagmus) and those studies in which indicators of *central* vestibular processing are measured (circularvection, time course of vestibular nystagmus, duration of optokinetic afternystagmus, and postural control under conditions of sensory conflict). *Sensory integration dysfunction is thought to be a central processing disorder.* Therefore, the results of each of these investigations provide support for the validity of sensory integration theory.

## Proprioception

Proprioception, as defined by Sherrington (1906), refers to perception of joint and body movement as well as position of the body, or body segments, in space. More specifically, proprioception enables us to check on the spatial orientation of our bodies or body parts in space, the rate and timing of our movements, how much force our muscles are exerting, and how much and how fast a muscle is being stretched (Kalaska, 1988; Matthews, 1988; McCloskey, 1985). Although Sherrington (1906) identified the muscle afferents, joint receptors, and vestibular labyrinth as proprioceptors, we have considered the vestibular receptors as a special class of proprioceptors and will confine our discussion in this section to the nonvestibular proprioceptors.

Prior to the early 1970s, a classic differentiation was made between conscious joint proprioception (kinesthesia), thought to arise primarily from joint receptors; and unconscious proprioception, thought to arise from the muscle-spindle and tendon receptors. A recent trend, however, is to use the terms proprioception and kinesthesia synonymously. For the purpose of our discussion, it is important that we recognize that this controversy exists. However, we will be more concerned with the distinction between *proprioceptors* (proprioceptive receptors) and *proprioception* (proprioception feedback and perception of joint and body movement). As we will see, not all proprioception is derived from proprioceptive receptors. Internal correlates of motor signals that are sent to the muscles once an action is planned (corollary discharge) also are an important source of proprioception. Corollary discharge is important for (a) differentiating between our active (internally generated) movements and passive movement generated by an external stimulus, (b) identifying if we have programmed an appropriate level of motor activity, (c) the development of body scheme, and (d) our perception of force (Jones, 1988). This knowledge of our body and our movements is important in motor planning.

## ACTIVE VERSUS PASSIVE MOVEMENT

As was discussed in Chapter 1, active movement provides the basis for developing neuronal models that are then used to plan more complex movements. Thus, the *active participation* of the individual in treatment has obvious implications. That is, passive movement imposed by external forces does not have the same effect on proprioceptors as does active movement (Evarts, 1985; Kalaska, 1988). Anyone questioning this need only extend all joints of the fingers except the proximal interphalangeal joint of the middle finger. When the proximal interphalangeal joint is flexed 90°, the extrinsic finger muscles are "disconnected" from their joint attachments, making it impossible to actively flex or extend the distal interphalangeal joint (McCloskey, 1985). However, the distal interphalangeal joint of the middle finger easily can be moved passively; doing so results in a markedly diminished sense of joint position or movement. Therefore, an important question for us to consider is how we know whether the sensory receptors are being stimulated as a result of our own active movements or by externally imposed passive movements.

When joint movement is active, it is hypothesized that an efferent copy (internal correlate or corollary discharge) of a centrally generated motor command is sent to sensory centers in the brain for comparison to a "reference of correctness" (Matthews, 1988). The reference of correctness is hypothesized to be a neuronal model or memory of "how it feels" to move in a particular way and "what is achieved" when we move in that w~v (Brooks, 1986). As shown in Figure 4–4, the motor command also is sent to ine muscles, the executors of active movement. When movement is passively imposed, no motor command is generated and no efference copy is sent to sensory centers.

## SOURCES OF PROPRIOCEPTION

It is now widely recognized that proprioceptive feedback arises primarily from muscle spindles, mechanoreceptors of the skin, and the centrally generated motor commands just discussed. Joint receptors, once thought to be a major source of proprioception, now are considered to be much less important. Moreover, experimental evidence now indicates that all proprioceptive inputs can contribute to conscious proprioception (Matthews, 1988; McCloskey, 1985; McCloskey, Cross, Hunter, & Potter, 1983; Moberg, 1983; Tracey, 1985).

The effective stimulus for the primary and secondary endings of the *muscle spindle* is stretch. Active stretch occurs when higher-level motor commands descend to produce alpha-gamma coactivation and when a muscle contracts against resistance. Therefore, evincing an adaptive behavior against resistance may be the most effective means available for generating proprioceptive feedback. For example, when we extend the head and upper trunk against gravity from the prone-lying position, extend our weight-bearing limbs to jump on a trampoline, or flex our arms to swing on a suspended trapeze, we are contracting against the resistance of gravity acting on our bodies. Moreover, when a weak muscle contracts against gravity, stretch of the muscle results in recruitment of more motor units so that the muscle can contract harder and become stronger. Stimulation of *cutaneous or skin mechanoreceptors* and *joint receptors* by active joint movement is believed to be particularly important in

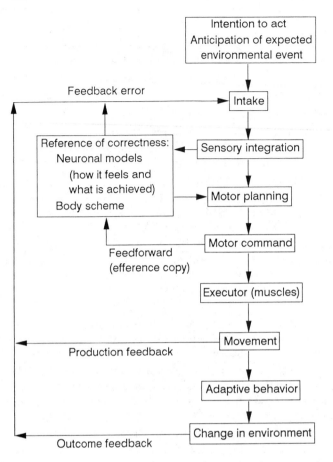

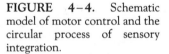

FIGURE 4-4. Schematic model of motor control and the circular process of sensory integration.

perception of movement of the fingers. In other joints, loss of joint and skin receptors results in no decline of proprioception (Matthews, 1988; McCloskey et al., 1983; Moberg, 1983). The therapeutic implication is that joint compression and traction probably are less effective sources of proprioception than is an active muscle contraction against resistance.

It also is important not to confuse cutaneous-generated proprioception with tactile sensation. Proprioception refers to sensations of movement or position that arise as a result of the individual's own movement. Tactile sensation pertains to awareness or perception of the location, or change in position, of an external stimulus applied to the skin. Tactile sensation provides an individual with information about the external environment. Often, tactile information is gathered as the individual moves his or her body or joints within the external environment. However, by definition, deep touch-pressure and other tactile inputs that are externally applied are not sources of proprioceptive inputs. As with active vs. passive movement, efference copy enables us to differentiate between stimulation of skin mechanoreceptors by active joint movement, and stimulation of skin mechanoreceptors by externally imposed tactile stimuli (Matthews, 1988). Again, active participation of the individual may have implications for treatment.

As we discussed earlier, *centrally generated motor commands* and efference copy also are sources of proprioceptive feedback. They are thought to be responsible for our sense of effort or conscious awareness that "proprioception is happening" (Brooks, 1986; Jones, 1988; Matthews, 1988; McCloskey, 1985).

> We have all experienced the sensation of increasing heaviness of a suitcase which we carry with progressively fatiguing muscles. Ultimately we put down such a load and rest when it has 'become too heavy'. But the load has not really become heavier: the pressure and tensions in the supporting limbs have not increased, and there is no reason to assume that the discharges from sensory receptors signalling pressures or tensions will have increased either. What makes the load seem heavier is that one perceives the greater effort, the greater efferent barrage of voluntarily-generated command signals, which has been necessary to maintain a contraction with progressively fatiguing and so less responsive muscles. Similar sensations of heaviness or increased muscular force accompany all other states of muscular weakness whether caused experimentally . . . , or by disease. (McCloskey, 1985, p. 152)

As we have already discussed, centrally generated motor commands and efference copy from motor centers are speculated to be necessary for the accurate interpretation of afferent sensory inputs. Centrally generated motor commands and efference copy also are important in motor control, that is, in the planning and producing of an adaptive motor behavior (see Fig. 4–4).

## Introduction to Motor Control

In order to understand the hypothesized role of proprioception in motor planning, some frequently used terms (e.g., closed-loop, open-loop, feedback, feedforward) must be defined. While there is general agreement concerning the use of these terms, some theorists and researchers continue to apply the terms inconsistently, sometimes within a single discussion of motor control. Establishing a common understanding of how we use these terms will provide the background for discussing the hypothesized contribution of proprioceptive processing deficits to vestibular-proprioceptive and bilateral integration and sequencing disorders of sensory integration.

### THEORIES OF MOTOR CONTROL

There are many theories of motor control, for example, closed-loop, open-loop, schema theory, and hierarchical control (see Brooks, 1986; Kelso, 1982; Schmidt, 1988; Stelmach, 1976; Zaichkowsky & Fuchs, 1986 for more comprehensive reviews). At one extreme is the peripheralist *closed-loop* view, which proposes that response-produced feedback is compared to a reference of correctness, the extent of error determined, and correction made. At the other extreme is the centralist *open loop* view, which proposes that muscle commands are preprogrammed (exist before a movement sequence even begins), and, once triggered, run their course without the possibility of correction from sensory feedback. Most theorists, however, recognize that neither of these views is entirely satisfactory, and instead adopt a more hybrid view of human motor control. These hybrid views acknowledge various forms of response-produced feedback as well as open-loop conditions under which no feedback occurs (Schmidt, 1988).

Schmidt (1988) postulated three types of response-produced feedback: (a) feedback that arises from the muscles as they contract, (b) feedback that arises from movement of the body or body parts in space, and (c) feedback from the environment. The first two arise from the response itself (how it feels to move or *production feedback*), and the latter arises from the change that occurs in the environment as a result of the response (what happens or *outcome feedback*) (see Fig. 4–4). In closed-loop movements, response-produced feedback is compared to the feedback that was expected. If there is a discrepancy between the feedback received and what was expected, an error is detected, and the need for a correction is signaled.

Kelso and Stelmach (1976) described an additional type of feedback, *internal feedback*, which is derived from information processed before the action begins. Whereas the peripheral theorists originally did not acknowledge the possible existence of internal feedback loops, most theorists now do. Within these internal feedback loops, a copy of the centrally generated motor command signal (corollary discharge or efference copy) is "fed forward" and compared to a sensory reference of correctness (Schmidt, 1988). Thus, efference copy may be a special type of internal feedback (*feedforward*) which, when compared to the reference of correctness, can be used to correct errors that are detected *prior to* the actual production of the action. Therefore, feedforward appears to be particularly important for actions that involve anticipation (Schmidt, 1988). Recall our earlier discussion of the role of corollary discharge in proprioception, and recall Todd, who had difficulty anticipating where to place his hands to catch a bounced ball. We might speculate that he has difficulty planning anticipatory projected action sequences because of poor proprioceptive feedback associated with corollary discharge.

This feedforward, or internal feedback, is differentiated from the response-produced feedback that comes from the movement. However, the term "feedforward" sometimes is used instead to refer to open-loop control systems; this is a major source of the confusion in the motor control literature. In both instances, the term is used to specify that there is no peripheral, response-produced feedback. Yet, the former is technically a closed-loop system because efference copy *does* provide a source of feedback. In open-loop systems, there is no feedback, internal or external. Therefore, we will use the terms feedback, feedforward, and open-loop to differentiate between the three hypothesized modes of motor control.

Feedback control appears to be particularly important in learning new skills. Once the skill is learned, increased reliance on feedforward becomes possible (Brooks, 1986; Kelso & Stelmach, 1976). From this, we might speculate that feedforward control represents a higher-level ability or skill on the spiral process of development. Further, individuals who have deficits only in feedforward motor control may be thought to be less severely involved than are those individuals who have both feedback and feedforward motor control deficits.

In support of this speculation, we note that Ayres (1978) found that children with vestibular bilateral integration disorders (see Chapter 1) are among the least affected of children with sensory integrative disorders. Further, factor and cluster analyses of the SIPT data suggest that bilateral integration deficits are associated with deficits in planning and executing projected action sequences (Ayres, 1989). These two observations, taken together, might suggest that children with bilateral integration and sequencing deficits are less involved than are children with other types of sensory integrative motor planning disorders because they only have deficits in proprioceptive-dependent feedforward motor control. Todd was identified as having a bilateral integration and sequencing disorder. Is it possible that Todd's problems with performing projected action sequences, such as jumping in a series of squares on the floor, are related to deficits in feedforward motor control? We will propose that cortical projections of vestibular-proprioceptive inputs are important for the planning and executing of bilateral and sequenced movements, and that the ability to plan projected action sequences is dependent on feedfoward motor control.

## CORTICAL PROJECTIONS OF VESTIBULAR-PROPRIOCEPTIVE INPUTS

Although the exact site of the primary vestibular cortex in humans remains controversial, there is evidence that labyrinthine and proprioceptive signals converge at cortical levels to provide conscious awareness of body orientation. One possible site for this convergence is *area 3a*, a transition area located between the primary motor and primary sensory cortex near the base of the central sulcus. Area 3a is known to be a major target for muscle spindle afferents, and recent research suggests that inputs to area 3a contribute to conscious awareness of movement, but not to motor planning (Dykes, Herron, & Lin, 1986; Gardner, 1988; Jones & Porter, 1980; Kalaska, 1988; Tuohimaa, Schneider, & Crosby, 1987).

Area 5 of the parietal cortex is another major site of convergence of bilateral proprioceptive inputs from muscle, cutaneous, and joint receptors of the body. Indirect vestibular signals also may project to area 5. As Jones and Porter (1980) indicated, there is a close association between sensation and motion. Although we do not know if conscious perception is necessarily separate from feedback to higher centers that control movement, there is evidence that cells in area 5 begin firing before movement is initiated, and continue to fire even under conditions of deafferentation and immobilization of joints. This suggests that some of these cells may play a role in planning active movement. Area 5 has reciprocal connections with precentral motor areas, including the *supplementary motor area* (Kalaska, 1988), further suggesting a role of proprioceptive inputs in motor planning.

## SUPPLEMENTARY MOTOR AREA

There are two premotor areas, the lateral arcuate premotor area and the medial supplementary motor area. This medial premotor area, which is proprioceptive-dependent, may be of particular significance in understanding deficits in bilateral integration and sequencing such as those exhibited by Todd (Table 4–1). Goldberg (1985) hypothesized that "the medial [premotor] system operates in 'projectional' action or action that is driven forward by prediction derived from an internal model of the world composed from previous experience which permits the creation of a probabilistic model of the future" (p. 568). In other words, the medial supplementary motor area appears to be involved in planning the very projected action sequences Todd finds so difficult. This is in contrast to the polymodal lateral arcuate premotor system that "operates in a responsive mode in which each action is dependent upon explicit external input" (p. 568). The hypothesized function of the two premotor areas is summarized in Table 4–1.

Goldberg (1985) described the individual with parkinsonism as being a "prototypical" example of impairment of the medial control system. Remarkably reminiscent of the problems Todd displays, individuals with Parkinson's disease characteristically have difficulty initiating, sequencing, and terminating projected action sequences. As a result, they become increasingly reliant on polymodal, especially visual, feedback for the guidance of movement. They also demonstrate characteristic deficits in *bilateral motor coordination.* Bilateral limb movements, such as those required in the Bilateral Motor Coordination subtest of the SIPT, are no longer executed as smooth reciprocal and continuous sequences. Rather, each hand moves independently of the other.

In the case of the individual with brain damage or Parkinson's disease, these deficits are the result of known lesions of medial supplementary motor area or the closely related basal ganglia. However, in Todd's case, we can speculate that if

TABLE 4–1. A COMPARISON OF FEATURES OF THE MEDIAL AND LATERAL MOTOR
PROGRAMMING SYSTEMS

|  | Medial | Lateral |
|---|---|---|
| "Premotor" center | Supplementary motor area | Arcuate premotor area |
| Sensory dependence | Primarily proprioceptive | Polymodal (including vision) |
| Control mode | Predictive (feedforward) | Responsive (feedback) |
| Skilled movement performance | Fluent execution of extended sequences of component actions | Input-dependent, slow, segmented execution |
| Bimanual control | Simultaneous (parallel or reciprocal) | Alternating (serial or segmental) |
| Callosal dependence | High | Low |
| Reaching to target | Trajectory (navigating) | Acquisition (piloting) |
| Action mode | Projectional (anticipatory) | Responsive (interactive) |
| Context sensitivity | Internal | External |
| Subcortical dependence | Basal ganglia | Cerebellum |

*Source:* Adapted from Goldberg (1985).

vestibular-proprioceptive processing deficits result in diminished or abnormal inputs to the proprioceptive-dependent supplementary motor area, the behavioral manifestation of vestibular-proprioceptive processing deficits at lower levels could result in behavioral deficits that are not unlike those seen in patients with known higher-level lesions.

> The medial system predominates when rapid, well learned, "skilled" movement sequences are executed using primarily [proprioceptive] information, independent of the requirements of ongoing visual feedback monitoring. The medial system is thus capable of using a model- or hypothesis-driven, feed-forward, predictive mode of control which may rely on efference copy for internal error correction and internal monitoring as the movement unfolds. (Goldberg, 1985, pp. 581–582)

## The Role of Vestibular-Proprioception in Body Scheme

If we now recall Chris, we remember that her most remarkable problem was her poor sense of her body position in space. Based on our discussion thus far of the contributions of vestibular-proprioception to awareness of body position and movement, it seems reasonable to postulate that Chris, with her severely impaired sense of body position in space, has deficits in integrating or interpreting vestibular-proprioceptive inputs.

Fisher and Bundy (1989; Fisher, unpublished data) described another subject who, based on an in-depth interview, also was found to have a poor sense of her body in space. This subject's sensory integrative deficits in central processing of vestibular inputs were confirmed through laboratory testing (Fisher, et al., 1986). She experienced "sensory overload" or "sensory disorientation" following a period of visual-vestibular stimulation that included visual-vestibular conflict; we now prefer the term *sensory disorientation*, which more accurately describes her response. Approximately 3 hours after stimulation, the subject began to experience the feeling that her head, arms, and legs had become detached from her body and were floating in space. When she attempted to walk on a level surface, she felt as if she were walking on an uneven, unpredictable surface. Sometimes the surface would seem to be higher than she expected it to be, and sometimes the ground would be lower than she expected it to be.

We also have suggested that vestibular-proprioceptive feedback from movements contributes to the development of neuronal models or the memory of how it feels to perform a given movement (see also Chapter 1). According to Brooks (1986), this information "is used in two ways: it regulates ongoing, present activity, and it guides, as part of the motor memory, the execution of such a task in the future. Thus our sense of effort and its memory are essential to both the execution and planning of motor action" (Brooks, 1986, p. 6). Brooks also appears to suggest that body scheme is important to the ability to plan projected movement sequences.

Matthews (1988) reviewed the existing evidence of the contribution of proprioception to body scheme and our awareness of our relationship to the external environment. Most of this research has involved the use of high-frequency vibration to provide abnormal proprioceptive inputs to the primary endings of the muscle spindle. The overwhelming evidence is that the system is easily confused, and our "central maps" of our body are readily modified (see also Jones, 1988). As a case in point, Matthews reported an unpublished study by J. R. Lackner.

> [Lackner] vibrated the biceps while the subject was holding onto his nose and who, as usual, felt that his elbow was extending. But since the stationary nose was still being held this produced sensory conflict, arising from the contradictory information as to where his arm was. Some subjects solved this problem very simply and logically, but by entirely unconscious nervous operations acting on their internal body map, and had the clear subjective impression that their nose was growing out and elongating so as to remain in contact with the apparently moving arm. As one said, "I feel like Pinocchio." (Matthews, 1988, p. 436)

Vibratory input can similarly alter the subjective sense of body position relative to objects in the environment, and active movement against increased gravity results not only in an increased sense of effort, but also in a sense that the external environment moves in reference to the moving body. For example, when the subject steps up onto a stool, "he has the illusion that the stool sinks down as he steps onto it" (Matthews, 1988, p. 437).

Matthews (1988) concluded that in normal conditions, the role of proprioception was to provide the motor system with a clear and unambiguous map of the external environment and of the body. Similarly, Nashner (1982) hypothesized that in conditions of visual-vestibular-somatosensory sensory conflict during balance control, the vestibular system provides accurate information that can be used to resolve the conflict. This suggestion that the vestibular-proprioceptors normally provide a *stable frame of reference against which other sensory inputs are interpreted* leads us to speculate about the possible effect that impaired central processing of vestibular-proprioceptive inputs might have on an individual subjected to conflicting or unfamiliar sensory experiences.

## Aversive Responses to Vestibular-Proprioceptive Inputs and Gravitational Insecurity

As we proceed, recall Chris, who described childhood memories of a pervasive fear of movement, who became tense and anxious on the suspended equipment used in treatment and who easily becomes nauseated when she rides in the car. Recall also that Chris has a very poor sense of her body and where it is in space. Chris' poor body scheme and possible impaired ability to resolve sensory conflict, because of her diminished or distorted vestibular-proprioceptive frame of reference, might be manifested behaviorally in her *aversive response* to vestibular-proprioceptive inputs and her *gravitational insecurity*. Aversive response to vestibular-proprioceptive inputs are characterized by nausea, vomiting, dizziness or vertigo, and other feelings of discomfort associated with autonomic (sympathetic) nervous system stimulation. Gravitational insecurity is characterized by excessive emotional reactions or fear that is out of proportion to the real threat or actual danger arising from vestibular-proprioceptive stimuli or position of the body in space. While neither disorder is well understood, both are hypothesized to be due to hyperresponsiveness or poor modulation of vestibular-proprioceptive inputs (Fisher & Bundy, 1989), and there is some evidence that increased sensitivity to vestibular stimulation or visual-vestibular conflict can result in motion sickness (Baloh & Honrubia, 1979).

## The Role of Vestibular-Proprioceptive Inputs in Postural Control

Both Chris and Todd, as you recall, had poor equilibrium. The results of testing children with learning disabilities and central deficits in integrating vestibular inputs suggest that central vestibular processing disorders may have a profound impact on balance (Horak et al. 1988; Shumway-Cook et al., 1987). In fact, Allum and Keshner (1986) suggested that while both vestibular and proprioceptive inputs are important in the control of postural sway, vestibular contributions predominate. This is in contrast to Nashner and his colleagues, who hypothesized that visual and somatosensory inputs predominate in balance control, and that the role of the vestibular system is to provide a stable frame of reference for resolving sensory conflict (Horak et al., 1988; Nashner, 1982; Shumway-Cook et al., 1987).

## Summary

We have presented evidence supporting vestibular and proprioceptive contributions to such diverse functions as the perception of position and active movement of the body in space, development of body scheme, ocular control (vestibular nystagmus and velocity storage), and postural responses (especially those involving tonic postural extensor muscles). We also have postulated that impairments of vestibular-proprioceptive processing that impact negatively on body scheme or the resolution of sensory conflicts encountered in everyday life may contribute to aversive responses to vestibular-proprioceptive inputs, or to gravitational insecurity. Finally, we presented recent research suggesting that proprioceptive (and possibly vestibular) inputs are involved in the programming and planning of bilateral projected action sequences. Although we have tried to differentiate between vestibular and proprioceptive contributions (which is possible only in laboratory settings), our clinical assessments do not enable us to determine whether the deficits we see in individuals with sensory integrative deficits are associated with impaired vestibular processing, impaired proprioceptive processing, or both. Therefore, when we evaluate individuals in clinical settings, we are unable to differentiate fully between vestibular and proprioceptive functioning. Consequently, we have emphasized the use of the term vestibular-proprioceptive. Future instrument development may enable us to be more precise.

## VESTIBULAR-PROPRIOCEPTIVE DISORDERS

Building on our discussion of the neurobehavioral aspects of vestibular-proprioception, we now will describe the types of vestibular-proprioceptive dysfunction seen in individuals with sensory integrative dysfunction. This will be followed by a discussion of the various methods used in the clinic to evaluate for the presence of vestibular-proprioceptive dysfunction. Where they are appropriate, standardized tests from the SIPT (Ayres, 1989) are included. However, in large part, evaluation is based on clinical observation of neuromotor behavior and client interview.

We wish to emphasize that the *identification of vestibular-proprioceptive sensory integrative dysfunction is based on a meaningful cluster of test scores or clinical observations that have in common a possible vestibular-proprioceptive basis.* Few of the assessments available clinically are direct measures of vestibular-proprioceptive function, and there are reasons other than poor central processing of vestibular-proprioceptive inputs why an individual might demonstrate low scores. However, the one factor that they all have in common is a vestibular-proprioceptive component. Therefore, when several scores are low, the probability increases that the low scores reflect central vestibular-proprioceptive processing deficits. There is some empirical evidence to support the validity of identifying central processing deficits based on a meaningful cluster of low scores on indirect measures of vestibular-proprioceptive functioning (Fisher et al., 1986).

Traditionally, Ayres (1972, 1976, 1978, 1979, 1980) hypothesized three disorders of sensory integration related to deficits in vestibular-proprioceptive processing. These are (a) postural-ocular movement disorder; (b) gravitational insecurity; and (c) intolerance of, or aversive response to, movement. (Duration of postrotary nystagmus is sometimes viewed as a separate domain of function because both shortened and prolonged durations are considered indicative of dysfunction; however, because postrotary nystagmus is a vestibular-ocular response, we have considered *shortened durations* of postrotary nystagmus to be one indicator of a postural-ocular disorder. We now will discuss each of the three types of vestibular-proprioceptive disorders in some detail.

## Postural-Ocular Movement Disorder

As the name implies, the major identifying characteristic of a postural-ocular movement disorder is evidence of several test scores and related clinical observations suggestive of poor postural and ocular control. More specifically, postural-ocular movement disorder is defined by the presence of a meaningful cluster of the following:

1. Inability to assume or maintain the prone extension posture
2. Difficulty flexing the neck when assuming the supine flexion position
3. Hypotonicity of extensor muscles
4. Poor proximal joint stability
5. Deficient postural adjustments or background movements
6. Poor equilibrium and support reactions, including depressed scores on Standing and Walking Balance of the SIPT
7. Depressed scores on Kinesthesia of the SIPT
8. Depressed scores on Postrotary Nystagmus of the SIPT

The emphasis is on postural control; Postrotary Nystagmus is the only clinical measure of ocular control. Smooth pursuits, saccades or quick localization, and convergence are *not* measures of vestibular-proprioceptive control of eye movements. As was the case with Chris, careful interview often will reveal evidence of concomitant deficits in body scheme and awareness of body position or movement in space. Finally, postural-ocular movement disorder is the vestibular-proprioceptive sensory integrative disorder thought to be associated with deficits in bilateral integration and sequencing (A. J. Ayres, personal communication, March 11, 1988).

## EVALUATION OF PRONE EXTENSION

The ability to assume and maintain the prone extension posture is an indicator of the strength of tonic postural extension. Ayres stated that the ability to assume and maintain the prone extension posture is a strong indicator of vestibular-proprioceptive functioning (A. J. Ayres, personal communication March 11, 1988). When vestibular-proprioceptive inputs to extensor muscles, especially of the neck and upper trunk, are diminished, the ability to assume the prone extension posture may be affected. Prone extension is evaluated first by demonstrating the desired posture, and then by asking the individual to assume the position independently (Fig. 4–5). Verbal and physical assistance may be given to ensure that the individual understands what is expected. The quality of the response is graded based on the ability to (a) assume the whole position quickly, that is, nonsegmentally; (b) hold the head steady and within 45° of vertical; (c) lift the shoulders, chest, and arms off the floor; (d) raise the distal one-third of both thighs off the floor; (e) maintain the knees in less than 30° of flexion; and (f) talk out loud. Individuals 6 years of age and older should be able to assume a full prone extension posture and hold it for 30 seconds; however, individuals with tight hip flexors may have difficulty lifting their thighs or assuming the position without flexing their knees more than 30° (Fisher & Bundy, 1989).

## EVALUATION OF NECK FLEXION DURING SUPINE FLEXION

When an individual assumes a supine position, vestibular-proprioceptive inputs (especially those originating from the utricle) descend to facilitate righting of the head and upper trunk. Although individuals with poor vestibular-proprioceptive processing usually demonstrate relatively fewer problems assuming the supine flexion position than the prone extension posture, a tendency to lead with the chin (or the presence of head lag) may reflect diminished vestibular-proprioceptive inputs to neck flexors.

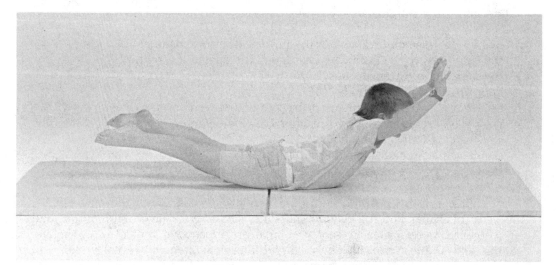

FIGURE 4–5. Normal prone extension position.

## EVALUATION OF EXTENSOR MUSCLE HYPOTONICITY

Hypotonicity, especially of extensor muscles, is influenced by descending vestibular-proprioceptive inputs. Hypotonicity cannot be measured directly. Therefore, the identification of extensor hypotonicity is based on a meaningful cluster of the following: (a) hyperextensibility of distal joints, (b) a standing posture characterized by lordosis and hyperextended or locked knees ("hypotonic posture"), and (c) "mushiness" of muscles when palpated. Before concluding that the individual is hypotonic, it is necessary to rule out the presence of joint laxity, lordosis compensatory to tight hip flexors, and lordotic posture normally seen in toddlers (Fisher & Bundy, 1989).

## EVALUATION OF PROXIMAL JOINT STABILITY

Joint stability refers to the ability of tonic postural extensor muscles to contract so as to stabilize proximal joints during weight-bearing. One of the best ways to evaluate for proximal stability is to ask the individual to assume a quadruped position, and to observe for persistence of (a) lordosis, (b) hyperextension or locking of the elbows, (c) raising of the medial border of the scapula, and (d) excessive scapular abduction (Fisher & Bundy, 1989). As with the evaluation of prone extension, verbal and physical cues may be given to ensure that the individual understands what is expected. While the ability to stabilize proximal joints is sometimes referred to as *cocontraction*, the use of this term may be misleading because simultaneous contraction of flexor and extensor muscles is not necessary for joint stability.

## EVALUATION OF POSTURAL ADJUSTMENTS OR BACKGROUND MOVEMENTS

Postural background movements are the appropriate postural adjustments made by the individual during the performance of adaptive behaviors. Poor postural background movements are exaggerated, awkward, inappropriate, or diminished postural adjustments. Poor postural background movements can be associated with low postural tone, deficient equilibrium reactions, or poor tonic proximal stability. There are no standard methods of evaluating postural background movements. However, they are readily observed during the performance of adaptive behaviors (Fisher & Bundy, 1989).

## EVALUATION OF EQUILIBRIUM AND SUPPORT REACTIONS

One of the best methods of assessing vestibular-proprioceptive contributions to postural control is through the evaluation of equilibrium and support reactions. However, because of the low correlations among different assessments of equilibrium, thorough evaluation requires that a variety of equilibrium tests be administered (Fisher, Wietlisbach, & Wilbarger, 1988). The Standing and Walking Balance Test of the SIPT is a standardized test of the ability to perform a series of balance tasks (Ayres, 1989). Similar standardized measures appropriate for older children and adults include the Bruininks-Oseretsky balance subtest (Bruininks, 1978) and the floor ataxia test battery (Fregly & Graybiel, 1968). While these assessments are standardized, they are limited in their ability to assess the qualitative aspects of equilibrium.

Fisher and colleagues (Fisher, 1989; Fisher & Bundy, 1989; Fisher et al., 1988) have developed three objective tests of the quality of equilibrium that have been shown to be useful in identifying individuals with vestibular-proprioceptive deficits.

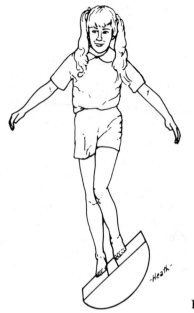

FIGURE 4–6. Normal response on the Tilt Board Tip test.

The three tests are Tilt Board Tip, Flat Board Reach, and Tilt Board Reach. On the Tilt Board Tip test, normal individuals of at least 5 years of age should maintain the head and upper trunk in the upright position, demonstrate an increased support reaction in the downhill leg, and flex the hip and knee of the uphill leg (Figs. 4–6, 4–7, and 4–8). Flat Board Reach and Tilt Board Reach are measures of the ability to maintain balance during lateral reach while standing on a stable and an unstable surface, respectively. Children younger than 7 years of age may not lift the uphill foot from the support surface (Fig. 4–9). By 7 years of age, normal individuals extend and

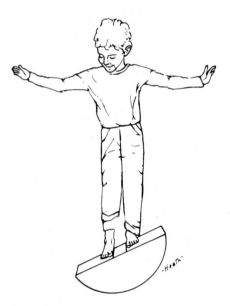

FIGURE 4–7. Abnormal or immature response on the Tilt Board Tip test: arms raised in a "high guard" position, uphill hip and knee not flexed, and gaze directed toward the floor.

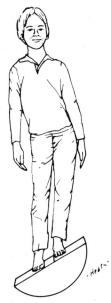

**FIGURE 4–8.** Abnormal or immature response on the Tilt Board Tip test with lack of hip and knee flexion of the uphill leg.

abduct the uphill arm and lift the uphill foot from the support surface; most individuals extend and abduct the uphill leg at least 30° from the original starting position (Fig. 4–10). Persistence in not lifting the uphill foot from the support surface, or the presence of uphill arm or leg flexion is suggestive of dysfunction, as shown in Figure 4–11 (Fisher, 1989). Interrater reliability of all three tests is high ($r > 0.90$); test-retest reliability of the reaching tasks is also high ($r > 0.90$), and may be better than the test-retest reliability of a tilt board test suggested by Atwater, Crowe, Deitz, and Richardson (1990).

Another promising battery of equilibrium tests for clinicians is being developed

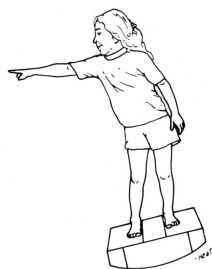

**FIGURE 4–9.** Uphill foot remains in contact with the support surface of the Tilt (or Flat) Board Reach test.

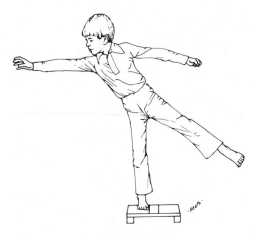

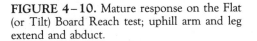

**FIGURE 4–10.** Mature response on the Flat (or Tilt) Board Reach test; uphill arm and leg extend and abduct.

by Crowe and colleagues (Crowe, Deitz, Richardson, & Atwater, in press). This Clinical Test of Sensory Interaction for Balance was adapted for clinical use by Horak and Shumway-Cook (Horak et al., 1988; Horak & Shumway-Cook, 1986; Shumway-Cook et al., 1987). This test is an assessment of the ability to maintain balance under conditions of sensory conflict. In this assessment, the amount of postural sway and duration of maintaining a particular position is measured under conditions of normal, absent, and altered (present, but distorted) visual or support surface information. For example, the ability to stand on a compliant foam surface (support surface input altered) when the eyes are closed (vision absent) depends on the ability to use vestibular information for resolution of the visual–support-surface–vestibular conflict for accurate orientation in space.

## KINESTHESIA

The Kinesthesia test of the SIPT (Ayres, 1989) is an assessment of the ability of a child to move his or her finger to the position where the finger had passively been placed by the examiner (see also Chapter 8). This test is questionable as a valid test of proprioception. By definition, proprioception (kinesthesia) is conscious aware-

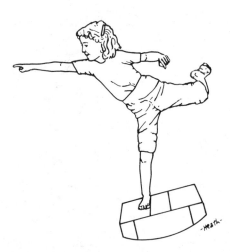

**FIGURE 4–11.** Abnormal response on the Tilt (or Flat) Board Reach test; the uphill arm and leg flex more than 30°.

ness of active, and not passive, movement of one's own body. Since movement of the child's arm is externally imposed by the examiner, no efference copy is generated. Further, the test-retest reliability of this test is the lowest of the SIPT ($r = 0.33$ for children with learning disabilities). Finally, the Kinesthesia test did not load on the factors that included the other vestibular-proprioceptive assessments (Ayres, 1989; see also Chapter 1 and Chapter 8). Ayres, in recognition of the limitations of the Kinesthesia test, stated: "I suspect one of the reasons Kinesthesia of the SIPT does not show a stronger loading is that it is not really a good test. I don't know how to make it better, though. It is too dependent upon the ability to focus attention on tactile-kinesthetic input. Standing and Walking Balance is a better measure of proprioception but it also reflects vestibular processing" (A. J. Ayres, personal communication, March 11, 1988).

## POSTROTARY NYSTAGMUS

Depressed duration of postrotary nystagmus is defined as a score on the Postrotary Nystagmus Test that is more than 1.0 standard deviation below the mean (Ayres, 1989). Because an inordinate amount of attention has been given to the evaluation of postrotary nystagmus, we believe that it is important for occupational therapists to understand the basis of the controversy in order to interpret the literature and test results appropriately. Accordingly, the validity of the Postrotary Nystagmus Test will be discussed in some detail.

Polatajko (1983), and more recently, Cohen (1989) have questioned the validity of the Postrotary Nystagmus Test. Because the Postrotary Nystagmus Test is administered in the light, both the vestibulo-ocular reflex and optokinetic nystagmus are elicited. As a result, perrotary vestibular nystagmus combines with optokinetic nystagmus to increase slow-phase eye velocity to match the speed of head rotation for the duration of the perrotary period (Fig. 4–12). In the postrotary phase, slow-phase eye velocity of optokinetic afternystagmus (which would normally be generated in the same direction as the perrotary nystagmus) is subtracted from the slow-phase eye velocity of postrotary nystagmus that is generated in the opposite direction. Thus, the time course of postrotary nystagmus, when tested in the light, is shorter than when it is tested in the dark. Further, when subjects are tested in the light, postrotary nystagmus can be suppressed by visual fixation. Other factors that might contribute to a shortened time course of postrotary nystagmus (whether tested in the light or in the dark) include habituation as a result of repeated vestibular stimulation, alertness, or tilt suppression (neck flexion upon termination of the perrotary stage of testing). We believe that Polatajko (1983) and Cohen (1989) present several valid reasons why a *normal* child could have depressed scores on the Postrotary Nystagmus Test. *Thus, when depressed scores occur in the presence of other vestibular-proprioceptive scores that are within normal limits, the shortened duration should not be taken as evidence of vestibular dysfunction.* Such a conservative interpretation of the Postrotary Nystagmus Test is also warranted by its relatively low test-retest reliability (Ayres, 1989; Morrison & Sublett, 1983).

Nonetheless, the various factors that can attenuate durations of postrotary nystagmus fail to explain adequately why children with learning disabilities have mean durations of postrotary nystagmus that are *even shorter than* the mean durations seen in normal children (Ayres, 1975, 1989). Individuals with impaired central processing of vestibular inputs demonstrate markedly reduced or absent velocity storage (Fisher et al., 1986). Thus, the time course of postrotary nystagmus can be expected to be shortened to match that of the cupular afferents. However, since

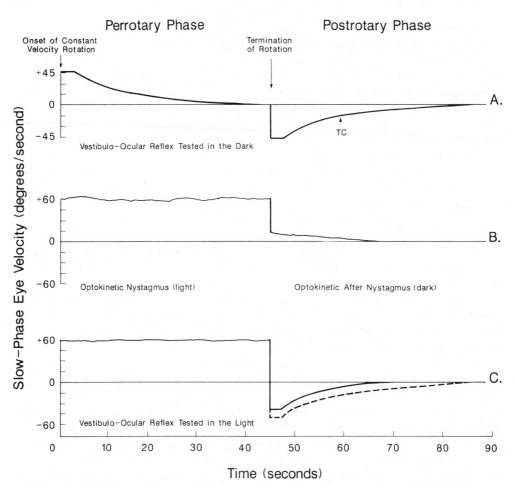

FIGURE 4–12. Schematic diagram of the time course of slow-phase eye velocity. *(A)* Vestibulo-ocular reflex, tested by rotating the subject in the dark. *(B)* Optokinetic nystagmus (perrotary phase) and optokinetic afternsytagmus (postrotary phase), tested with the subject stationary and with a striped visual surround rotated around the subject. In the postrotary phase, the subject sits in the dark, so there is no more movement of the visual surround. *(C)* Summative effects of the vestibulo-ocular reflex and optokinetic stimulation, tested by rotating the subject in the light within a stationary visual surround. Slow-phase eye velocity of optokinetic afternystagmus (*B*, above the line) is subtracted from the slow-phase eye velocity of vestibular postrotary nystagmus (*A*, below the line). The result is an attenuation of duration of postrotary nystagmus (*C*, solid line). The difference between the broken line and the solid line reflects the effects of subtracting optokinetic afternystagmus (in one direction) from postrotary nystagmus (in the opposite direction).

velocity storage is diminished, optokinetic afternystagmus is not generated in the postrotary phase and does not shorten further the time course of postrotary vestibular nystagmus.

Although head tilt (increased neck flexion) or fixation can result in "dumping" of velocity storage in normal individuals (Raphan et al., 1979; Koenig & Dichgans, 1981), once again we have a situation where the individual with central vestibular processing deficits does not store the velocity signal, and therefore, has none to "dump." In fact it seems more appropriate to speculate that decreased, rather than enhanced, fixation suppression would be associated with immaturity or inadequate functioning of brainstem velocity storage mechanisms (Ornitz & Honrubia, 1988).

Therefore, when the duration of postrotary nystagmus is depressed beyond that seen in normal individuals who demonstrate normal velocity storage and fixation suppression, and when such depression scores occur in the presence of sufficient related evidence of impaired vestibular-proprioceptive functioning, duration of postrotary nystagmus may provide supporting evidence for the presence of dysfunction. In most cases, however, the clinical determination of the presence or absence of vestibular-proprioceptive processing deficits can be made in the absence of Postrotary Nystagmus scores (Fisher et al., 1986).

## Gravitational Insecurity

Gravitational insecurity is a distinct disorder that may occur in individuals with normal postural-ocular responses. Further, we believe that gravitational insecurity also may be viewed as a sensory modulation disorder, even when it occurs in individuals with frank neurological disorders and in the absence of other sensory integrative deficits. At the very least, sensory integration theory is the only model of practice that has addressed this disorder.

Gravitational insecurity is defined as an emotional or fear reaction that is out of proportion to the actual threat or danger of the vestibular-proprioceptive stimuli or the position of the body in space (especially those body positions in which the feet are no longer in contact with the floor). Gravitational insecurity has been hypothesized to be due to poor modulation of otolithic inputs (Fisher & Bundy, 1989). We speculated earlier that another possible basis for gravitational insecurity pertains to the contribution of vestibular-proprioceptive inputs to the development of body scheme and the resolution of sensory conflict. Further research is needed to clarify the basis of the disorder.

Currently, evaluation of gravitational insecurity must be based on interview of the individual as well as clinical observation of excessive fear reactions during evaluation of other postural responses. Gravitational insecurity also may be observed during treatment when the individual assumes a position on unstable or suspended equipment.

A promising new objective observational assessment has been piloted and found to be able to differentiate between normal children and children who are gravitationally insecure. In the pilot version, individuals were observed performing 15 potentially fear-inducing activities that were scored on a three-point scale for each of three domains: avoidance, emotional responses, and postural responses (May-Benson, 1988).

## Intolerance or Aversive Response to Movement

Intolerance or aversive response to movement is closely associated with gravitational insecurity, and the two disorders often occur in the same individual. Like gravitational insecurity, intolerance or an aversive response to movement is viewed as a distinct disorder. Unlike gravitational insecurity, it is not considered a sensory modulation disorder unless other possible causes (e.g., peripheral vestibular disease, traumatic head injury) can be ruled out (cf. Baloh & Honrubia, 1979). Whereas aversive responses are hypothesized to be due to poor modulation of semicircular canal inputs (Fisher & Bundy, 1989), we also speculated earlier in this chapter (as we did with gravitational insecurity) about a possible contribution of normal processing of vestibular-proprioceptive inputs to the resolution of sensory conflict.

Evaluation is best accomplished by interview for evidence of a history of inordinate autonomic nervous system reactions to movement stimuli (e.g., car rides, playground and carnival rides, rotation). Intolerance or aversive responses to movement also may be observed during administration of the Postrotary Nystagmus test, or during treatment. When aversive responses occur, the source of the aversive stimulus should be removed immediately.

# BILATERAL INTEGRATION AND SEQUENCING

Bilateral integration deficits (the inability to use two sides of the body together in a coordinated manner) traditionally have been associated with deficits in central processing of vestibular-proprioceptive inputs (cf. Ayres, 1972, 1976, 1979). Although factor-analytic studies linked postural-ocular movement disorder with deficits in bilateral integration (see Chapter 1), Ayres never was "able to find neurophysiological support for the relationship of vestibular function to bilateral integration" (A. J. Ayres, personal communication, March 11, 1988).

More recently, deficits in bilateral integration were linked with deficits in sequencing (Ayres, 1989), and we have presented evidence suggesting a possible neurobehavioral link between vestibular-proprioceptive functioning and bilateral integration and sequencing. Although a postural-ocular movement disorder, which is the behavioral manifestation of a vestibular-proprioceptive processing disorder, is hypothesized to be the basis for the bilateral integration and sequencing deficits, further research may lead to revision of this hypothesis.

Deficits in bilateral integration and sequencing are indicated by a meaningful cluster of the following:

1. Depressed scores on Bilateral Motor Coordination, Sequencing Praxis, Graphesthesia, and Oral Praxis of the SIPT (Postural Praxis also may be low, but is not considered an indicator of bilateral integration and sequencing unless tests of tactile discrimination are within normal limits)
2. Depressed scores on Space Visualization Contralateral Use and Preferred Hand Use scores from the SIPT
3. Clinical observation of poor bilateral coordination, right-left confusion, or avoidance of moving one arm across the midline of the body into contralateral space
4. Clinical observation of poor sequencing or projected movements, especially bilateral projected action sequences

## SIPT ASSESSMENTS OF BILATERAL INTEGRATION AND SEQUENCING

Bilateral Motor Coordination, Sequencing Praxis, Graphesthesia, and Oral Praxis are unique among the SIPT in that each requires that the child plan and execute movements without the benefit of response-produced feedback. That is, there is no opportunity to correct errors once they have occurred. Postural Praxis can be performed without the benefit of response-produced feedback, but the child does have 3 seconds to correct response errors before points are deducted. The Standing and Walking Test of the SIPT, which was discussed earlier, has been statistically associated with these other SIPT scores. It is assumed to reflect the vestibular-proprioceptive contributions to bilateral integration and sequencing, rather than to be a measure of bilateral integration and sequencing, per se.

The Space Visualization Contralateral Use score from the SIPT is a measure of the number of times the child spontaneously crosses the midline to pick up a test item from contralateral space. Low scores indicate that the child used the ipsilateral hand to pick up test items more frequently than expected. It should be noted that the test-retest reliability for the Space Visualization Contralateral Use score was low ($r = .049$ for children with learning disabilities). The Preferred Hand Use score is a measure of the number of times the child uses his or her preferred hand to pick up test items (from ipsilateral or contralateral space). The "preferred" hand is defined as the one the child prefers to use for writing. Low scores indicate that the preferred hand was used less frequently than expected, and thus may be an indicator that hand preference is not well established.

## CLINICAL EVALUATION OF BILATERAL INTEGRATION

Deficits in bilateral integration are supported by clinical observation of deficits in coordinating the two sides of the body, and possibly by right-left confusion, avoidance of crossing the midline of the body, and failure to develop a more skilled or preferred hand. Bilateral motor control can be observed in a variety of tasks, but observation of age-appropriate hopping, skipping, and jumping with both feet together are among the better measures of bilateral motor coordination. Jumping jacks, symmetrical stride jumping, and reciprocal stride jumping also are helpful tools used to evaluate bilateral motor coordination. Magalhaes, Koomar, and Cermak (1989) reported preliminary norms and a rating scale for evaluating 5- to 9-year-old children. The ability to perform jumping jacks, the most reliable of the assessments, appears to mature by age 7 years. Reciprocal stride jumps were found to be the most difficult; few of the 9-year-old children obtained near-perfect scores.

Avoidance of crossing the midline of the body and right-left confusion are best observed during performance of unstructured tasks. Observation of midline crossing also should avoid "contrived" situations. For example, placing cones on the floor on either side of a child seated on a piece of suspended equipment, and asking the child to place rings over the cones, is not likely to elicit midline crossing. Most children choose the easier option and use their right hands to place rings over the cone positioned on the right side, and use their left hands to place rings over the cone positioned on the left side. If, on the other hand, the child already has one hand engaged in activity (e.g., holding on to the suspension rope), he or she will be unable to transfer the ring from one hand to the other.

Right-left confusion may be a relatively poor indicator of deficits of bilateral integration. First, right-left confusion is easily mistaken for difficulty in assigning a verbal label to the right or left side of the body. Second, Fisher and Camenzuli (1987) questioned the hypothesis that right-left confusion reflects bilateral symmetry of the nervous system; sensory integration theory has hypothesized that deficits in bilateral integration are associated with deficits in lateralization within the nervous system (Ayres, 1976, 1979, 1989). Lateralization is discussed in more detail in Chapter 7.

Related to lateralization is the development of hand preference. "Handedness is now considered to be stable in most children by at least 5 years of age, although earlier work had formerly been interpreted as indicating it was not fixed until about 9 years (Tan, 1985). Children as young as 4 years of age who have not yet established a clear hand preference (mixed handedness) demonstrate lower overall scores on tests of gross and fine motor coordination when compared to children with established right or left hand preference (Tan, 1985). These results support the observation that mixed handedness may be associated with motor incoordination.

CLINICAL EVALUATION OF PROJECTED ACTION SEQUENCES

Two of the better methods of evaluating the ability to plan and produce projected action sequences are those that were administered to Todd: catching a bounced ball and jumping in a series of squares placed on the floor. In the latter case, bilateral motor coordination is indicated by the ability to jump with both feet together. Poor sequencing of projected movements is indicated by difficulty initiating, sequencing, and terminating the series of jumps. In both the ball catching and jumping tasks, anticipation is an important factor. Difficulty learning to perform jumping jacks, symmetrical stride jumping, and reciprocal stride jumping, even with demonstration, also may reflect deficits in planning and producing projected action sequences (Magalhaes et al., 1989). Other methods that can be used to evaluate the ability to plan and produce projected action sequences include kicking a rolling soccer ball or stepping over a rolling bolster. These two tasks are especially difficult if the task requires that *both* the object (ball or bolster) and the child be moving (see also Chapter 10).

# THEORETICAL ISSUES FOR TREATMENT PLANNING

As we consider theoretical issues of treatment planning, let us return to Todd. When Todd was evaluated, we found that he had poor balance, poor prone extension, poor postural stabilization, and hypotonicity or weakness of his extensor muscles. Based on a cluster of clinical observations that have been linked to a postural-ocular movement disorder, we conclude that Todd has central deficits in processing vestibular-proprioceptive information. In part, we base this conclusion on the absence of any other apparent cause of his postural deficits.

As we begin to link theory with practice, we consider the postulate of sensory integration theory which states that the provision of enhanced opportunities for sensory intake, provided within the context of a meaningful activity, will enhance sensory integration (see Chapter 1). We conclude that treatment activities for Todd should emphasize vestibular-proprioceptive stimulation. Further, since Todd demonstrates tonic postural deficits, we conclude that we should begin with activities which emphasize sustained, linear vestibular stimulation in combination with activities which require that Todd evince tonic postural responses against resistance. Finally, in order to stimulate all possible combinations of hair cells within the vestibular receptors, we consider activities which will require Todd to assume a variety of head positions. But, since our focus is on developing his tonic postural extensors, we emphasize the prone position.

If we now consider Todd's motor coordination problems, we recall that he had problems producing bilateral projected action sequences, and low scores on Bilateral Motor Coordination and Sequencing Praxis. While less clear, his right-to-left reversals also may be related to the evidence suggesting that Todd has deficits in bilateral integration and sequencing.

Because our treatment postulate further indicates that the provision of opportunities for sensory intake be provided within the context of planning and producing an adaptive behavior, we decide to stress activities that involve bilateral motor control, sequencing, and anticipation (projected action sequences). Thus, when we put it all together, we select, or guide Todd to select, treatment activities which he will enjoy and find motivating, which provide utricular vestibular stimulation, and which involve the planning and production of projected action sequences against resistance.

Clearly, the provision of sensory integration treatment programs is an art as well as a science. The "art" of actually selecting and implementing treatment programs based on the theory is discussed in Chapters 10 and 12.

# REFERENCES

Allum, J. H. J., & Keshner, E. A. (1986). Vestibular and proprioceptive control of sway stabilization. In W. Bles & T. Brandt (Eds.), *Disorders of posture and gait* (pp. 83–97). New York: Elsevier.

Atwater, S. W., Crowe, T. K., Deitz, J. C., & Richardson, P. K. (1990). Interrater and test-retester reliability of two pediatric balance tests. *Physical Therapy, 70,* 79–87.

Ayres, A. J. (1972). *Sensory integration and learning disorders.* Los Angeles: Western Psychological Services.

Ayres, A. J. (1975). *Southern California Postrotary Nystagmus Test.* Los Angeles: Western Psychological Services.

Ayres, A. J. (1976). *Interpreting the Southern California Sensory Integration Tests.* Los Angeles: Western Psychological Services.

Ayres, A. J. (1978). Learning disabilities and the vestibular system. *Journal of Learning Disabilities, 12,* 18–29.

Ayres, A. J. (1979). *Sensory integration and the child.* Los Angeles: Western Psychological Services.

Ayres, A. J. (1980). *Southern California Sensory Integration Tests manual: Revised 1980.* Los Angeles: Western Psychological Services.

Ayres, A. J. (1989). *Sensory Integration and Praxis Tests.* Los Angeles: Western Psychological Services.

Baloh, R. W., & Honrubia, V. (1979). *Clinical neurophysiology of the vestibular system.* Philadelphia: F. A. Davis.

Bonder, B. R., & Fisher, A. G. (1989). Sensory integration and treatment of the elderly. *Gerontology Special Interest Section News, 12*(1), 2–4.

Brooks, V. B. (1986). *The neural basis of motor control.* New York: Oxford University.

Brown, B., Haegerstrom-Portnoy, G., Yingling, C. D., Herron, J., Galin, D., & Marcus, M. (1983). Dyslexic children have normal vestibular responses to rotation. *Archives of Neurology, 40,* 370–373.

Bruininks, R. H. (1978). *Bruininks-Oseretsky Test of Motor Proficiency examiner's manual.* Circle Pines, MN: American Guidance Service.

Cazals, Y., & Aurousseau, C. (1987). Saccular acoustic responses in the guinea pig involve superior olive but not inferior colliculus. In M. D. Graham & J. L. Kemink, *The vestibular system: Neurophysiologic and clinical research* (pp. 601–606). New York: Raven.

Clark, F., Mailloux, Z., & Parham, D. (1989). Sensory integration and children with learning disabilities. In P. N. Pratt & A. S. Allen, *Occupational therapy for children* (2nd ed., pp. 457–507). St. Louis: C. V. Mosby.

Cohen, B., Henn, V., Raphan, T., & Dennett, D. (1981). Velocity storage, nystagmus, and visual-vestibular interactions in humans. *Annals of the New York Academy of Sciences, 374,* 421–433.

Cohen, H. (1989). Testing vestibular function: Problems with the Southern California Postrotary Nystagmus Test. *American Journal of Occupational Therapy, 43,* 475–477.

Crowe, T. K., Deitz, J. C., Richardson, P. K., & Atwater, S. W. (in press). Interrater reliability of the Clinical Test of Sensory Interaction for Balance. *Physical and Occupational Therapy in Pediatrics.*

deQuiros, J. B., & Schrager, O. L. (1979). *Neuropsychological fundamentals in learning disabilities* (rev. ed). Novato, CA: Academic Therapy.

Dykes, R. W., Herron, P., & Lin, C. (1986). Ventroposterior thalamic regions projecting to cytoarchitectonic areas 3a and 3b in the cat. *Journal of Neurophysiology, 56,* 1521–1541.

Evarts, E. V. (1985). Sherrington's concept of proprioception. In E. V. Evarts, S. P. Wise, & B. Bousfield (Eds)., *The motor system in neurobiology* (pp. 183–186). New York: Elsevier.

Fisher, A. G. (1989). Objective assessment of the quality of response during two equilibrium tests. *Physical and Occupational Therapy in Pediatrics, 9*(3), 57–78.

Fisher, A. G., & Bundy, A. C. (1989). Vestibular stimulation in the treatment of postural and related disorders. In O. D. Payton, R. P. DiFabio, S. V. Paris, E. J. Protas, & A. F. VanSant (Eds.), *Manual of Physical Therapy Techniques* (pp. 239–258). New York: Churchill Livingstone.

Fisher, A. G., Mixon, J., & Herman, R. (1986). The validity of the clinical diagnosis of vestibular dysfunction. *Occupational Therapy Journal of Research, 6,* 3–20.

Fisher, A. G., Wietlisbach, S. E., & Wilbarger, J. L. (1988). Adult performance on three tests of equilibrium. *American Journal of Occupational Therapy, 42,* 30–35.

Fisher, C. B., & Camenzuli, C. A. (1987). Influence of body rotation on children's left-right confusion: A challenge to bilateral symmetry theory. *Developmental Psychology, 23,* 187–189.

Frank, J., & Levinson, H. N. (1975–76). Dysmetric dyslexia and dyspraxia. *Academic Therapy, 11,* 133–143.

Frank, J. M., & Levinson, H. N. (1976–77). Seasickness mechanisms in dysmetric dyslexia and dyspraxia. *Academic Therapy, 12,* 133–152.

Fregly, A. R., & Graybiel, A. (1968). An ataxia test battery not requiring rails. *Aerospace Medicine, 39,* 277–282.

Gardner, E. P. (1988). Somatosensory cortical mechanisms of feature detection in tactile and kinesthetic discrimination. *Canadian Journal of Physiology and Pharmacology, 66,* 439–454.

Goldberg, G. (1985). Supplementary motor area structure and function: Review and hypotheses. *Behavioral and Brain Sciences, 8,* 567–616.

Heide, W., Schrader, V., Koenig, E., & Dichgans, J. (1988). Impaired discharge of the eye velocity storage mechanism in patients with lesions of the vestibulo-cerebellum. In E. Pirodda & O. Pompeiano (Eds.), *Advances in oto-rhino-laryngology: Vol. 41. Neurophysiology of the vestibular system* (pp. 44–48). New York: Karger.

Horak, F. B., Shumway-Cook, A., Crowe, T. K., Black, F. O. (1988). Vestibular function and motor proficiency in children with impaired hearing, or with learning disability and motor impairments. *Developmental Medicine and Child Neurology, 30,* 64–79.

Jell, R. M., Phillips, H. D., Lafortune, S. H., & Ireland, D. J. (1988). Comparison of caloric and OKAN tests in patients with vestibular deficits. In E. Pirodda & O. Pompeiano (Eds.), *Advances in oto-rhino-laryngology: Vol. 41. Neurophysiology of the vestibular system* (pp. 201–205). New York: Karger.

Jones, L. A. (1988). Motor illusions: What do they reveal about proprioception? *Psychological Bulletin, 103,* 72–86.

Jones, E. G., & Porter, R. (1980). What is area 3a? *Brain Research Review, 2,* 1–43.

Kalaska, J. F. (1988). The representation of arm movements in postcentral and parietal cortex. *Canadian Journal of Physiology and Pharmacology, 66,* 455–463.

Kelso, J. A. S. (Ed.). (1982). *Human motor behavior: An introduction.* Hillsdale, NJ: Lawrence Erlbaum Associates.

Kelso, J. A. S., & Stelmach, G. E. (1976). Central and peripheral mechanisms in motor control. In G. E. Stelmach (Ed.), *Motor control: Issues and trends* (pp. 1–40). New York: Academic Press.

Koenig, E., & Dichgans, J. (1981). Aftereffects of vestibular and optokinetic stimulation and their interaction. *Annals of the New York Academy of Sciences, 374,* 434–445.

Leigh, R. J., & Zee, D. S. (1983). *The neurology of eye movements.* Philadelphia: F. A. Davis.

Magnusson, M., Pyykko, I., Schalen, L, & Enbom, H. (1988). The effect of alertness on the velocity storage mechanism. In E. Pirodda & O. Pompeiano (Eds.), *Advances in oto-rhino-laryngology: Vol. 41. Neurophysiology of the vestibular system* (pp. 53–57). New York: Karger.

Matthews, P. B. C. (1988). Proprioceptors and their contribution to somatosensory mapping: Complex messages require complex processing. *Canadian Journal of Physiology and Pharmacology, 66,* 430–438.

May-Benson, T. A. (1988). *Identifying gravitational insecurity in children with sensory integrative dysfunction: A pilot study.* Unpublished master's thesis, Boston University.

McCloskey, D. I. (1985). Knowledge about muscular contractions. In E. V. Evarts, S. P. Wise, & B. Bousfield (Eds.), *The motor system in neurobiology* (pp. 149–153). New York: Elsevier.

McCloskey, D. I., Cross, M. J., Honner, R., & Potter, E. K. (1983). Sensory effects of pulling or vibrating exposed tendons in man. *Brain, 106,* 21–37.

Magalhaes, L. C., Koomar, J., & Cermak, S. A. (1989). Bilateral motor coordination in 5- to 9-year-old children: A pilot study. *American Journal of Occupational Therapy, 43,* 437–443.

Moberg, E. (1983). The role of cutaneous afferents in position sense, kinaesthesia, and motor function of the hand. *Brain, 106,* 1–19.

Morrison D., & Sublett, J. (1983). Reliability of the Southern California Postrotary Nystagmus Test with learning disabled children. *American Journal of Occupational Therapy, 37,* 694–698.

Nashner, L. M. (1982). Adaptation of human movement to altered environments. *Trends in Neuroscience, 5,* 351–361.

Ornitz, E. M., & Honrubia, V. (1988). Developmental modulation of vestibular-ocular function. In E. Pirodda & O. Pompeiano (Eds.), *Advances in oto-rhino-laryngology: Vol. 41. Neurophysiology of the vestibular system* (pp. 36–39). New York: Karger.

Polatajko, H. J. (1983). The Southern California Postrotary Nystagmus Test: A validity study. *Canadian Journal of Occupational Therapy, 50,* 119–123.

Polatajko, H. J. (1985). A critical look at vestibular dysfunction in learning-disabled children. *Developmental Medicine and Child Neurology, 27,* 283–292.

Raphan, T., Matsuo, V., & Cohen, B. (1979). Velocity storage in the vestibulo-ocular reflex arc (VOR). *Experimental Brain Research, 35,* 229–248.

Roberts, T. D. M. (1978). *Neurophysiology of postural mechanisms* (2nd ed.). Boston: Butterworths.

Schmidt, R. A. (1988). *Motor control and learning: A behavioral emphasis* (2nd ed.). Champaign, IL: Human Kinetics.

Sherrington, C. S. (1906). *The integrative action of the nervous system.* New Haven: Yale University Press.

Shumway-Cook, A. (1989). Equilibrium deficits in children. In M. H. Woollacott & A. Shumway-Cook (Eds.), *Development of posture and gait across the lifespan* (pp. 229–252). Columbia, SC: University of South Carolina.

Shumway-Cook, A., & Horak, F. B. (1986). Assessing the influence of sensory interaction on balance: Suggestions from the field. *Physical Therapy, 66,* 1548–1550.

Shumway-Cook, A., Horak, F., & Black, F. O. (1987). A critical examination of vestibular function in motor-impaired learning disabled children. *International Journal of Pediatric Otorhinolaryngology, 14,* 21–30.

Stelmach, G. E. (Ed.). (1976). *Motor control: Issues and trends.* New York: Academic.

Tan, L. E. (1985). Laterality and motor skills in four-year-olds. *Child Development, 56,* 119–124.

Tuohimaa, P., Schneider, R. C., & Crosby, E. C. (1987). Cerebral cortical lesions and vestibular disturbances: An experimental study on the monkey. In M. D. Graham & J. L. Kemink, *The vestibular system: Neurophysiologic and clinical research* (pp. 411–419). New York: Raven.

Tracey, D. J. (1985). Joint receptors and the control of movement. In E. V. Evarts, S. P. Wise, & B. Bousfield (Eds.), *The motor system in neurobiology* (pp. 178–182). New York: Elsevier.

Wilson, V. J., & Melvill Jones, G. (1979). *Mammalian vestibular physiology.* New York: Plenum.

Zaichkowsky, L. D., & Fuchs, C. Z. (Eds). (1986). *The psychology of motor behavior: Development, control, learning and performance.* Ithaca, NY: Mouvement.

# CHAPTER 5

# Tactile Processing and Sensory Defensiveness

**Charlotte Brasic Royeen, PhD, OTR**
**Shelly J. Lane, PhD, OTR**

*Touching involves risk. It is a form of nonverbal communication and, therefore, may be misunderstood by one or both parties involved. It invades intimate space and may be a threat. If we are not in tune with ourselves and the one we touch, it may be inappropriate. However, non-touch may be just as devastating at a time when words are insufficient or cannot be processed appropriately because of disintegration of the individual.*

*Huss, 1977, p. 305*

Touch is our first language. It is the first system to function in utero, and it mediates our first experiences in this world. We are nourished, we are calmed, and we first become attached to others (bonding) through touch (Montagu, 1978). The sensation of touch is, in fact, the "oldest and most primitive expressive channel" (Collier, 1985, p. 29), and it is a primary system for "making contact" with the external world. We are extremely dependent on touch until language, motor skills, and cognitive processes develop and can guide us in experiencing and interacting with the environment (Collier, 1985).

Sensory integration theory postulates certain relationships between the central processing of tactile inputs and behavior. These postulated relationships help us to understand normal and abnormal behavior because they help us to understand how and why we react to stimuli and situations in the manner that we do. More specifically, sensory integration theory provides explanations for (a) the observed relationship between problems of *tactile discrimination* that impair tactile, including haptic, perception and motor planning; and (b) the tendency of certain people to respond negatively or aversively to certain types of tactile stimuli. This latter problem, known as *tactile defensiveness*, can potentially and negatively affect almost all aspects of human occupation or activity across the life span, but most especially the affective domain and related social development.

Tactile receptors are found throughout the skin and, generally speaking, are activated by externally applied stimuli such as touch, pressure, pain, and temperature. Discussions of tactile input often include mention of proprioceptive sensations arising from movement of the body and limbs. This combination of tactile and proprioceptive inputs is sometimes referred to as somatosensory processing (cf. Ayres, 1989). Because there is frequently a close interaction between touch, and joint and body movement, it sometimes is difficult to separate the influence of these two sensory systems. Both tactile and proprioceptive systems are considered to play a primary role in early development, serving as foundations for subsequent social, emotional, and possibly academic development (Suomi, 1984; Reite, 1984; Gottfried, 1984; Satz, Fletcher, Morris, & Taylor, 1984). Both sensory systems are, therefore, of paramount concern in sensory integration theory and practice.

## PURPOSE AND SCOPE

The purpose of this chapter is to acquaint the reader with the fundamental principles, theory, and functions of the tactile system as they relate to sensory integration theory and practice. Proprioception was discussed in Chapter 4. Here we will begin by presenting clinical examples that depict the various ways in which tactile processing deficits can manifest themselves and can affect behavior and development. These clinical descriptions are intended to give the reader a "working knowledge" of deficits in tactile processing.

We will follow the case examples with definitions and clinical descriptions of the problems of *tactile defensiveness* and *poor tactile discrimination*. Then we will review the pertinent neuroanatomical and neurophysiological constructs associated with the structure and function of the tactile system. This section will emphasize aspects of neurobiology that are particularly helpful in understanding tactile processing disorders. As with previous chapters, prior understanding of tactile system neuroanatomy is assumed.

Although the behavioral manifestations of tactile defensiveness have been clearly delineated since 1964, when Ayres first defined tactile defensiveness, the theoretical basis of this disorder has remained vague or unclear. During the interim period, the postulated theoretical basis has continued to change as numerous occupational therapists have developed theoretical explanations of tactile defensiveness based on existing neurobiological and pain literature. In the next section, we will review these perspectives, beginning with Ayres' early thoughts regarding the etiology of the problem and proceeding to the most current theoretical explanation of tactile defensiveness. In fact, our view of tactile defensiveness proposes that tactile defensiveness is one manifestation of *sensory defensiveness*, a sensory modulation disorder that also includes the gravitational insecurity and aversive responses to vestibular-proprioceptive stimuli discussed in Chapter 4. After discussing concepts important to sensory defensiveness, we will turn our attention to deficits in tactile discrimination. We will address the neurobehavioral aspects and implications of poor tactile discrimination. We will also introduce the hypothesized relationship of tactile discrimination to the development of praxis. The relationship between somatosensation and praxis is, however, the focus of Chapter 6.

Next, we will discuss the evaluation of tactile processing disorders. Unlike most other disorders of sensory integration, the identification of tactile defensiveness relies primarily on nonstandardized tools, observation, and clinical judgement skills. Therefore, methods useful for identifying these problems and their behavioral sequelae are presented. The Sensory Integration and Praxis Tests (SIPT) (Ayres, 1989) provide a basis for identifying diminished tactile discrimination, and they are discussed briefly. Finally, we will examine theoretical constructs for treating both tactile defensiveness and poor tactile discrimination.

## CLINICAL PICTURE OF TACTILE DYSFUNCTION

The behavioral or observable manifestations of tactile dysfunction vary depending on the type of tactile system processing deficit. Moreover, the behavioral manifestations of tactile dysfunction can vary between individuals and even within a particular individual over time. Despite the variations in the behavioral manifestations of tactile processing dysfunction, two patterns of dysfunction have been identified through research and clinical practice, tactile defensiveness and poor tactile perception. These are two *different* types of dysfunction that may or may not occur concomitantly.

### Lydia

Lydia was born to a 36-year-old, first-time mother after a long, difficult labor. When fetal distress occurred in the 35th hour of labor, Lydia was delivered by cesarean section. Her mother, Mrs. A, received a number of medications during labor, including Nembutal, Pitocin, morphine, and a spinal anesthetic. Mrs. A reacted negatively to the morphine, and her blood pressure dropped severely during the cesarean section.

Although the baby's Apgar score was 7 (Apgar, 1953), Lydia was oxygenated and placed in a neonatal intensive care unit. She had excessive fluid in her lungs, as well as an unspecified infection due to rupture of the amniotic membranes at least 40 hours prior to actual delivery. Lydia stayed in intensive care for 7 days. She nursed well and was discharged home.

Six weeks postpartum, Mrs. A told her pediatrician she felt overwhelmed with the care of Lydia. She was concerned about Lydia's irritability and distressed that she slept only 2 to 3 hours at a time. Lydia's pediatrician explained that this was not unusual for a baby her age and assured Mrs. A that things would improve.

When Lydia was 6 months of age and her behavior still had not improved, Mrs. A contacted Julie, an occupational therapist. Through an interview, Julie explored Lydia's home behavior, and its impact on Mrs. A, by asking Mrs. A such questions as, "How and when does Lydia sleep?" "Tell me about your daily routine, and taking care of Lydia." "What activities do you do from breakfast to lunch?"

Mrs. A said that Lydia nursed well, but refused a pacifier. Any attempt to insert a pacifier into her mouth resulted in Lydia forcefully spitting it out. Julie also learned that Lydia needed to be held in close physical contact during all waking hours. Attempts to put her down resulted in loud screaming. Thus, Lydia was either held or worn in a snugly as Mrs. A performed all of her household and shopping activities. Baths were also a source of distress for mother and baby. Finally, Julie learned that Lydia was still sleeping only 2 to 3 hours at a time, awakening repeatedly throughout the night.

Lydia's need for constant physical contact (i.e., always needing to be held), her aversion to the pacifier, her irritability, and her poor regulation of her sleep/wake cycles, caused Julie to suspect that Lydia had a tactile processing dysfunction. She specifically suspected that the baby was tactually defensive and that this tactile processing disorder was interfering with Lydia's ability to self-regulate sleep/wake cycles.

## Rick

Rick is a 5-year, 6-month-old child enrolled in a special education program. Rick had been medically diagnosed as developmentally delayed; his IQ is a little below average, but well within normal limits. The classroom teacher, Mr. D, referred Rick for occupational therapy evaluation because his behavior, and delays in fine motor skills, were interfering with his classroom performance. Rick's fine motor problems pertained to coloring, managing the fastenings (buttons, zippers, shoe laces) on his clothing, opening containers, and manipulating small objects during play.

Occupational therapy evaluation included the administration of the Sensory Integration and Praxis Tests (SIPT) (Ayres, 1989). Rick's scores on the tests that involved tactile discrimination were consistently well below age expectations. Rick had difficulty (a) identifying which finger was touched by the examiner (Finger Identification), (b) localizing where he was touched on his forearm or hand (Localization of Tactile Stimuli), (c) reproducing geometric designs drawn on the back of his hand (Graphesthesia), and (d) matching shapes through active manipulation (haptic perception; Manual Form Perception). Whereas Rick was able to tolerate the testing reasonably well, he frequently expressed dislike of these tactile tests. He often rubbed his hands or arms where he had been touched by the examiner, and toward the end of the third tactile test, he became restless and began to ask, "Are you almost done? Can I go back to my room now?"

Other tests on which Rick's scores were particularly low included those tests that involved visuomotor coordination. One of these tests, Motor Accuracy, involved tracing a printed line with a pen. The other test, Design Copying, required that Rick use a pencil to copy print geometric designs.

Additional evaluation data were obtained through an interview with Rick's teacher and observation of Rick in the classroom and during play. Observation revealed that severe falls, bumps, or similar events produced no noticeable response in Rick. Rick's teacher, Mr. D, said, "Rick doesn't seem to know when he should feel hurt. At times, he knocks his head against the wall and he doesn't seem to even notice." In fact, Mr. D felt that he sometimes sought out painful sensory stimuli. Yet, Mr. D also had noticed that at other times, Rick seemed to overreact to incidental, seemingly insignificant tactile input, such as when a classmate bumped into him. At these moments, Rick would withdraw from touch and sometimes get angry at the person touching him.

Additional observation revealed that Rick did not appear to respond to simple verbal directions and failed to react, or orient, to many environmental stimuli. At times, he acted as if he were oblivious to things going on around him. In contrast, he often became agitated and overreacted to loud sounds and lights going on or off.

Steve, the occupational therapist, postulated that Rick was experiencing a variety of tactile processing disorders. Rick's low scores on the tactile tests of the SIPT suggested poor tactile discrimination. That Rick sought out painful stimuli suggested that he had a desire for strong tactile sensations, but his responses to inadvertent touch, lights, and sounds suggested an exaggerated reaction or aversion to many types of sensory experiences. Consequently, Steve suspected that Rick was tactually defensive and that he also had a more general sensory modulation disorder. Steve wondered if Rick's significant problems in fine motor coordination might have been related to poor tactile discrimination.

Lydia and Rick are examples of two children with very different deficits in tactile processing. Lydia exemplifies the type of child who would be identified as *tactually defensive*. Her case indicates that these problems can be identified and treated at very young ages using non-standardized assessment tools. Older children or adults with tactile defensiveness might demonstrate a different but related pattern of behaviors. Rick's problems lay in his (a) *inability to modulate sensory input*, resulting in considerable lability in his response to sensory stimuli, and (b) poor *tactile discrimination*. Deficits in tactile discrimination are usually identified along with other problems, especially poor gross and fine motor planning (Ayres 1972b, 1979). As we mentioned earlier, Chapter 6 provides an in-depth discussion of motor planning deficits associated with poor tactile discrimination.

Let us now turn our attention to defining sensory integrative deficits in tactile processing.

## TACTILE DEFENSIVENESS

Tactile defensiveness refers to observable aversive or negative behavioral responses to certain types of tactile stimuli that most people would find to be non-noxious (nonpainful). Simply stated, tactile defensiveness is the inability to interpret appropriately the affective (rather than perceptual) meaning of touch or touch experiences within the context of the situation and in a way meaningful for use by the organism (A. J. Ayres, personal communication, March 17, 1988). Tactile defensiveness is hypothesized to be a disorder in the modulation or regulation of tactile sensory input (Clark, Mailloux, & Parham, 1989). It is characterized by a meaningful collection of the following behaviors (Ayres, 1979; Larson, 1982; Royeen, 1985):

1 Avoidance of touch
   a Avoidance of certain styles or textures (e.g., scratchy or rough) of clothing, or conversely, an unusual preference for certain styles or textures of clothing (e.g., soft materials, long pants, or sleeves)
   b Preference for standing at the end of a line to avoid contact with other children
   c Tendency to pull away from anticipated touch or from interactions involving touch, including avoidance of touch to the face
   d Avoidance of play activities that involve body contact, sometimes manifested by a tendency to prefer solitary play
2 Aversive responses to non-noxious touch
   a Aversion or struggle when picked up, hugged, or cuddled
   b Aversion to certain daily living tasks, including baths or showers, cutting of fingernails, haircuts, and face washing
   c Aversion to dental care
   d Aversion to art materials, including avoidance of finger paints, paste, or sand
3 Atypical affective responses to non-noxious tactile stimuli
   a Responding with aggression to light touch to arms, face, or legs
   b Increased stress in response to being physically close to people
   c Objection, withdrawal, or negative responses to touch contact, including that encountered in the context of intimate relationships

Royeen (1985) has used these symptoms of tactile defensiveness to develop a detailed domain specification of tactile defensiveness for what she has described as the syndrome of tactile defensiveness. The reader is referred to this work for more detail.

Tactile defensiveness is rarely found in isolation. There are also a wide range of behaviors that, *when they occur in the presence of a characteristic pattern of primary indicators of tactile defensiveness*, are hypothesized to be secondary deficits or seque-lae to the tactile defensiveness. These behaviors are not themselves indicative of tactile defensiveness, but they are often closely associated with it. Empirical work by Ayres (1965, 1966b, 1969) has established a correlation between tactile defensive-ness and distractibility, increased levels of activity, and perceptual-motor problems in learning-disabled children. Bauer (1977) also substantiated a relationship be-tween tactile sensitivity and increased levels of activity. More recently, it has been speculated that tactile defensiveness can be a predisposing factor for irregular emotional tone, lability, extreme need for personal space, and disruption in personal care (Wilbarger & Royeen, 1987). Finally, touch is a critical component of developing intimate relationships. This led Scardina (1986) to hypothesize that tactile defen-siveness may interfere with the ability to establish or maintain intimate relation-ships. Thus, a child or adult with tactile defensiveness may experience a myriad of additional secondary deficits.

We cannot provide a complete list of all of the possible situations that might elicit defensive reactions to touch, nor is tactile defensiveness the only reason that a person might show an aversive or negative reaction to touch. As with all disorders of sensory integration, the identification of tactile defensiveness is based on the pres-ence of a consistent pattern, or a sufficient number of aversive or negative reactions to touch, to confirm that it is indeed the response to touch that provides the basis of the reaction. This is particularly important when we consider the affective or emo-tional overlay that may occur with tactile defensiveness. That is, certain of these behaviors could have an emotional disorder as the *primary* cause of the behavior. This is in contrast to the "pervasive emotional sequelae" that can result from the primary problem of tactile defensiveness. Therefore, whenever possible, it is impera-tive that the therapist differentiate between emotional reactions that are the result of tactile defensiveness and those that are the result of primary emotional disorders.

## POOR TACTILE DISCRIMINATION

Poor tactile discrimination refers to the inability to identify the temporal and spatial qualities of tactile stimuli (A. J. Ayres, personal communication, March 17, 1988). It is the inability to optimally perceive and organize incoming discriminative touch information for use. Thus, poor tactile discrimination is a *disorder of tactile perception*. Like tactile defensiveness, it is hypothesized to be a *central* processing disorder.

Poor tactile perception may include difficulty in discriminating where and how many times one is being touched, as in tactile localization, two-point discrimination, and finger identification (Sinclair, 1981); impaired ability to *recognize* the shape of an object through active manipulation, as in haptic perception or stereognosis (Chusid, 1979); and inefficiency in how one tactually explores an object or environment to solicit additional cues which give meaning about that object or environment, as in active touch (Gibson, 1962; Haron & Henderson, 1985). Poor tactile discrimination also may contribute to an impaired awareness of self, that is, body scheme (Ayres, 1972b, 1989).

As will be discussed in detail in Chapter 6, poor tactile perception is hypothesized to contribute to somatodyspraxia, a specific disorder in motor planning. Further, tactile discrimination deficits, like all disorders of sensory integration, can be associated with a wide variety of related motor, perceptual, and psychosocial (affective) problems or difficulties. Thus, the overall clinical picture of the client with poor tactile perception can be extremely varied.

# NEUROBEHAVIORAL BASIS OF TACTILE DYSFUNCTION

A number of important neurobehavioral constructs provide the theoretical foundation of tactile processing disorders. As we will see, some of these constructs help us to understand the relationship between tactile discrimination and motor planning, while others provide an understanding of tactile defensiveness within the more global problem of sensory defensiveness. We will include in our summary a discussion of those neural structures hypothesized to be related to the mediation and modulation of pain, because pain control pathways have been implicated in the theoretical basis of both tactile defensiveness and sensory defensiveness. Information that is helpful in understanding the behaviors observed in children with tactile dysfunction will be presented. However, a detailed account of the anatomy and physiology of the systems associated with tactile processing is beyond the scope of this chapter. The reader who is interested in more detailed information is referred to several good sources (Kandel & Schwartz, 1985; deGroot & Chusid, 1988; Noback & Demerest, 1981). Much of the information presented below is derived from Kandel and Schwartz (1985).

## Tactile Receptors

The skin is the sensory organ subserving the tactile system (Montagu, 1978). Within the skin are housed many specific receptors, but viewing the total skin surface as a receptive organ encourages us to appreciate the pervasive nature of the tactile system (Montagu, 1978). Table 5–1 describes the various receptors housed

**TABLE 5–1. LOCATIONS, MODALITIES OF SENSATION, ADAPTATION RATES, AND FIBER TYPES ASSOCIATED WITH SKIN RECEPTORS**

| Type | Location | Stimulus | Fiber Type | Adaptation |
|------|----------|----------|------------|------------|
| Free nerve ending | Dermis, joint capsules, tendons, ligaments | Pain, temperature | A-delta, C | Slow |
| Hair follicle plexus | Deep dermis | Hair displacement; pain | A-beta | Fast |
| Meissner's corpuscles (tactile corpuscles) | Papillae of skin, mucous membranes of tongue tip | Touch | A-beta | Fast |
| Pacinian corpuscles | Subcutaneous tissue | Pressure, vibration | A-beta | Fast |
| Krause's end bulb | Papillae of hairless skin; near hair follicle plexus | Cold? | A-delta, C | Below 20°C; no adaptation |
| Merkel's disc | Epidermis of hairless skin; hair follicles | | A-beta | Slow |
| Ruffini ending | Joint capsules; connective tissue | Touch | A-beta | Slow |

within the skin, their locations, *primary* modalities of stimulation, adaptation rates, and fiber types associated with the skin receptor. Fibers are typed by diameter, which is related to fiber conduction speed. Large, heavily myelinated fibers (A-beta) conduct faster than small, lightly myelinated fibers (C). Although all receptors respond to all inputs, only the stimuli to which the receptor responds *optimally* is listed.

## Dorsal Column Medial Lemniscal System

Tactile stimuli received by a peripheral receptor are carried to the spinal cord through afferent fibers and transmitted to the brain via either the dorsal column medial lemniscal system or the anterolateral system. The dorsal column medial lemniscal system transmits primarily tactile, vibratory, touch-pressure, and proprioceptive information. The dorsal column pathways consistently are associated with the functions inherent in tactile discrimination or perception: detection of size, form, texture, and movement across the skin. Recent studies indicate that temporal coding of tactile information is an additional function of dorsal column pathways (Vierck, Cohen, & Cooper, 1985).

Clinicians and researchers have hypothesized that poor tactile perception may be related to difficulties in manipulative hand skills (Haron & Henderson, 1985; Nathan, Smith, & Cook, 1986). We may speculate that difficulty in perceiving the size and form of an object during the process of *active* manipulation results in difficulty handling the object. We also may speculate that difficulty in perceiving the boundaries of the hand and the relationship of the fingers to one another impacts on manipulation skills. Because Rick had low scores on the tactile tests of the SIPT, and he has deficits in fine motor skill, we might hypothesize that these two problems are related.

In the brain, dorsal column fibers synapse in both the ventral posterior lateral nucleus of the thalamus and within the reticular formation. Thalamic interpretation is thought to permit vague conscious discrimination of tactile input. Further definition of this input requires cortical processing. Cortical reception areas for the dorsal column medial lemniscal system include the primary and secondary somatic sensory cortex as well as areas 5 and 7 of the posterior parietal lobe. Areas 5 and 7 are both associated with the *manipulation of objects* and are important in discerning their tactile qualities (haptic perception). Any clinician who has tried to evaluate stereognosis in a client who does not automatically manipulate the object in his or her hand can appreciate the importance of manipulation for tactile perception. Also within the parietal lobe, aspects of tactile and proprioceptive input converge and subsequently project to anterior *motor planning areas* of the brain (see Table 4–1). Thus, the dorsal column medial lemniscal system could be expected to have an impact on both object manipulation and motor planning. And, in Rick's case, we might consider the possibility of a relationship between his problems with tactile discrimination and his difficulty in planning and producing coordinated fine motor output (see Chapter 6).

Another role of the dorsal column medial lemniscal system may be in modulating arousal. Clinically, certain types of sensory information have been observed to have a calming effect. Deep touch-pressure and proprioceptive information can have this quality (Ayres, 1972b; Farber, 1982; Knickerbocker, 1980) and both are carried to the central nervous system via the dorsal columns. Since the reticular formation mediates arousal, the reticular projections of the dorsal column pathway may be related to the efficacy of these inputs in decreasing arousal and producing calming.

## Anterolateral System

The anterolateral system is composed of three separate pathways that function primarily to mediate pain, crude touch (the detection of an object's *position*, but not its movement across the skin), and temperature. Mediation of both neutral warmth and the "tickle" sensation also are related to transmission within these anterolateral pathways. These pathways are spinothalamic, spinoreticular, and spinotectal. Projections from this system are found within the thalamus, the reticular system, and the tectum. Interestingly, most fibers within the anterolateral system terminate within the reticular formation. Diffuse pain input and pain associated with chronic problems are thought to be projected to this area of the brain.

Localization of sharp or acute pain relies on projections to the ventral posterior lateral nucleus of the thalamus. Because the dorsal column medial lemniscal system also projects to the ventral posterior lateral nucleus, and because there is some degree of convergence in this nucleus of anterolateral and dorsal column inputs, this nucleus is thought to be an important area for interaction of information from the two tactile systems. Dorsal column input is thought to inhibit transmission in the anterolateral pathways, and the thalamus may be one site for this interaction (Peele, 1977). This may partially explain why deep touch-pressure and proprioception have been observed clinically to diminish the sensation of pain. It may also help to explain why deep-pressure and other vestibular-proprioceptive inputs seem to alleviate some aspects of tactile defensiveness (Fisher & Dunn, 1983). Projections from the ventral posterior lateral nucleus go to the somatic sensory cortices (both primary and secondary) which, therefore, are other *potential* anatomical sites for interaction between these two tactile systems.

Another brain region receiving information via the anterolateral pathway is the periaqueductal grey area, an important brain center for pain interpretation. The periaqueductal grey area has many connections with the *limbic system* via the hypothalamus. This center is believed to be important in modulating pain within different emotional contexts.

The third projection area, the tectum, is often associated with the visual (superior colliculus) and auditory (inferior colliculus) systems. The tectum is also, however, an important pain reception center.

Many aspects of touch associated with tactile defensiveness are hypothetically associated with transmission through the anterolateral pathways and with the central interpretation of the input (Ayres, 1972b). Given that the anterolateral system projects to the regions of the brain responsible for arousal (reticular system), emotional tone (limbic structures), and autonomic regulation (hypothalamus), one can postulate that tactile defensive behaviors, such as those observed in Lydia and Rick, may be related to the connections among these systems and brain regions. Hypothesized relationships between these structures and tactile defensiveness will be discussed in more detail below.

## Functional Overlap

Although past researchers hypothesized that the dorsal column medial lemniscal system and the anterolateral system were separate and discrete, current understanding delineates considerable functional overlap between them (Melzack & Wall, 1973). For example, the dorsal column medial lemniscal system plays an important role in the localization of pain. Further, clients with lesions in this system retain some skill in tactile discrimination. Thus, some aspects of pain are transmitted through the dorsal column medial lemniscal system, and some aspects of tactile discrimination must be carried in the anterolateral system. Kandel and Schwartz (1985) described this redundancy in terms of parallel pathways.

> Parallel pathways are advantageous for two reasons: they add subtlety and richness to a perceptual experience by allowing the same information to be handled in different ways, and they offer a measure of insurance. If one pathway is damaged, the other can provide residual perceptual capability. (Kandel & Schwartz, 1985, p. 307)

Such functional redundancy in the organization of the nervous system may play a role in the efficacy of intervention.

## TACTILE DEFENSIVENESS: HISTORICAL PERSPECTIVES

Since 1964, when Ayres first described tactile defensiveness, few occupational therapists have questioned the existence of the disorder. However, the neurobiological basis for the disorder has remained unclear, and thus controversial. As new research on the nature and function of the tactile system has become available, occupational therapists have incorporated this knowledge with existing sensory integration theory in an attempt to develop a more adequate theoretical explanation of tactile defensiveness. Still, it must be recognized that the proposed theories related to tactile defensiveness continue to be revised and further developed.

A historical review of our understanding of tactile defensiveness begins with the ideas originally proposed by Ayres (1964) and proceeds to current perspectives proposed by Wilbarger and Royeen (1987). Over time, a common theme that has persisted through many revisions of our thinking has been a postulated *continuum of function* within the tactile system. We will see that this concept has been generalized from Ayres (1972b) and others to currently proposed explanations of sensory defensiveness, and the concept of sensory registration. Another common theme across perspectives has been the concept of a *lack of inhibition* of sensory input. Thus, the development of our understanding of tactile defensiveness probably represents a refinement of our thinking over time, rather than the proposal of radically different views of tactile defensiveness.

### Ayres: Tactile Defensiveness

In 1964, Ayres proposed a "provisional theory" to explain a clinical syndrome comprised of deficits in tactile defensiveness, distractibility, and increased level of activity.

> The concept of tactile defensiveness has its seeds in the earlier observations of Henry Head (1920), whose insights into the function of the nervous system formed a precursor to these postulates. It is not reasonable to expect the technical aspects of his work—now over a half century old—to be completely congruent with current neurophysiological data, but many of his concepts have proved useful insights into the understanding of human function.
> Central to Head's theory of tactile functions were the dual functional afferent systems, the protopathic and epicritic. (Ayres, 1972b, p. 211)

Ayres (1972b) viewed the dualism of these two systems as a *continuum* rather than a strict dichotomy. They interact "to provide a continuum of information and response with a need-for-defense interpretation and reaction at one end of the continuum and a discriminative interpretation and discrete response at the other end." (p. 214)

Tactile defensiveness was hypothesized to be the result of an imbalance between these two systems; duality of function was generalized from a protopathic-epicritic continuum to an anterolateral-dorsal column continuum (Ayres, 1964, 1972b). According to Ayres (1972b), tactile defensiveness occurred when the discriminative dorsal column medial lemniscal system failed to exert its normal *inhibitory influence* over the anterolateral system. As a result, light touch evoked protective, escape-like behavior and strong emotional responses.

> It may be, then, that the tactile defensive response and other defensive responses to nociceptive qualities in sensory stimuli represent an insufficient amount of the inhibitory component in a functional system designed to monitor a certain type of impulse control. Thus, the behavioral response system designed for protection and survival predominates over a system designed to allow the organism to respond to the spatial temporal qualities of the tactile stimuli. (Ayres, 1972b, p. 215)

Ayres (1964) further suggested that adrenaline (epinephrine), released from the sympathetic nervous system during stress, played a role in the behavioral manifestations of tactile defensiveness, in that the reticular activating system was sensitive to the effects of adrenaline and the dorsal column medial lemniscal pathway was not. Ayres theorized that anxiety was both a cause and an effect of the predominance of the protective system and that the problem was self-perpetuating. Furthermore, a child chronically controlled by the protective system would be offered little opportunity for appropriate environmental exploration, and this might lead to delays in perceptual-motor development.

As early as 1972, Ayres (1972b) recognized that the gate control theory of Melzack and Wall (1965) "unified" various historical perspectives on the duality of the tactile system. Further, she proposed that the gate control theory provided a conceptual model for tactile defensiveness. Briefly stated, this theory suggests that "gate" neurons present in the dorsal horn of the spinal cord control the passage of impulses to the central nervous system. Control of these gate cells is influenced both by incoming tactile inputs and by cortical influences. Tactile inputs carried in large A-beta fibers that are commonly associated with touch-pressure and other inputs mediated by the dorsal column medial lemniscal pathway, activate the gate cells, which in turn prevent the transmission of pain to the central nervous system. By contrast, inputs mediated by small A-delta and C (pain) fibers inhibit the gate cell. Thus, because the "gate is open" when the gate cell is inhibited, transmission of pain impulses is permitted. Importantly, cortical influences such as anxiety, attention, and anticipation, as well as sensory input over other channels, also mediate gate activity. All of these play a role in determining whether the gate cell is activated (gate closed) or inhibited (gate opened) and, therefore, whether pain transmission can proceed (Melzack & Wall, 1973).

Thus, Ayres (1972b) believed that the provision of specific (discriminative) tactile and proprioceptive stimuli would activate the dorsal column medial lemniscal system to "close the gating mechanism" so as to block the protective response to touch, and diminish associated increased levels of activity and distractibility. Moreover, she believed that tactile stimuli that elicited a defensive response inhibited the gate cell, thereby permitting transmission of stimuli to the central nervous system, and resulting in a defensive response. Deep touch-pressure and other sensations mediated by the dorsal column may result in gate cell activation, decreasing transmission of defense-eliciting stimuli and thereby diminishing the defensive response. These hypotheses also explain the ability of previous stimuli, moods, and so forth, to influence the responses of the child with tactile defensiveness. These factors would be a component of the descending cortical influences on the gate, whereby stressful states, for example, might result in gate cell inhibition and thus permit transmission of defense-eliciting stimuli.

## Evolving Perspectives

Unfortunately, some aspects of the gate control theory have not been confirmed by research, while others are poorly understood and controversial. For instance, no actual gate neurons have been found in the spinal cord. It is known, however, that descending central pain controls exist and that stimulation of the dorsal column will lead to pain relief (Kandel & Schwartz, 1985).

### TACTILE DEFENSIVENESS AND POOR TACTILE DISCRIMINATION AS DISTINCT DISORDERS OF TACTILE PROCESSING

In 1983, Fisher and Dunn published a review of these recent advances in pain control theory, including recent perspectives on the gate control theory of Melzack and Wall (1973), and more recent evidence of inhibitory pain pathways. An important contribution of Fisher and Dunn (1983) was the recognition that the reduction of tactile defensiveness would not lead to improved tactile discrimination. Rather, they stressed that tactile defensiveness and poor tactile discrimination are *separate disorders of tactile processing* and not two ends of the same continuum; both tactile defensiveness and poor tactile discrimination can, and often do, occur in isolation (Fisher & Dunn, 1983). As we will discuss later in this chapter, the hypothesized continuum pertains to variability in behavior *within* the disorder of tactile defensiveness.

### LACK OF HIGHER-LEVEL INHIBITION AS A SOURCE OF POOR MODULATION

One year earlier, Larson (1982) hypothesized that tactile defensiveness may be the result of a filtering deficit resulting from too little inhibition. The high arousal, distractibility, and defensiveness observed in children with tactile defensiveness is explained by a lack of inhibition of irrelevant input.

> [O]ne possible explanation of tactile defensiveness is based on the interconnections between the somatic afferent system and the central nervous system, especially the reticular activating system. To function effectively, the central nervous system must be able to filter or inhibit much of the sensory bombardment from the environment that is irrelevant at that specific moment (Luria, 1973). It is postulated that in the tactually defensive child, central influences from higher levels may result in an imbalance in descending mechanisms of the reticular system with a lack of or a predominance of the excitatory component, resulting in too much or not enough inhibition. This leads to an inability to appropriately respond to or suppress differentially the stimuli within the perceptual field. (Larson, 1982, p. 592)

Fisher and Dunn (1983) subsequently suggested that the application of the phrase "lack of inhibition" to the child with tactile defensiveness is appropriate in describing the failure of higher central nervous system structures to *modulate* incoming tactile stimuli. They pointed out that "clinical descriptions of 'lack of inhibition' in children who display [tactile defensiveness] seem to be compatible with the concept that higher-level influences are not adequately modulating tactile inputs" (p. 2). Thus, they advocated the use of treatment techniques to decrease arousal, including touch-pressure, proprioception, and linear vestibular stimulation.

Although Larson (1982), and Fisher and Dunn (1983) limited themselves to discussions of children with tactile defensiveness, their arguments could readily be applied to children with other than tactile defensiveness. It is interesting to note that, while Larson (1982) emphasized a lack of inhibition resulting in tactile defensiveness, she actually described an *imbalance in descending mechanisms*, resulting in either too little or too much inhibition. "This imbalance decreases the ability to perceive incoming stimuli from tactile and *other sensory modalities* [italics added]" (Larson, 1982, p. 592).

## SENSORY DEFENSIVENESS AND SENSORY DORMANCY

The term *sensory defensiveness* was first introduced by Knickerbocker (1980) and applied to a more generalized problem reflecting increased sensitivity of the tactile and other sensory systems. She postulated that a disorganized response to sensory input may result from an imbalance between inhibition and excitation within the nervous system, leading to too little inhibition and a consequent flood of input reaching higher central nervous system structures. Knickerbocker suggested that such defensiveness may be observed in the olfactory (O), tactile (T), and auditory (A) systems, and called this the "OTA Triad." Children with such sensory defensiveness are characterized as being overly active, hyperverbal, distractible, and disorganized, that is, similar in many respects to children like Lydia and Rick, who are tactually defensive.

Ayres (1972b) previously had alluded to the concept of such a triad in her 1972 work, stating,

> [I]t is proposed that tactile defensiveness is part of a more generalized "set" of the nervous system toward interpreting stimuli in terms of "danger, attend to these stimuli, and prepare for fight or flight," or at least, "I can't stand these stimuli." Over-responsiveness to auditory and olfactory and even some visual stimuli is seen occasionally in the tactually defensive child. (Ayres, 1972b, p. 209)

Knickerbocker also described a situation she called *sensory dormancy*. This, too, is characterized by behavior which is disorganized and may seem immature, but which results from excessive inhibition of incoming sensory input and a lack of sensory arousal. Dormancy was observed in the olfactory, tactile, and auditory systems. Knickerbocker described a child experiencing sensory dormancy as being quiet and compliant.

Recall the description of Rick at the beginning of this chapter. Rick was identified as developmentally delayed, and both his teacher and occupational therapist observed that he failed to notice when he was hurt and that he seemed to seek out painful stimuli. This pattern may be characteristic of sensory dormancy and may suggest a modulation failure. In addition, when Rick did respond to incoming sensation, he tended to overrespond and become agitated. Perhaps, for these children, there is no middle ground and their response is all or none. This interesting "flip side" of sensory defensiveness will require much more study.

Knickerbocker (1980) thus expanded on Ayres' (1964, 1972b) theory of tactile defensiveness by *explicitly* extending the concept to other sensory systems. She also introduced the concept of sensory dormancy to describe children who demonstrated a lack of arousal. However, she did not indicate that these two conditions could be present in the same child, such as we see in Rick. Further, she did not propose a neuroanatomical or a neurophyisological model to account for either sensory defensiveness or sensory dormancy.

## Current View: Sensory Defensiveness and Sensory Modulation Disorders

Our current perspective on tactile defensiveness views this disorder as one component within a broader dysfunctional category of sensory defensiveness, which includes auditory and visual defensiveness. Sensory defensiveness, in turn, is one type of sensory modulation disorder that also includes gravitational insecurity and aversive responses to vestibular stimuli (see Chapter 4). Wilbarger (Wilbarger & Royeen, 1987) emphasized the hypothesized emotional difficulties that may result from sensory defensiveness by calling certain manifestations of the dysfunction *sensory affective disorder.* Our clinical experience suggests that a child like Lydia, if untreated, can develop emotional difficulty later in life; thus the descriptor sensory affective disorder.

Royeen (1989a) has elaborated this theory and hypothesized that sensory defensiveness and sensory dormancy, together, may be considered *sensory modulation disorders* that are at opposite ends of a sensory responsivity/registration continuum, with overorientation at one end and a failure to orient at the other. Figure 5–1 depicts this continuum.

Royeen suggested that sensory registration undergoes normal variation in the course of a day or an hour in all individuals. It is when this variation is extreme, when an individual spends excessive time at one end of the continuum or the other, or shifts from one extreme to the other, that a problem is indicated.

Inherent within this concept is the ability to speculate about human behavior that is both normal and atypical. In discussing application of this theory, Cermak (1988) stated, "many children seem to swing to either or both ends of this continuum and have difficulty attending or maintaining the midrange" (p. 2). This theory of sensory modulation disorders, then, may explain the inconsistencies we observed in Rick.

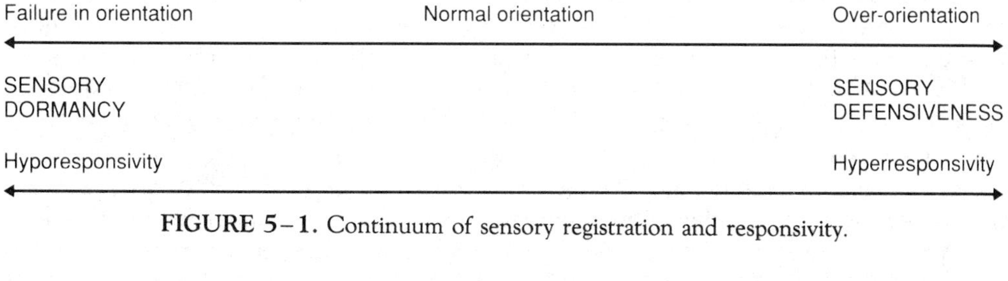

| Failure in orientation | Normal orientation | Over-orientation |
|---|---|---|
| SENSORY DORMANCY | | SENSORY DEFENSIVENESS |
| Hyporesponsivity | | Hyperresponsivity |

FIGURE 5–1. Continuum of sensory registration and responsivity.

It may be more precise to hypothesize that deficient *modulation* mechanisms within the central nervous system, rather than simply deficient inhibitory mechanisms, underlie both sensory defensiveness and sensory dormancy. Accordingly, the developing theory of sensory modulation disorders *emphasizes* the role of the limbic system as a modulation center for sensory input. Emphasis on this role (a) provides an explanation for the emotional or social difficulties often accompanying tactile and sensory defensiveness, (b) accounts for the presence of defensiveness or dormancy across sensory systems, and (c) allows for extreme shifts or inconsistencies in responsivity (from defensiveness to dormancy) that may be observed in an individual either with regard to a single sensory system or across sensory systems.

Rick typifies the child who is simultaneously overresonding to some tactile stimuli (tactile defensiveness), while seemingly underresponding to others, such as pain. Accordingly, Rick could be charted or placed at both ends of the continuum in terms of sensory system processing or registration, and thus could be said to have a sensory modulation disorder. Because of this, Royeen (1989a) further speculated that the ends of the continuum "meet" and that the continuum is in fact circular, implying that sensory defensiveness and sensory dormancy are adjacent and related phenomena under the rubric of a sensory modulation disorder. Such a theoretical model allows for an "atypical" individual to shift from defensiveness to dormancy (or vice versa) without ever being in the midrange or within normal limits, an observation that is consistent with our clinical experience.

The suggestion that deficiencies in sensory modulation, rather than deficiencies in sensory inhibition, underlie both sensory defensiveness and dormancy directs inquiry to a center for modulation across all sensory systems. Such a system has been identified as critical in related theoretical development pertaining to pain perception (Casey, 1973). This is the limbic system.

## Sensory Modulation and The Limbic System

The limbic system is a complex set of structures with a vast array of associated functions. From a broad perspective, it can be said to contribute to self-preservation (deGroot & Chusid, 1988). It plays a role in learning and memory, eating and drinking behaviors, aggression, sexual behavior, and, importantly, expression of emotion (Isaacson, 1982). The septohippocampal circuitry of the limbic system and the hypothalamus have been incorporated into a theory of sensory defensiveness and sensory modulation disorders (Wilbarger & Royeen, 1987).

Like many studies of the limbic system, the septal region has been investigated largely through lesion and stimulation studies. Lesions of the septal region have been shown to result in *transient hyperemotionality* in many rodents and in humans (Isaacson, 1982). The increased emotionality can be reduced with handling and is less severe when the animals experience the lesion during their youth. In addition, some lesioned animals appear to demonstrate *exaggerated defensive reactions* and are *hyperresponsive* to handling, light touch (air puffs), poking with a stick, temperature changes, light, and sounds (Grossman, 1978; Fried, 1972; Olton & Gage, 1974; Donovick, 1968; Green & Schwartzbaum, 1968). This hyperresponsivity is characterized by increases in motor activity. *Increased levels of activity* have been elicited with small lesions in some animals. Many parallels can be seen here between these lesion-induced behaviors and behaviors identified in children exhibiting sensory defensiveness. Of particular interest is the fact that identical lesions in two different species *may not* result in the same behavioral outcome. The outcome appears to be related to the genetic background of the animal as well as prelesion experiences and the testing environment. Thus, in generalizing this information to children with problems, we must be extremely careful!

In addition to lesion studies, stimulation studies of the septal area have indicated that this region plays a role in the modulation of pleasure and exerts an inhibitory influence on the autonomic nervous system. Generally, the septal area is thought to play a role in an organism's use of environmental stimulation. It permits the organism to attend to any stimulus in the environment, even those having low stimulus value (Isaacson, 1982). Thus, in a normal state, this part of the limbic system may be said to *contribute to our ability to interact successfully with the environment.*

Hippocampal lesions can result in a wide variety of behavioral alterations that seem to be related to an animal's genetic background and to the conditions under which a behavior is elicited. Here, too, extreme caution must be taken in generalizing from animal studies to humans. It is interesting to note, however, that hippocampal lesions may result in animals who *fail to persist* in new tasks. They will readily begin a goal-oriented task, but will not stay with it to completion. There is also an *increase in activity* in some situations, especially during "open-field" testing. This increased movement, however, is not associated with increased exploration; the animal seems to move about a great deal, but fails to effectively use the environmental information available from this increased movement. There is also a *decreased fear intensity* elicited by threatening stimuli and reduced aggression in lesioned animals (Isaacson, 1982), as well as *sleep disturbance* in that the duration of sleep episodes is shortened (Kim, Choi, Kim, Kim, Huh, & Moon, 1971). Again, we can observe certain parallel behaviors in some children experiencing sensory modulation deficits. According to Isaacson (1982), the hippocampus is less closely associated with the autonomic nervous system, mood, and emotion than are other components of the limbic system, and it is more involved with happenings in the world outside the body. The hippocampus appears to act as "a gatekeeper for both sensory and motor activities" (p. 236).

The hypothalamus maintains an important and reciprocal relationship with the limbic structures and is often included in discussions of this system. The hypothalamus is a control center for autonomic nervous system mechanisms. According to Isaacson (1982), this structure interacts with nearly every other central structure to maintain "suitable conditions for mental actions and for behavior" (p. 108).

The role of all these structures in sensory modulation disorders in children is still extremely speculative. Many of the functions described, however, can be well integrated with a theory of sensory modulation disorders.

One additional aspect of the relationship between sensory modulation and the limbic system deserves attention. Clinicians have long suspected that anxiety resulting from stress can amplify tactile and sensory defensiveness. The anxiety resulting from stress may be associated with unfounded apprehension or fear, as well as with concentration difficulties, restlessness, and other symptoms in almost any system of the body (Ashton, 1987). These manifestations of stress and anxiety have been associated with limbic structures and components of the reticular system, hypothalamus, and cortex, as well as with the action of the neurotransmitters norepinephrine, epinephrine, and serotonin, which are associated with these regions (Ashton, 1987). Antianxiety drugs that disrupt the action of these neurotransmitters reduce anxiety-induced behaviors. Activation of this anxiety system, which Gray (1982) calls the behavioral inhibition system, depends upon the organism's ability to compare actual input with expected input. Put differently, in any situation we all have certain *expectations* of what will occur. We expect a hug from a friend to feel good and a shot to be only slightly painful. If the friendly hug turns into an uncomfortable squeeze, or the injection has a burning quality not previously experienced, then our *expectation* does not *match* the real situation and we find ourselves with increased arousal and anxiety. Gray stated that if a *match* occurs between expected and actual input, the behavioral inhibition system is not activated and general behavior is not altered. If a *mismatch* occurs, the behavioral inhibition system is activated and takes control of behavior, leading to increased arousal and attention to the incoming stimuli. This theory of anxiety and stress behavior has been questioned, but is now fairly well accepted (Gray, 1982).

If one accepts the concept of limbic involvement in sensory modulation, of which tactile defensiveness is a component, then these stress behaviors may play a role in the manifestation of tactile defensiveness. When incoming and expected inputs are mismatched, Gray's (1982) behavioral inhibition system takes over, leading to increased arousal and attention to the sensory stimuli, and perhaps resulting in an increase in the defensive response. These concepts of sensory modulation are extremely hypothetical, however, and require considerably more study.

## Summary

By borrowing from other theories of nervous system function and dysfunction, we can begin to describe a mechanism that may underlie tactile defensiveness and disorders of sensory modulation. An important construct developed during the past 25 years involves viewing the registration of sensory input as a continuum and recognizing that sensory input is, at least in part, centrally modulated. Such modulation depends not only on incoming sensation, but also on previous input and the current state of the nervous system. This working model can be used to treat tactile defensiveness, with the caveat that the theory will be further modified as understanding and knowledge increase.

## POOR TACTILE PERCEPTION

Based on the neuroanatomical and neurophysiological characteristics previously described, tactile perception is a function that relates to *interpretation of temporal and spatial aspects of tactile stimuli*, and that is associated mainly with the dorsal column medial lemniscal system (Kandel & Schwartz, 1985). Poor tactile perception can be viewed as a deficit in processing, primarily within this system and its neuroanatomical correlates.

Unlike tactile defensiveness, no cogent hypotheses of the etiology of poor tactile perception has actually been proposed. Instead, there are discussions of the development of tactile perception, references to the existence of deficits in tactile perception, and consideration of the relationship between these deficits and other skills, such as praxis and visual perception (Ayres, 1972b; Snow, 1989). Concepts important to understanding tactile perception are presented in this section.

Passive touch is defined as touch applied to the skin or body, whereas active touch implies manipulation and is a volitional act. Touch in general is considered important to normal development. Tactile perception develops gradually after birth. Both active and passive touch are likely to play a role in the development of skills (Snow, 1989).

Initial responses to tactile information (passive touch) by an infant are likely to be generalized, and interpretation of the stimuli are likely to be diffuse (Lowrey, 1986). Research in tactile processing suggests that early tactile information may be important not only for the development of tactile perception, but also for the development of parent-infant attachment, stress coping mechanisms, sociability, and cognitive development (Gottfried, 1984).

The oral areas are the first to respond to touch in utero (Lowrey, 1986), and the mouth is the first source of tactile information available to the infant after birth (Getman, 1985). The mouth has also been said to be one of the more precise tactile discriminators in infants. As early as 25 to 33 days postterm, infants can orally detect differences in the shapes of pacifiers (Meltzoff & Borton, 1979). Knowledge of the qualities of an object often comes from mouthing until objects of interest are too large and complex for adequate oral exploration (Getman, 1985).

Tactile exploration of body parts by the fingers develops gradually. Kravitz, Goldenberg, & Neyhus (1978) indicated that infants explore their head and face within hours after birth, their fingers at a median age of 12 weeks, their body at a median age of 15 weeks, their legs at 16 weeks, and their feet at 19 weeks. Temperature discrimination has been identified in babies as young as 6 months of age (Bushnell, Shaw, & Strauss, 1985); and haptic shape discrimination, as determined by manual exploration, is said to be present in 9-month-old babies (Gottfried & Rose, 1980). Tactile exploration becomes associated with visual exploration early in infancy, and the baby comes to rely on both forms of exploration for successful environmental interaction (Getman, 1985). Tactile perception skills continue to mature and become more refined through adolescence (cf. Heydorn, 1985).

Tactile perception and proprioceptive input are believed to make important contributions to the development of a body scheme. Both somatosensory inputs and body scheme are hypothesized to provide the basis for the development of praxis. The important role of proprioception in body scheme and praxis was discussed in Chapter 4. The combined contributions of tactile perception and proprioception to praxis are expanded in Chapter 6.

According to Ayres (1972b), the ability to integrate tactile information may be more important to the development of tactile discrimination than is the quantity of input. She stated that children experiencing sensory integrative deficits in tactile discrimination probably have sufficient *quantity* of input, but are having difficulty processing or integrating the input (Ayres, 1972b). Such difficulty not only results in poor tactile discrimination, but also can interfere with the development of praxis. Ayres (1972b) also hypothesized that poor tactile discrimination may underlie inadequate fine motor skills because of its possible interference with manipulative skills.

Several factor analyses of scores from the Southern California Sensory Integration Tests (Ayres, 1980) indicated that tactile discrimination skills are not associated with tactile defensiveness (Ayres 1965, 1966a, 1969, 1977). In fact, in several factor analyses, tactile defensiveness appeared as an independent factor, whereas tactile discrimination abilities were associated with praxis (Ayres, 1965, 1966a, 1969, 1977) and, in some instances, with visual perception (Ayres, 1965, 1972b, 1977). This failure to identify tactile discrimination as a separate factor in any analysis may support the proposition that this function subserves the development of many other skills.

# EVALUATION OF TACTILE DYSFUNCTION

Evaluation of tactile processing is discussed in three parts: (a) relevant information from the client family, and other professionals; (b) SIPT (Ayres, 1989) measures related to poor tactile discrimination; and (c) other standardized tests and non-standardized evaluation methods.

One preliminary comment should be made. Because of the primary and pervasive role of the tactile system in human activity, any disorder in the central nervous system is likely to affect tactile system processing in some way (Grimm, 1976). However, the tactile disorders associated with nervous system disease or damage may not be the same as the types of tactile dysfunction that are related to sensory integrative dysfunction. The following sections on evaluation and treatment are focused on sensory-integrative-based tactile processing dysfunction. The evaluation of related motor and perceptual deficits is discussed in subsequent chapters.

The evaluation of tactile or sensory defensiveness is based primarily on interview, non-standardized evaluation, and observation of behavior. More specifically, the interview and observation of behavior may cover daily living, school, and play behaviors. The goal of the interview is to determine whether a meaningful cluster of the behaviors indicative of tactile defensiveness, listed earlier in this chapter, is present. The evaluation of tactile discrimination can be based primarily on SIPT scores.

## Relevant Information from Client, Family, and Others

Relevant information from persons involved in the life of the client is of primary importance in identifying tactile or sensory defensiveness. In the case of a child, these persons may be parents, primary caregivers, and teachers. In the case of an adult, they may be a spouse, colleagues, or parents. In all instances, the major source of information is the client.

The foremost issue is, Why has the client been referred? What behaviors, problems, or factors precipitated the events which led to referral of the client for assessment? Is the primary reason for referral anything that suggests tactile defensiveness?

In this process of interviewing the client and other individuals familiar with his or her behavior, it is important to differentiate between those symptoms that reflect tactile or sensory defensiveness and those which reflect the hypothesized secondary deficits or sequelae. The latter, while commonly associated with tactile or sensory defensiveness, cannot be considered to be primary indicators of the presence of a disorder. Among the most commonly observed sequelae are an increased level of activity and distractibility.

## Sensory Integration and Praxis Tests

Interpretation of tactile tests is complex and must include consideration of all the test scores of the SIPT, as well as related clinical observations of neuromotor behavior. Currently, the identification of tactile defensiveness relies on behaviors observed during testing rather than on test scores per se. Specific SIPT that evaluate tactile discrimination include Finger Identification, Localization of Tactile Stimuli, Manual Form Perception, and Graphesthesia (see Chapter 8).

## Other Evaluation Tools

Royeen (1985, 1986, 1987, 1989a, 1989b; Royeen & Fortune, 1990) has executed programmatic research toward developing an attitude scale for screening tactile defensiveness in school-aged children and has completed related work assessing tactile defensiveness in preschoolers. This work is the first systematic attempt to measure the construct "tactile defensiveness" using attitudes related to this problem. A copy of Royeen's scale for tactile defensiveness is included in Appendix 5 – A.

Another way to assess tactile system processing is through the use of a sensory history (e.g., Larson, 1982). Various versions of sensory histories are used in clinical practice. A sensory history allows a therapist to explore the developmental history of an individual in relation to how the individual responds to sensory stimuli. A sensory history can yield meaningful data on tactile discrimination but is a most useful in exploring individual development related to sensory responsivity. Sample questions on tactile processing, compiled by Wilbarger and Oetter (1989) from various sensory histories, include the following:

1 Does the child:
   **a** Seem overly sensitive to rough food textures?
   **b** Over- or underdress?
   **c** Seem unaware of cuts, bruises, and so forth?
   **d** Avoid using his or her hands?
   **e** Mouth objects or clothes excessively?
   **f** Hurt him- or herself or others?
   **g** Seem to pick fights?
   **h** Seem overly sensitive to food or water temperature?
2 Did the child:
   **a** Cry excessively during infancy?
   **b** Have difficulty establishing sleep/wake cycles during infancy?

If the client is a young child, tactually based play activities may be an excellent way to assess tactile perception or tactile defensiveness, as well as their possible effects on function and performance. This format is most useful when combined with other testing and interview. Exploratory play that is targeted to further identify a tactile processing deficit involves the therapist playing with a child in an environment rich with textures and tactually based activities (e.g., finger painting, bubbles, "drawing" with shaving cream). While engaging the child in these activities, the therapist should note the child's (a) reactions to tactile sensations, (b) initiation of touch (or lack thereof), (c) ability to engage in active touch, and (d) "emotional tone" during various activities and situations.

A *protocol* or procedure *for assessing responsivity* (underreaction or overreaction to certain sensory stimuli) was presented by Ayres and Tickle (1980) as part of a research investigation into the effectiveness of sensory integration therapy. This protocol provides an approach for evaluating overall responsivity and registration across sensory systems. However, it was designed for use with autistic children and may not be appropriate for higher-level functioning children.

Informal activities that might be used to assess tactile discrimination can include tasks requiring haptic shape discrimination (see Chapter 6), texture discrimination, and the ability to recognize how or where the client has been touched.

## Data Interpretation

Interpretation of the data that leads the occupational therapist to suspect the presence of tactile defensiveness or poor tactile perception is a complex process. For the most part, the identification of either disorder should be based on *patterns* or *clusters of behaviors* indicative of possible dysfunction. The identification of a problem should *not* be based on data from a single source.

If a therapist suspects tactile defensiveness or poor tactile perception, the next step in the evaluation is to relate the dysfunction to the occupational role of the individual. It is not sufficient just to identify the client, whether child or adult, as tactually defensive. The therapist also must determine if the tactile defensiveness is interfering with the occupational role of the individual. If tactile defensiveness does appear to be an interfering factor, the next step is to discover how and why it is affecting the individual's life, and how the dysfunction is related to the reason for referral. The interpretation process is discussed in more detail in Chapter 9.

# INTERVENTION

The differences between tactile defensiveness and poor tactile perception require different therapeutic interventions. We will discuss each separately.

## Tactile Defensiveness

Intervention for tactile defensiveness may be most effective using the threefold approach of (a) recognition and explanation of the nature of the dysfunction and how it is interfering with the client's life, (b) modification of the environment as much as possible to reduce stress and limit aversive stimuli, and (c) direct intervention. The components of this approach are discussed below.

### EXPLANATION OF THE PROBLEM

Sometimes understanding the problem is the single most important aspect of intervention. Imagine what it is like to know that you are different from other people, but not to be able to articulate how or why! Professional recognition of tactile defensiveness is 30 years old, yet, it is neither understood nor accepted by the general population. As a result, individuals with tactile defensiveness can spend their entire lives without understanding how or why they are different from others. In fact, many individuals with tactile defensiveness may have been "misdiagnosed" as having behavior disorders or being overly aggressive.

Therefore, an occupational therapist who can identify the nature of the problem and help the client understand his or her own behavior provides a significant service. Clinical experience suggests that it can be helpful for the client to understand that he or she is tactually defensive, and that many idiosyncratic habits are not simply neurotic, but are attempts to cope with the stresses of tactile defensiveness. Problem recognition is a particularly important part of therapy when tactile defensiveness is severe. In this case, the occupational therapist may wish to work in conjunction with a psychologist, psychiatrist, social worker, or counselor in helping the client understand what impact tactile defensiveness is having on his or her behavior.

## ENVIRONMENTAL MODIFICATION

Modifying aspects of the individual's environment is critical to a comprehensive approach to treating tactile defensiveness. Environmental modifications include (a) reducing extraneous stimuli in the environment, (b) reorganizing patterns and habits to reduce the likelihood of experiencing unexpected touch, and (c) increasing activities designed to provide more soothing or appropriate types of sensory experiences. Farber (1989) suggested that when stimulation is therapeutically controlled, behavior may become more adaptive. This concept may well apply to the tactually defensive individual.

Sears (1981) delineated such an environmentally based approach for special education personnel to use with tactually defensive children in the classroom. She discussed how the occupational therapist can work with members of other disciplines to effect environmental change in a comprehensive approach to intervention for tactile defensiveness. Her suggestions include approaching the child from the front, approaching the child at the child's eye level, seating the child in the back of the classroom, and allowing the child to stand at the end of lines. (Refer to Chapter 11 for more detailed information on consultation.)

Additionally, the client can be encouraged to make his or her own modifications, based on the client's specific responses to tactile stimulation.

## DIRECT INTERVENTION

The purpose of direct intervention is to "reset" or modulate the defensive orientation of the client's nervous system, using the environment and prescribed sensory experiences, and to couple this with elicitation of an appropriate adaptive behavior. Such intervention is theorized to promote more balanced responses to sensory events.

Direct intervention for tactile defensiveness centers on three treatment principles hypothesized to promote improved balance between inhibition and excitation within the nervous system, or simply to promote enhanced central nervous system functioning. These principles are (a) to provide enhanced opportunities for the individual to take in deep touch-pressure, proprioceptive, and linear vestibular information (Ayres, 1972b; Fisher & Dunn, 1983), (b) to facilitate functioning of the parasympathetic autonomic nervous system, that is, decreased arousal (Farber, 1982), and (c) to increase self-initiated tactile activities (Sears, 1981).

The emotional tone conveyed by the occupational therapist should be positive and should show acceptance within appropriate limits. The tactually defensive individual may benefit from a warm, open emotional tone that reduces the stress that is thought to exacerbate defensiveness. Such an approach may increase the client's comfort with tactile experiences, whether self-administered or initiated by the occupational therapist. Moreover, the environmental tone of the room should be inviting, without visual clutter and noise. The "sparse" room in treatment and at home may be the most comforting environmental situation for a tactually defensive individual.

Clinical experience reveals a common misunderstanding about intervention for tactile defensiveness. Because tactile defensiveness is a tactile processing dysfunction, many individuals believe that tactile stimulation is the treatment of choice for tactile defensiveness. Such an approach may be misguided, according to the postulate that, in treatment, it is not the stimulation per se that promotes improved sensory processing, but rather, the organization of sensory input for use which promotes central nervous system maturation. In fact, sensory stimulation in cases of tactile defensiveness may be contraindicated. As Farber said, "it is even conceivable that overstimulation . . . may actually cause a rebound effect yielding more maladaptive behavior" (1982, p. 126).

Clinical experience has also shown that treatment of skin hypersensitivity due to nerve lesion or disease may differ from treatment of tactile defensiveness. In cases of hypersensitivity, desensitization techniques may be appropriate and effective (Robinson & McPhee, 1986), but they are not thought to be effective and may be contraindicated for tactile defensiveness.

One exception may be a new, experimental approach for the treatment of sensory defensiveness that has been delineated by Wilbarger (Wilbarger & Royeen, 1987). Wilbarger proposed a radical alteration of the balance between excitation and inhibition within the nervous system in a short amount of time compared to more traditional approaches. Wilbarger's approach is a modification of Rood's technique of brushing and employs a *non-scratching* surgical scrub brush, used in conjunction with gentle joint compression to the upper and lower extremities and trunk. Although continued research into its effectiveness is necessary, preliminary clinical results are promising. Lydia provides one such example.

Lydia was placed on a "sensory diet" for tactile defensiveness as described by Wilbarger (Wilbarger & Royeen, 1987). The sensory diet consisted of baby massage and gentle joint compression at each diaper change. Lydia received her extra "sensory food" approximately six to seven times a day, corresponding to the number of diaper changes she required. The sensory diet also included deep touch-pressure to Lydia's tongue and upper palate (Farber, 1982) prior to each breastfeeding during the day.

Within 3 months of referral, Lydia regulated herself to sleeping 8 hours each night and taking two daytime naps. By 10 months of age, Lydia no longer required constant physical contact during waking hours. Also, she began to use a pacifier vigorously for non-nutritive sucking, and eventually began to use her thumb for that purpose.

The Test of Sensory Functions in Infants (DeGangi & Greenspan, 1989) was administered at 11 months by an occupational therapist unfamiliar with Lydia's history. At that time, Lydia was found to be within normal limits in all areas, except that she exhibited mild tactile defensiveness. Informal clinical observations by a group of physicians and psychologists 1 month later found Lydia to be a happy and healthy baby.

## Poor Tactile Perception

A therapist would rarely, if ever, be treating an isolated problem in tactile discrimination. The provision of enhanced opportunities to take in tactile information derived from active participation in meaningful activity, coupled with appropriate environmental demands, are generally recommended as a component of the overall treatment program.

## SUMMARY

Throughout the chapter, we have referred to the cases of Lydia and Rick for illustrations of disorders of tactile system processing. It is easy to see the importance of the tactile system in their development. Although the tactile system is by no means the only system functioning at birth, we do have reason to believe that its function is important. We have discussed the various expressions of problems within the tactile system, and through a review of the hypothesized neurobiological basis of these disorders, we have attempted to understand tactile processing deficits. We also have examined the means of assessing these problems, both by using standardized tests such as the SIPT, and by using non-standardized methods such as interview and sensory history taking. In our experience, standardized tests often are limited in their ability to identify tactile processing disorders. Finally, treatment concepts were presented to provide the reader with a foundation for developing specific intervention strategies; the use of a "sensory diet" to reduce tactile defensiveness was illustrated by the experience with Lydia.

# REFERENCES

Apgar, V. (1953). A proposal for a new method of evaluation of the newborn infant. *Current Research in Anesthesia and Analgesia, 32*, 260–267.

Ashton, J. (1987). *Brain disorders and psychotropic drugs*. New York: Oxford University Press.

Ayres, A. J. (1964). Tactile functions: Their relations to hyperactive and perceptual motor behavior. *American Journal of Occupational Therapy, 18*, 6–11.

Ayres, A. J. (1965). Patterns of perceptual-motor dysfunction in children. *Perceptual and Motor Skills, 20*, 335–369.

Ayres, A. J. (1966a). Interactions among perceptual-motor function in a group of normal children. *American Journal of Occupational Therapy, 20*, 288–292.

Ayres, A. J. (1966b). Interrelationships among perceptual-motor functions in children. *American Journal of Occupational Therapy, 20*, 68–71.

Ayres, A. J. (1969). Deficits in sensory integration in educationally handicapped children. *Journal of Learning Disabilities, 2*, 160–168.

Ayres, A. J. (1972a). Improving academic scores through sensory integration. *Journal of Learning Disabilities, 5*, 336–343.

Ayres, A. J. (1972b). *Sensory integration and learning disorders*. Los Angeles: Western Psychological Services.

Ayres, A. J. (1977). Cluster analyses of measure of sensory integration. *American Journal of Occupational Therapy, 31*, 362–366.

Ayres, A. J. (1979). *Sensory integration and the child*. Los Angeles: Western Psychological Services.

Ayres, A. J. (1980). *Southern California Sensory Integration Tests manual: Revised 1980*. Los Angeles: Western Psychological Services.

Ayres, A. J. (1989). *Sensory Integration and Praxis Tests*. Los Angeles: Western Psychological Services.

Ayres, A. J., & Tickle, L. (1980). Hyper-responsivity to touch and vestibular stimulation as a predictor of responsivity to sensory integrative procedures by autistic children. *American Journal of Occupational Therapy, 34*, 375–381.

Bauer, B. (1977). Tactile-sensitive behavior in hyperactive and non-hyperactive children. *American Journal of Occupational Therapy, 31*, 447–450.

Bushnell, E. W., Shaw, L., & Strauss, D. (1985). Relationship between visual and tactual exploration by 6-month-olds. *Developmental Psychology, 21*, 591–600.

Casey (1973). The neurophysiological basis of pain. *Postgraduate Medicine, 53*, 62.

Cermak, S. (1988). The relationship between attention deficits and sensory integration disorders (Part I). *Sensory Integration Special Interest Section Newsletter, 11*(2), 1–4.

Chusid, J. G. (1979). *Correlative neuroanatomy and functional neurology* (17th ed.). Los Altos, CA: Lange Medical Publishers.

Clark, F. A., Mailloux, S., & Parham, D. (1989). Sensory integration and learning disabilities. In P.N. Pratt & A.S. Allen (Eds.), *Occupational Therapy for Children* (2nd ed., pp. 457–507). St. Louis, MO: C.V. Mosby.

Collier, G. (1985). *Emotional expression*. Hillsdale, NJ: Lawrence Erlbaum Associates.

DeGangi, G., & Greenspan, S. I. (1989). *Test of Sensory Functions in Infants*. Los Angeles: Western Psychological Services.

deGroot, J. & Chusid, J. G. (1988). *Correlative neuroanatomy* (12th ed.). Connecticut: Appleton and Lange.

Donovick, P. J. (1968). Effects of localized septal lesions on hippocampal EEG activity in behavior in rats. *Journal of Comparative and Physiological Psychology, 66*, 569–578.

Farber, S. D. (1982). *Neurorehabilitation: A multisensory approach*. Philadelphia: W.B. Saunders.

Farber, S. D. (1989, May). *Neuroscience and occupational therapy: Vital connections*. Eleanor Clark Slagle Lectureship at the American Occupational Therapy Association Annual Conference, Baltimore, MD.

Fisher, A. G., & Dunn, W. (1983). Tactile defensiveness: Historical perspectives, new research: A theory grows. *Sensory Integration Special Interest Section Newsletter, 6*(2), 1–2.

Fried, P. A. (1972). The effect of differential hippocampal lesions and pre- and post-operative training on extinction. *Revenue Canadienne de Psychologie, 26*, 61–70.

Getman, G. N. (1985). Hand-eye coordinations. *Academic Therapy, 20*, 261–275.

Gibson, J. J. (1962). Observations of active touch. *Psychological Review, 69*, 477–491.

Gottfried, A. W. (1984). Touch as an organizer for learning and development. In C.C. Brown (Ed.), *The many facets of touch* (pp. 114–122). Skillman, NJ: Johnson and Johnson Baby Products.

Gottfried, A. W., & Rose, S. A. (1980). Tactile recognition in infants. *Child Development, 51*, 69–74.

Gray, J. A. (1982). *The neurophyschology of anxiety.* New York: Claredon.

Green, R. H., & Schwartzbaum, J. S. (1968). Effects of unilateral septal lesions on avoidance behavior discrimination reversal and hippocampal EEG. *Journal of Comparative and Physiological Psychology, 65*, 388–396.

Grossman, S. P. (1978). An experimental "dissection" of the septal syndrome. *Functions of the septo-hippocampal system* (pp. 227–273). Ciba Foundation Symposium 58 (new series). New York: Elsevier.

Haron, M., & Henderson, A. (1985). Active and passive touch in developmentally dyspraxic and normal boys. *Occupational Therapy Journal of Research, 5*, 102–112.

Head, H. (1920). *Studies in neurology: Vol. 2.* New York: Oxford University Press.

Heydorn, B. L. (1985). A psychometric study of developmental changes in stereognostic ability. *Perceptual and Motor Skills, 61*, 1206.

Huss, A. J. (1977). Touch with care or a caring touch. *American Journal of Occupational Therapy, 31*, 295–309.

Isaacson, R. L. (1982). *The limbic system* (2nd ed.). New York: W.B. Saunders.

Kandel, E. R., & Schwartz, J. H. (1985). *Principles of neural science.* New York: Elsevier.

Kim, C., Choi, H., Kim, J. K., Kim, M. S., Huh, M. K., & Moon, Y. B. (1971). General behavioral activity and its component patterns in hippocampectomized rats. *Brain Research, 19*, 379–394.

Knickerbocker, B. M. (1980). *A holistic approach to learning disabilities.* Thorofare, NJ: C.B. Slack.

Kravitz, H., Goldenberg, D., & Neyhaus, A. (1978). Tactual exploration by normal infants. *Developmental Medicine and Child Neurology, 20*, 720–726.

Larson, K. A. (1982). The sensory history of developmentally delayed children with and without tactile defensiveness. *American Journal of Occupational Therapy, 36*, 590–596.

Lowrey, G. H. (1986). *Growth and development of children* (8th ed.). Chicago: Yearbook.

Luria, A. R.. (1973). *The working brain: An introduction to neuropsychology.* New York: Basic Books.

Meltzoff, A. N., & Borton, R. W. (1979). Intermodal matching by human neonates. *Nature, 22*, 403–404.

Melzack, R., & Wall P. D. (1965). Pain mechanisms: A new theory. *Science, 150*, 971–979.

Melzack, R., & Wall, P. D. (1973). *The challenge of pain.* New York: Basic Books.

Montagu, A. (1978). *Touching: The human significance of the skin.* New York: Harper and Row.

Nathan, P. W., Smith, M. C., & Cook, A. W. (1986). Sensory effects in man of lesions of the posterior columns and of some other afferent pathways. *Brain, 109*(pt. 5), 1003–1041.

Noback, C., & Demerest, R. (1981). *The human nervous system.* New York: McGraw-Hill.

Olton, D. S., & Gage, F. H. (1974). Role of the fornix in the septal syndrome. *Physiology and Behavior, 13*, 269–279.

Peele, T. L. (1977). *The neuroanatomic basis for clinical neurology,* (3rd ed., pp. 436–455). New York: McGraw-Hill.

Reite, M. L. (1984). Touch, attachment and health—Is there a relationship? In C. C. Brown (Ed.), *The many facets of touch* (pp. 58–65). Skillman, NJ: Johnson and Johnson Baby Products.

Robinson, A., & McPhee, S. D. (1986). Case report: Treating the patient with digital hypersensitivity. *American Journal of Occupational Therapy, 40*, 285–287.

Royeen, C. B. (1985). Domain specifications of the construct tactile defensiveness. *American Journal of Occupational Therapy, 39*(9), 596–599.

Royeen, C. B. (1986). Development of a scale measuring tactile defensiveness in children. *American Journal of Occupational Therapy, 46*, 414–419.

Royeen, C. B. (1987). Test-retest reliability of a touch scale for tactile defensiveness. *Physical and Occupational Therapy in Pediatrics, 7*(3), 45–52.

Royeen, C. B. (1989a). Commentary on "tactile functions in learning-disabled and normal children: Reliability and validity considerations." *Occupational Therapy Journal of Research, 9*, 16–23.

Royeen, C. B. (1989b, August). *Tactile defensiveness: An overview of the construct.* Paper presented at the International Society for Social Pediatrics, Brixen, Italy.

Royeen, C. B., & Fortune, J. C. (1990). TIE: Touch inventory for school aged children. *American Journal of Occupational Therapy, 44*, 155–160.

Satz, P., Fletcher, J. M., Morris, R., Taylor, H. G. (1984). Finger localization and reading achievement. In C. C. Brown (Ed.), *The many facets of touch* (pp. 123–130). Skillman, NJ: Johnson and Johnson Baby Products.

Scardina, V. (1986). A. Jean Ayres Lectureship. *Sensory Integration Newsletter, 14*(3), 2–10.

Sears, C. (1981). The tactilely defensive child. *Academic Therapy, 16*, 563–569.

Sinclair, D. (1981). *Mechanisms of cutaneous sensation.* New York: Oxford University Press.

Snow, C. W. (1989). *Infant development.* Englewood Cliffs, NJ: Prentice Hall.

Suomi, S. J. (1984). The role of touch in rhesus monkey social development. In C.C. Brown (Ed.), *The many facets of touch* (pp. 41–50). Skillman, NJ: Johnson and Johnson Baby Products.

Vierck, C. J., Cohen, R. H., & Cooper, B. Y. (1985). Effects of spinal lesions on temporal resolution of cutaneous sensations. *Somatosensory Research, 3,* 45–46.

Wilbarger, P., & Royeen, C. B. (1987, May). *Tactile defensiveness: Theory, applications and treatment.* Annual Interdisciplinary Doctoral Conference, Sargent College, Boston University.

Wilbarger, P., & Oetter, P. (1989, October). *Sensory processing disorders.* Paper presented at the American Occupational Therapy Association Practice Symposium, St. Louis, MO.

# TIE:Touch Inventory for Elementary School-Aged Children*

## EQUIPMENT

Two chairs and a table are required, as well as a copy of the instrument and three blocks made of poster board. Each block has one of the response choices inscribed on it with large black letters: "No" on a 2-inch by 2-inch response card, "A little" on a 2-inch by 3-inch response card, and "A lot" on a 2-inch by 4-inch response card.

## PROCEDURE

The scale takes less than 10 minutes to administer. The subject (S) and the examiner (Ex) sit across from each other. Ex uses a shield to cover the instrument in order to reduce distraction for S.

Ex orients S to the task. Ex explains that they will be playing a game in which there are no "right" answers and no "wrong" answers. The game is being played so that the Ex can learn more about S.

Ex explains the response format to S. Ex says:

"I will ask you questions and you are to answer them saying either 'No,' 'A little,' or 'A lot'."

Ex is to point to each of the three blocks inscribed with the phrases while saying them aloud. Ex continues, saying:

"Let's practice the game for you to learn how to play it. I will ask you a question—'Do you like ice cream?' You answer by saying either 'No,' 'A little,' or 'A lot'."

Ex points to the blocks again when stating choices for response. Ex continues:

"Remember to point to the block that is your choice. You don't have to say which one it is, just point to it."

In the beginning, S is required to point to the block which is his or her choice. S may also state his or her answer aloud but this is not required. The purpose of the blocks is to aid S in remembering the three response items. Thus, it is all right if after

---

*Source: Royeen, C.B., & Fortune, J.C. (1990). TIE: Touch inventory for school aged children. *American Journal of Occupational Therapy, 44*, 165–170, with permission.

## TOUCH INVENTORY FOR ELEMENTARY SCHOOL–AGED CHILDREN (TIE)
### by Charlotte Brasic Royeen

Date: _____

Subject: _____

Examiner: _____

Procedure: Administer the scale according to standard instructions. Response of "No" is scored "1"; a response of "A Little" is scored "2"; and a response of "A Lot" is scored "3".

| Response (Check) 1 | 2 | 3 | No. | Question |
|---|---|---|---|---|
| [ ] | [ ] | [ ] | 1. | Does it bother you to go barefooted? |
| [ ] | [ ] | [ ] | 2. | Do fuzzy shirts bother you? |
| [ ] | [ ] | [ ] | 3. | Do fuzzy socks bother you? |
| [ ] | [ ] | [ ] | 4. | Do turtleneck shirts bother you? |
| [ ] | [ ] | [ ] | 5. | Does it bother you to have your face washed? |
| [ ] | [ ] | [ ] | 6. | Does it bother you to have your nails cut? |
| [ ] | [ ] | [ ] | 7. | Does it bother you to have your hair combed by someone else? |
| [ ] | [ ] | [ ] | 8. | Does it bother you to play on a carpet? |
| [ ] | [ ] | [ ] | 9. | After someone touches you, do you feel like scratching that spot? |
| [ ] | [ ] | [ ] | 10. | After someone touches you, do you feel like rubbing that spot? |
| [ ] | [ ] | [ ] | 11. | Does it bother you to walk barefooted in the grass and sand? |
| [ ] | [ ] | [ ] | 12. | Does getting dirty bother you? |
| [ ] | [ ] | [ ] | 13. | Do you find it hard to pay attention? |
| [ ] | [ ] | [ ] | 14. | Does it bother you if you cannot see who is touching you? |
| [ ] | [ ] | [ ] | 15. | Does fingerpainting bother you? |
| [ ] | [ ] | [ ] | 16. | Do rough bedsheets bother you? |
| [ ] | [ ] | [ ] | 17. | Do you like to touch people, but it bothers you when they touch you back? |
| [ ] | [ ] | [ ] | 18. | Does it bother you when people come from behind? |
| [ ] | [ ] | [ ] | 19. | Does it bother you to be kissed by someone other than your parents? |
| [ ] | [ ] | [ ] | 20. | Does it bother you to be hugged or held? |
| [ ] | [ ] | [ ] | 21. | Does it bother you to play games with your feet? |
| [ ] | [ ] | [ ] | 22. | Does it bother you to have your face touched? |
| [ ] | [ ] | [ ] | 23. | Does it bother you to be touched if you don't expect it? |
| [ ] | [ ] | [ ] | 24. | Do you have difficulty making friends? |
| [ ] | [ ] | [ ] | 25. | Does it bother you to stand in line? |
| [ ] | [ ] | [ ] | 26. | Does it bother you when someone is close by? |

[ ]                  (no. of responses scored "1") × 1 = [      ]

+ [ ]                (no. of responses scored "2") × 2 = [      ]

+ [ ]              (no. of responses scored "3") × 3 = [      ]

Total Score = [      ]

Percentile Score = [      ]

doing the test for a few items the subject stops pointing to the blocks. The purpose of the practice session is to teach the child the response format. Therefore, the procedures should be repeated until Ex is certain that S understands how to answer the questions. Suggested questions to use if further practice is required follow:

"Do you like snakes?", "Do you like turtles?", "Do you like vegetables?", "Do you like school?"

Once S understands the task and the required response style, Ex says: "Now we will play the game."

Ex may restate or explain the item until S understands it. If S asks Ex to repeat an item or states that he or she does not understand the question. Ex should read the question and wait for S to respond. If S does not respond and needs prompting, Ex may say:

"Which answer do you want?" and then point to the three answers on the response cards, "No," "A Little," or "A Lot."

Ex records S's answer and notes any pertinent observations. Upon completion of the session, Ex praises S for his participation.

## SCORING AND INTERPRETING THE TIE

The TIE is easily scored by summing the child's response scores (i.e., adding the scores from items 1 through 26). The child's score is then compared to the normative data supplied in Table 5–A.

Proper interpretation of Table 5–A is contingent upon understanding that a high raw score does not mean a better performance on part of the child. Recall that the response format for the TIE is 1 = no, 2 = a little, and 3 = a lot. Therefore, a child who responds with "a lot" for many of the test items will receive a higher raw score than the child who answers with "a little" for many of the test items. Thus, *the higher the score, the more the child's self-reported behaviors are associated with behaviors indicative of tactile defensiveness.* Conversely, *the lower the score, the less the subject's self-reported behaviors are associated with behaviors indicative of tactile defensiveness.*

Conversion of raw scores into corresponding percentile scores using Table 5–A provides a standard reference for how a given child responds to test items compared to the normative sample. Again, it is important to note that a higher percentile score does not mean a better test performance. Rather, a higher percentile score, for example, the range of the 75th percentile and above, means that at least 75 percent of the normative sample answered with responses *less* associated with tactile defensiveness: Only 25 percent of the normative sample answered with responses *more* associated with tactile defensiveness.

## TABLE 5–A. DATA FOR SCORING THE TIE

Mean score = 41
Standard Deviation = 7.8
Standard Error of the Mean = 0.38

| Percentile Score | Raw Score |
|---|---|
| 100 | 60 |
| 90 | 51 |
| 75 | 45 |
| 50 | 40 |
| 25 | 35 |
| 10 | 31 |
| 0 | 25 |

| Percentile Score | 0 | 10 | 25 | 50 | 75 | 90 | 100 |
|---|---|---|---|---|---|---|---|
| Raw Score | 25 | 30 | 35 | 40 | 45 | 50 | 60 |

CHAPTER **6**

# Somatodyspraxia

**Sharon A. Cermak, EdD, OTR**

*There is no typically clumsy child.*

*Gordon & McKinlay, 1980, p. 2*

The term *praxis* means "action based on will" and comes from the Greek word for "doing, acting, deed, practice" (W. Safire, NY Times, June, 1989). The client with dyspraxia has difficulty with performing in, and acting on, the environment (Ayres, 1985). What all clients with dyspraxia have in common is a deficit in motor planning that results in motor clumsiness. The focus of this chapter is the client with a specific type of developmental dyspraxia hypothesized to result from impaired tactile and proprioceptive processing. Ayres (1989) called this type of dyspraxia *somatodyspraxia* to reflect the somatosensory basis of the disorder.

When we use the theory of sensory integration to understand the client with dyspraxia, we hypothesize that somatodyspraxia is but one disorder of praxis. Not all clients who are dyspraxic have sensory integrative dysfunction. Moreover, much of the literature on developmental dyspraxia and clients with motor clumsiness refers to this group of clients collectively as "the clumsy child" (cf. Gubbay, 1975). In order to avoid confusion, we will use the term *dyspraxia* when we refer to the large group of clients with developmental disorders of motor planning. We will use the term *clumsy* when the authors did not explicitly specify if the clients studied were dyspraxic. We will use the term *somatodyspraxia* to refer to the subgroup of clients whose dyspraxia we hypothesize to be due to poor somatosensory processing. Finally, we prefer to use the term *dyspraxia* rather than *apraxia* when we refer to clients with developmental motor planning deficits. The prefix *a* means an inability whereas the prefix *dys* means an impairment in the ability. The client with developmental dyspraxia is able to motor plan, but this ability is impaired. This is in contrast to the client with adult-onset *apraxia* who has lost a once-intact motor planning behavior. Mario, whom we met in Chapter 1, is a child with somatodyspraxia. Like all clients with dyspraxia, he is clumsy, he has difficulty performing motor skills, and he needs more practice in order to learn motor tasks than do other children his age. Mario, like other children with somatodyspraxia, has never acquired normal adaptive motor behavior.

We observe praxis when we observe an individual's ability to interact with his or her physical world. We may therefore be tempted to assume that dyspraxia is *primarily* a motor problem. This belief is reinforced by the fact that the term dyspraxia has often been used synonymously with "motor planning" or "motor clumsiness." However, the occupational therapist interested in praxis is as concerned with an individual's sensory processing and conceptual abilities as with his or her neuromotor abilities (Ayres, 1985; Ayres, Mailloux, & Wendler, 1987). Thus, of primary concern in the client with somatodyspraxia is his or her ability to process sensory information. In this type of developmental dyspraxia, the ability to process and integrate sensory information is hypothesized to form the basis for the client's knowledge of his or her own body, which in turn forms the basis for the beginning conceptualizations necessary for motor planning (Ayres, 1972a, 1979, 1985).

As we mentioned earlier, somatodyspraxis is not the only disorder of praxis that has been associated with impaired sensory processing. Based on the results of factor and cluster analyses of Sensory Integration and Praxis Test (SIPT) scores, Ayres (1989) identified four major types of practic dysfunction: bilateral integration and sequencing, somatodyspraxia, dyspraxia on verbal command, and visuodyspraxia. The clinical pictures and hypothesized etiologies of these practic disorders are quite different. As was discussed in Chapter 4, deficits in bilateral integration and sequencing are hypothesized to reflect a practic disorder due to impaired processing of vestibular-proprioceptive information. Tactile discrimination abilities of children with bilateral integration and sequencing deficits are *normal*. Further, the motor planning deficits of these children often are subtle and confined to the ability to plan and produce bilateral and projected motor action sequences (see Chapter 4). Dyspraxia on verbal command and visuodyspraxia will be discussed in Chapter 7. Dyspraxia on verbal command is *not considered to be due to a disorder of sensory integration*. As was pointed out in Chapter 1 (see also Chapter 8), visuopraxis (or visuodyspraxia) is a label for a group of disorders that may have a common conceptual link with praxis, *but are not disorders of praxis*. Rather, this group of disorders, which include poor form and space perception, visuomotor coordination, and visual construction, may be associated with, or sequelae to, somatodyspraxia.

Ayres' (1989) attempt to designate reliable and valid subtypes of dyspraxia (bilateral integration and sequencing, somatodyspraxia, and dyspraxia on verbal command) constituted an important step toward the determination of the needs of clients with developmental dyspraxia (see also Chapter 8). The ability to identify distinct subtypes of clients with developmental dyspraxia, whose pattern of abilities and deficits may require different intervention styles and strategies, may serve as the foundation upon which to construct optimal methods for treatment. We feel that an important component of this effort is the differentiation between clients whose deficits in motor planning can be hypothesized to be due to disorders of sensory integration and those clients with dyspraxia who do not manifest disorders of sensory integration. Moreover, it should be recognized that the classification of clients into "homogeneous" subtypes does not imply that individuals classified within any given subgroup are identical. Rather, it is quite likely that clients would show fairly substantial individual differences. Additionally, clients with deficits in motor planning may show characteristics of more than one subtype of dyspraxia (Ayres, 1989).

## PURPOSE AND SCOPE

This chapter is intended to provide a comprehensive view of somatodyspraxia. It includes a definition and description of the disorder, discussion of the neuroanatomical bases and etiology of developmental dyspraxia, review of assessment tools, strategies for differential identification of somatodyspraxia from among other practic disorders, and finally, a discussion of theoretical implications for intervention. To assist us in the process of discussing the various aspects of this disorder, we will present the clinical picture of a child with somatodyspraxia. This will include a summary of her presenting problems, our evaluation, and our suggestions for occupational therapy intervention.

## KEISHA

### Reason for Referral

Keisha is a 6-year, 10-month-old girl who is currently in the 6th month of 1st grade. An occupational therapy evaluation was requested by Keisha's parents to investigate for possible sensory integrative problems and to clarify the difficulties Keisha is having in school. Keisha's teacher has reported that Keisha is having difficulty with pasting, coloring, and writing, and that she is not able to use scissors. Her teacher has also expressed concern about Keisha's poor pencil grasp, especially because she often presses so hard on the paper that the point of her pencil breaks.

When we evaluated Keisha, we gave her the SIPT (Ayres, 1989) and we observed her on a variety of nonstandardized clinical observations of neuromotor behavior. To supplement our evaluation, we also interviewed Keisha's mother and her teacher, and we observed her in her classroom. The following is a summary of the results of our occupational therapy evaluation.

### Parent Interview

Keisha's mother reported that Keisha was the product of a full-term normal pregnancy and delivery. She weighed 6 lb, 8 oz and did not experience neonatal difficulties. Developmental milestones were achieved within normal limits. She sat at 6 months, crawled at 8 months, and walked at 14 months. Speech also developed within normal limits. Keisha was able to say single words at 12 months, and she spoke in sentences at 18 months. Keisha's mother also told us that she really didn't notice that Keisha was different from other children until she began to notice persistent mild articulation problems. Because she was aware that mild articulation problems are relatively common, she really didn't become concerned until Keisha's teacher expressed concerns about Keisha's school performance. In fact, she had always been proud of Keisha as she seemed to be quite bright. According to her mother, a recent psychological assessment revealed that Keisha's IQ is 132.

When we talked further with Keisha's mother, we learned that Keisha is able to print her name; however, she is not able to copy simple words (e.g., friends' names) even when the letters are the same as those in her own name. Although she plays with other children in the neighborhood, many of her friends are younger than Keisha. When they play together, Keisha usually "directs" their play toward quiet indoor activities such as playing with puppets, dolls, and toy dishes. When her friends do not want to play "Keisha's games," Keisha often walks away and plays by herself. Thus, Keisha spends a lot of time playing alone. Her favorite activity is watching television. When her parents buy her toys that require fine motor skills, she creates fantasy games instead of using them for manipulative play.

Finally, Keisha's mother, thinking back on Keisha's motor development, expressed concern about Keisha's gross motor skills. She recalled that Keisha was not able to pedal a tricycle until she was 5 years of age. She still does not walk down stairs reciprocally, and she did not learn to pump the swing by herself until 2 months ago.

## Classroom Observation

When we observed Keisha in the classroom, we found that, indeed, many of the problems her teacher had described seemed to be problem areas for Keisha. Compared with the other children in her classroom, Keisha clearly had difficulty with writing, coloring, and cutting with scissors. When given a four-to-five single-piece puzzle, Keisha was able to locate the correct position for the puzzle piece, but was unable to manipulate it to fit it into its place. When getting ready to go outside, Keisha put her coat on upside down. She was unable to manage the zipper on her coat or to fasten the buttons on the front of her blouse. During recess, Keisha preferred to spend the entire time alone on the swings. At snack time, she was not able to open her milk carton and needed help opening her package of crackers.

Later, when we talked with her teacher, we learned that Keisha has excellent verbal skills and verbal memory; she also mentioned that Keisha is receiving speech therapy for her articulation problems.

## Clinical Observations and Related Measures

During our observations of her neuromotor behaviors, we noted that Keisha was hypotonic and that her proximal joint stability was poor. Equilibrium testing indicated that her responses were somewhat delayed when compared to other children of Keisha's age. Keisha tended to try to hold on to the examiner rather than use equilibrium reactions to maintain her balance. She was unable to assume the prone extension or the supine flexion positions. On paper and pencil tasks, Keisha showed a right hand preference and used a static tripod pencil grasp. Keisha was able to perform sequential thumb-to-finger touching with the right and left hands separately, although she needed to closely visually monitor her fingers. Keisha was unable to complete sequential thumb-to-finger touching with both hands simultaneously. Finally, she did not demonstrate any aversive or avoidance responses to touch during our evaluation. Her performance on the Touch Inventory for Elementary School Aged Children (Royeen & Fortune, 1990) (see also Chapter 5) also indicated that she did not have tactile defensiveness.

## SIPT

When we evaluated Keisha using the SIPT (Ayres, 1989), we found that she had significantly low scores on three of the four tactile tests. These three test scores reflect her ability to identify the finger that is touched by the examiner (Finger Identification), the ability to replicate designs that are drawn of the back of the hand (Graphesthesia), and the ability to recognize the shapes of objects through manipulation (haptic perception; Manual Form Perception). Only her ability to locate precisely the place on her arm where she was touched (Localization of Tactile Stimuli) was in the average range.

Her ability to remember the direction and extent of passive arm movements (Kinesthesia) was in the low-average range, but her static and dynamic balance abilities (Standing and Walking Balance) were below normal expectations for a child of Keisha's age. In contrast, the duration of her postrotary nystagmus was within the average range.

One of Keisha's lowest scores on the entire test battery was on Postural Praxis, a test of the ability to reproduce unusual postures assumed by the examiner, and an important indicator of somatodyspraxia. Her ability to copy sequenced arm and finger movements (Sequencing Praxis) also was low. On Bilateral Motor Coordination, a test of the ability to replicate bilateral projected action sequences, Keisha scored within the deficient range. Her ability to replicate positions and movements of the tongue, lips, and jaw (Oral Praxis) also was deficient. Keisha was able to carry out movements on verbal command and achieved a score within normal limits on Praxis on Verbal Command.

Her ability to trace a line with a pen (Motor Accuracy) and to reproduce two-dimensional forms (Design Copying) also were below age expectations. The rest of Keisha's scores suggested normal form and space perception and constructional abilities.

## Summary

The results of our evaluation indicated that Keisha had deficits in tactile discrimination (see Chapter 5). The presence of a postural-ocular movement disorder suggested deficits in central processing of vestibular-proprioceptive information (see Chapter 4). Her performance on the praxis tests of the SIPT suggested the presence of dyspraxia, and her difficulty with the drawing tasks indicated that she has poor visuomotor skills. Using the theory as our guide, we hypothesized that her primary problem was somatodyspraxia. Her somatodyspraxia appeared to be secondary to inadequate processing of tactile and vestibular-proprioceptive information. It appeared that Keisha's somatodyspraxia involved both gross and fine motor planning components, and was associated with impairment of visuomotor co-ordination.

## DEFINITION OF DEVELOPMENTAL DYSPRAXIA AND SOMATODYSPRAXIA

Dyspraxia is defined as difficulty in planning and carrying out skilled, nonhabitual motor acts in the correct sequence. It is not a primary problem in motor coordination (motor execution). Rather, the problem is hypothesized to be due to difficulty in formulating the plan of action. Praxis includes both knowing what to do and how to do it (Ayres, 1972a, 1979, 1985, 1989).

Ayres (1972a) defined somatosensory-based dyspraxia, or somatodyspraxia (Ayres, 1989), as a disorder of encoding a *new*, as opposed to a habitual, motor response strategy. That is, clients with somatodyspraxia have difficulty learning new tasks, but once learned and performed as a part of the client's daily life performance, the task can be performed with adequate skill. Although clients can acquire reasonable degrees of skill in specific activities with practice, the acquired skill remains highly specific to the particular tasks they have practiced and doesn't generalize to other similar activities. Thus, the client with somatodyspraxia must continuously learn each variant of a task as though it were a totally new task.

Other factors besides the ability to generalize skill from one specific task to another may affect the quality of movement. Walton, Ellis, and Court (1963) stated that "in children with developmental dyspraxia, movements are performed with an excessive expenditure of energy and with inaccurate judgement of the required force, tempo and amplitude of movement" (p. 606). Praxis also may include the ability to organize behaviors and develop or choose appropriate motor strategies to accomplish a task. Thus, clients with developmental dyspraxia often are disorganized in their approach to tasks and have poor work habits (Cermak, 1985).

Although definitions of developmental dyspraxia and somatodyspraxia are essentially equivalent with regard to the motor manifestations of the planning deficit, *a critical component of somatodyspraxia is the presence of a disorder in tactile discrimination.* Poor tactile discrimination is *not* necessarily a symptom of developmental dyspraxia. And if the motor planning deficits do not occur concurrently with poor tactile discrimination, the practic disorder cannot be considered somatodyspraxia.

# CLINICAL PICTURE OF SOMATODYSPRAXIA

Table 6–1 summarizes the problems that typify the client with somatodyspraxia, which we will discuss in the following sections. As we proceed, it is important to be aware that some of these problems are considered primary indicators of somatodys-

TABLE 6–1. CLINICAL PICTURE OF SOMATODYSPRAXIA

| Play, Developmental, and Educational Indices | Behavioral Characteristics | SIPT Performance | Clinical Observations |
|---|---|---|---|
| 1. Clumsy<br>2. Poor tactile discrimination abilities<br>3. Inadequate body scheme<br>4. Difficulty with sequencing and timing<br>5. Slowness in learning activities of daily living (especially fastenings)<br>6. Problems in gross motor skills and sports<br>7. Problems in constructive or manipulatory play and poor fine motor abilities<br>8. Handwriting deficits<br>9. Developmental articulatory deficit<br>10. Accompanying soft neurological signs<br>11. Accompanying learning disabilities | 1. Low self-esteem and poor self-concept<br>2. Easily frustrated; avoids new situations<br>3. Often manipulative<br>4. May prefer "talking" to "doing" (unless also language-impaired)<br>5. Often late and forgetful<br>6. Disorganized approach to tasks | 1. On tests indicative of poor praxis, low scores on:<br>a. Postural Praxis<br>b. Bilateral Motor Coordination<br>c. Sequencing Praxis<br>d. Oral Praxis<br>e. Possibly, Praxis on Verbal Command<br>2. On tests indicative of poor somatosensory processing, low scores on:<br>a. Finger Identification<br>b. Graphesthesia<br>c. Localization of Tactile Stimuli<br>d. Manual Form Perception<br>e. Standing and Walking Balance<br>f. Possibly, Kinesthesia | 1. Inadequate supine flexion<br>2. Difficulty with sequential finger touching<br>3. Other indications of poor motor skill, including:<br>a. Impaired ramp movements<br>b. Difficulty with rapid alternating movements<br>4. Sometimes, clinical observations indicative of poor vestibular-proprioceptive processing (see Chapter 4) |

praxia, whereas others are frequently associated problems that are more accurately viewed as *end products of, or sequelae to, dyspraxia*. Further, as we already mentioned, the clinical picture of clients with somatodyspraxia varies considerably. As we will see, if we compare these indicators with those manifested by Keisha, clients with somatodyspraxia generally do not show *all* these problems.

## Play, Developmental, and Educational Indices

Dyspraxia, in its milder forms, often will not be detected during the first few years of life, as the child usually achieves motor milestones within normal (albeit often low normal) limits (Gubbay, 1979, 1985). Although the child often may bump into things and need more help than do most other children of the same age, this is often dismissed by the child's parents as an "individual variation." However, when the parents of a child subsequently identified as dyspraxic look back at this period of their child's development, they often say that they "felt something was wrong," but they didn't know what it was.

In the preschool years, problems become more evident. The child often has difficulty with certain aspects of activities of daily living such as learning to fasten buttons, blowing his or her nose, and manipulating objects such as door handles. The child often has difficulty with puzzles, with cutting, coloring, and pasting, and with playground equipment. However, because many preschool programs provide children with individual activity choices, the child with developmental dyspraxia may avoid those activities he or she finds difficult. Again, this may be interpreted by the child's teacher as individual preference or style, and thus the child's problems may not always be recognized.

As was the case with Keisha, previously unrecognized problems become evident in the early school years; previously identified problems become more apparent. Two factors appear to contribute to this. First, many of the school, home, and play activities in which school-aged children participate are highly structured. For example, daily routines are to be completed within allotted time frames, organized sports are to be played according to specific rules, and school work is to be neat. Second, in many instances, the child no longer has the option of avoiding participation; often participation is required. For the child with developmental dyspraxia, continued problems in dressing (including managing fastenings such as zippers and shoe laces) may result in the morning routine of getting dressed for school becoming a "battleground" between parent and child. In school, the child may experience difficulty in handwriting and art projects that involve cutting, coloring, pasting, and assembling. Play skills such as learning to ride a bicycle, skipping rope, and ball activities are performed with difficulty. Finally, organized sports and physical education become increasingly important and the child often experiences difficulties in these areas.

In the third and fourth grades, there is a dramatic increase in demands for written output (Levine, 1987). Levine used the term *developmental output failure* to describe the problem of children whose academic *production* cannot keep pace with expectations. One reason for their "failure" is that the motor implementation of written work is deficient. According to Levine (1987), "writing becomes the sine qua non of academic productivity" (p. 224), and the demands for high output and for increasingly sophisticated visuomotor (graphomotor) implementation increase as the child progresses in school. Thus, the production or output failure may be due to poor visuomotor skills, fine motor dysfunction, or difficulties with the input or memory programs needed to plan or guide the written output. Failure to keep up with the amount of work required may result in a decline in grades, in motivation, and in self-esteem (Levine, 1984). Because problems in this area are one of the major reasons why school-aged children with sensory integrative dysfunction are referred for occupational therapy services, we have included in Appendix 6–A a more detailed discussion of fine motor and handwriting deficits.

Even in adulthood, developmental dyspraxia may limit career choices and influence choice of leisure activities. In a follow-up study of 24 clumsy children and matched controls, Knuckey and Gubbay (1983) found that the adults who had been clumsy as children had less skilled jobs (with regard to manual dexterity) than did normal control subjects. This applied particularly to those subjects who had been most clumsy as children. Thus, when a student manifests dysfunction in both academic and motor realms, it is even more likely to impact on his or her future work and play roles.

## Behavioral Characteristics

We introduced the relationship between dyspraxia and frequently accompanying behavioral manifestations in our discussion of the spiral process of self-actualization in Chapter 1. This was elaborated in Chapter 2 when we discussed the relationship between the mind and the brain-body. The client with developmental dyspraxia does not have adequate motor planning skills and therefore cannot effectively interact with, and influence, his or her environment. This impacts on the client's belief in his or her ability (belief in skill) and his or her sense of control, which influences the client's sense of mastery, self-confidence, and subsequent satisfaction. This in turn may impact on the client's "will to do" (described as "intention" by some authors, or as motivation, inner drive, and self-direction in Chapters 1 and 2).

Because the client with somatodyspraxia often has poor play or sports skills, he or she may be teased by peers and excluded from games. This frequently results in a low self-esteem and increased isolation. Shaw, Levine, and Belfer (1982) found that children with learning disabilities and poor motor coordination had more problems in self-esteem than did children with learning disabilities and adequate motor coordination. They stated that the children with both learning and motor problems were at particular risk for low self-esteem and named this phenomenon "developmental double jeopardy." We saw this phenomenon in Chapter 2 in our description of Joe, a boy who desperately wanted to play baseball well and yet knew that he was "no good" at playing the game. This *may* be less of a problem for Keisha because she seems to enjoy more quiet indoor games. We wonder, however, about her choosing to swing alone at recess rather than playing with the other children.

As was the case with Joe, many children with dyspraxia are aware of the things they cannot do. Unlike Joe, who persisted in trying to learn to play baseball despite a history of "bad" experiences playing baseball, they often try to avoid situations they find difficult. They may try to restructure tasks and "make deals" with peers or adults. As a result, children with dyspraxia often are seen as manipulative. Although we do not know for sure, this may be the case with Keisha. It does seem to be the case that she "manipulates" which play activities she and her friends choose.

## Patterns of Test Performance and Related Problems

### TESTS OF INTELLIGENCE

According to Gubbay (1975, 1985), the child with dyspraxia has normal intelligence. Dawdy (1981) favored a broader definition, stating "it is probably unrealistic and theoretically restrictive to assume normal or near-normal intellectual capacity as a diagnostic criterion" (p. 34). Thus, the issue of intelligence remains controversial. Can we consider a client with mental retardation to be dyspraxic? The client with mental retardation typically is delayed in all areas, including language. When a client's language delays are consistent with the delays manifested in other areas, we would not consider calling the client aphasic. Similarly, when the delays in motor planning are consistent with the client's cognitive and motor development, we would not consider the client to be dyspraxic. Furthermore, we must be careful not to consider delays in motor performance (as determined by standardized assessment) as necessarily indicative of poor motor planning. Therefore, we *only* consider a client with mental retardation to be dyspraxic if (a) the motor deficits are due to poor motor planning and not poor motor skill, per se; and (b) the motor planning deficits are *significantly below his or her performance in other areas.*

Gubbay (1975) also stated that the single most important diagnostic criterion of dyspraxia is a significantly lower performance IQ than verbal IQ score (usually considered to be a 15-point discrepancy) on the Revised Wechsler Intelligence Scale for Children. While this pattern is characteristic for many children with learning disabilities, and may be true for the child with good conceptual abilities but poor motor planning abilities, not all children with dyspraxia meet these criteria. For example, children with dysphasia and dyspraxia might manifest lower verbal IQ than performance IQ scores. Such a scoring pattern also is seen in most apraxic adults, in whom apraxia is usually associated with left hemisphere damage (Lezak, 1983). We do not have Keisha's verbal and performance IQ scores, but *if* she has a significant difference between her two IQ scores, we can guess, based on her good verbal skills and her poor visuomotor skills, that her performance IQ is the one that is lower.

### SIPT AND RELATED CLINICAL OBSERVATIONS

The child with somatodyspraxia shows a characteristic pattern of test scores on the SIPT and related clinical observations of neuromotor behavior that is highlighted in Table 6-1 (Ayres, 1972a, 1975, 1976, 1979, 1989). Recalling Keisha's SIPT performance, we note that she had deficient scores on the four major tests of praxis: Postural Praxis, Bilateral Motor Coordination, Sequencing Praxis, and Oral Praxis. As is often the case with children with dyspraxia and good verbal skills, her Praxis on Verbal Command score was normal. We also see that Keisha has low scores on all but one of the important tests of somatosensory processing. The results of her clinical observation revealed both (a) poor supine flexion and possibly poor sequential finger touching, and (b) a meaningful cluster of scores suggestive of poor vestibular-proprioceptive processing. *It is this overall test score pattern that leads us to identify a child such as Keisha as having somatodyspraxia.* In contrast, as we implied earlier, the other indices and behavioral characteristics we have discussed are more appropriately viewed as commonly occurring presenting problems or sequelae of the primary disorder of somatodyspraxia. This includes Keisha's poor performance on tests of visuomotor skill. Again, we want to emphasize that many children with somatodyspraxia will not show low scores on all of these tests. Moreover, low scores on many of these tests are not unique to the clinical picture of somatodyspraxia and may be seen with other types of dysfunction (see Table 1–1, which highlights this point).

# NEUROANATOMICAL BASIS OF APRAXIA

When we compare the literature on adult-onset apraxia to the literature on developmental dyspraxia, we find that much more has been done to explore the neuroanatomical basis of adult-onset practic disorders. While adult-onset practic disorders share some common characteristics with somatodyspraxia (e.g., hypothesized conceptual basis, impairments of sequencing, poor quality of motor execution), the two disorders are not synonymous. Nevertheless, provided that we remain cognizant of the fundamental differences between the two disorders, review of aspects of the neuroanatomical bases for adult-onset apraxia can provide us with insight into possible neuroanatomical and behavioral aspects of developmental dyspraxia. For example, in Chapter 4 we reviewed the roles in motor planning of the medial supplementary and lateral arcuate premotor areas, which were determined based on the study of adults with known brain lesions. Then, we speculated that similar symptoms *might occur* if sensory inputs to these cortical motor planning centers were impaired (see Table 4–1).

Additional research has further clarified the role of the supplementary medial motor area in motor planning. Based on (a) the results of two case studies in which the role of the left supplementary motor area was implicated in praxis (Watson, Fleet, Gonzalez-Rothi, & Heilman, 1986) and (b) the anatomical and physiological literature, which suggests that the supplementary motor area is involved in motor programming (Brinkman & Porter, 1979; Roland, Larsen, Lassen, & Skinhoj, 1980), Watson et al. (1986) concluded that the supplementary motor area is important for programming transitive movements of the limbs. Transitive movements are movements made in relationship to an object or instrument (e.g., hammer). Watson and colleagues stated that proper use of a tool requires a centrally generated command and sensory feedback. It has been proposed that the supplementary motor area may be important for generating central commands and influencing the level of activity in area 4 during the period of preparation.

Much of the literature on lesions producing adult-onset apraxia has emphasized the role of cortical structures and particularly the frontal (premotor cortex) and parietal lobes of left hemisphere (Faglioni & Basso, 1985; Geschwind, 1975; Gonzalez-Rothi, Mack, & Heilman, 1986; Luria, 1980). Yet, in spite of the focus on the role of the left hemisphere, it appears that there is not one specific area that is clearly responsible for adult-onset apraxia. Luria (1980) consistently stressed the importance of *functional systems* in most complex activities, including praxis. Other researchers elaborated on this view that the neuroanatomical substrate of praxis may be recognized as a functional system, and recognized the contribution of both the right hemisphere (Basso, Capitani, Laiacona, & Zanobio, 1985; DeRenzi, Motti, & Nichelli, 1980; Rapcsak, Gonzalez-Rothi, & Heilman, 1987) and deep structures (Agostoni, Coletti, Orlando, & Tredici, 1983; Kolb & Whishaw, 1985; Paillard, 1982).

Basso, Capitani, Sala, Laiacona, and Spinnler (1987) stated that "there must be some specific role of deep structures in the genesis of apraxia" (p. 145). However, they were not able to identify any crucial structure whose damage would separate neurologically impaired patients with practic disorders from neurologically impaired patients without practic disorders. This finding may be explained by widespread interconnections among brain areas.

The striatum has wide connections with the associative parietal cortex (ipsilateral and contralateral), and it is widely interconnected also with various parts of the thalamus, with the globus pallidus, subthalamus and especially with the substantia nigra. All these structures are links in complex feed-back circuits and it is therefore not surprising that apraxia can occur whatever the damaged structure is. (Agostoni et al., 1983, p. 807)

Finally, Agostoni and colleagues (1983) reported on seven patients with apraxia who had lesions of the basal ganglia or thalamus. They concluded that apraxia is not only a higher-level cortical function, but may depend also on the integrity of *subcortical* circuits and structures.

The hypothesized basis of somatodyspraxia focuses on impaired tactile, proprioceptive, and possibly vestibular (polymodal) processing in subcortical structures (Ayres, 1972a, 1979, 1989). Increased understanding of the role of these structures, similarly obtained from studies of adults with identified lesions, potentially can provide insight into the impact of neural dysfunction within these structures that may result from impaired processing of polymodal, somatosensory inputs.

For example, Brooks (1986) discussed the role of the *limbic system* in praxis and motor learning. He suggested that the limbic system may serve in a "comparator role" in the process of gaining insight into the solution of a task in motor learning. Brooks (1986) suggested that insightful behavior relates to "knowing what to do." He emphasized that learning to perform a task requires an understanding of its nature, and that knowing "what to do" precedes learning "how to do it." Based on research with monkeys, Brooks proposed a "limbic comparator hypothesis," in which he stated that "insightful learning is governed by comparison in various neural centers of two converging limbic projections, one from the relevance-sensitive amygdala and another from corollary recipients of amygdaloid information such as the cingulate cortex" (pp. 31–32).

In examining motor control mechanisms in skilled movement, Paillard (1982) suggested that learned programs are not prewired as are inborn programs, and that "command signals" from the cortex (inducing the parietal cortex) mobilize subcortical programs of learned motor acts (that may be found in the basal ganglia), which, in turn, activate the motor cortex. Kolb and Whishaw (1985) also noted the functional relationship between cortical and subcortical structures and suggested that damage to subcortical structures may be "essential to apraxia" (p. 211).

## ETIOLOGY OF DEVELOPMENTAL DYSPRAXIA

### Neuroanatomical Basis

Whereas it is apparent that many regions of the brain contribute to praxis, the "locus of lesion" in adult-onset apraxia is generally viewed as the left, language-dominant hemisphere (Poeck, 1982). In contrast, there is not a clear-cut, well-established, and agreed-upon neuroanatomical structure implicated in the cause of developmental dyspraxia. In fact, in 1979, Gubbay defined the clumsy child as one "whose ability to perform skilled movement is impaired despite normal intelligence and *normal findings on conventional neurological examination* [italics added]" (p. 146). Frank brain damage would therefore disqualify a client from the diagnosis of developmental dyspraxia. This view now may be changing, based on more sophisticated procedures such as computerized tomography (CT) scans, magnetic resonance imaging (MRI), positron emission tomography (PET) scans, and regional cerebral blood flow studies (rCBF) that enable us to more accurately examine the brain's structure and function.

Despite the existence of this new technology, few studies of children with developmental clumsiness have used it. Nevertheless, in a landmark study in which CT scans of clumsy children were examined, researchers found that 39 percent of the sample of clumsy children showed abnormal CT scans, compared to only 9 percent of the controls (Knuckey, Apsimon, & Gubbay, 1983). Furthermore, when the group of clumsy children was subdivided into clumsy and very clumsy children, the incidence of abnormal CT scans in the very clumsy children was 48 percent. Specific deficits noted included ventricular dilation, peripheral atrophy, and prominent brain regions. There also were several cases with more specific parenchymal abnormalities; however, in these cases a particular pattern of deficit was not evident. As opposed to adult-onset apraxia, the left hemisphere was not found to be most frequently involved in these children.

Because Knuckey and colleagues (1983) selected their subjects for "clumsiness" based on an eight-item screening test, and they did not evaluate the sensory integrative status of their subjects, it is not possible to know to what extent these results may be applied to the client with developmental dyspraxia or the specific subgroup with somatodyspraxia. Rather, difficulty in localizing a specific neurological "substrate" or "locus" for developmental dyspraxia favors the viewpoint posited by Luria (1963, 1980) and others (Basso, Luzzatti, & Spinnler, 1980; DeRenzi, Faglioni, & Sorgato, 1982) that praxis is dependent upon a complex functional system or network involving cortical and subcortical structures. Conrad, Cermak, and Drake (1983) suggested a similar concept in their study with children.

## Significant Birth History

Gubbay (1978, 1985) examined the birth histories of children with dyspraxia and noted that, in 50 percent of the cases, there was a significant history of prenatal, perinatal, or neonatal factors. He also noted that the ratio of males to females was two to one and that there was a higher percentage of firstborn children. Whereas problems at birth might be a factor in the cause of developmental dyspraxia, half of the children with dyspraxia did not have significant birth histories. Further, similar findings of significant birth histories have been reported for individuals with any of a number of other disabilities, such as learning disabilities, autism, and mental retardation (Geschwind & Galaburda, 1985), indicating that such histories are not unique to clients with developmental dyspraxia.

## An Important Historical Aside

Before we begin to discuss the role of somatosensation in the next section of this chapter, it is important to clarify a number of critical issues. All of these have been discussed earlier, either in this chapter or in previous chapters. All of them converge when we apply them to the disorder we now know as somatodyspraxia.

First, when Ayres (1972a, 1979, 1989) considered the role of somatosensation in praxis, she *emphasized* tactile information (discriminative touch). Only *secondarily* did she consider proprioception (and possibly vestibular-proprioception). Yet, because both discriminative touch and proprioception are conveyed to cortical structures via the dorsal column medial lemniscal pathway, researchers who have studied the effects of dorsal column lesions have not clarified whether the deficits we observe are due to impaired tactile discrimination, impaired proprioception, or both (impaired somatosensation). We now recognize, however, that when we consider the role of tactile and proprioceptive information in motor planning, this distinction may become very important. In Chapter 4, we summarized the role of the medial and lateral premotor areas in motor planning. Whereas the medial supplementary motor area is proprioceptive-dependent, the lateral arcuate premotor area is polymodal. Tactile and visual, as well as proprioceptive, information is projected to the lateral arcuate premotor area (Goldberg, 1985) (see also Table 4–1).

In Chapter 4, we proposed that bilateral integration and sequencing deficits were generally subtle, and primarily confined to impairments of bilateral and projected action sequences. Anticipation, or the ability to project into the future, is a critical component of this more subtle motor planning deficit. It is hypothesized that bilateral integration and sequence of deficits have their basis in vestibular-proprioceptive, *but not tactile*, processing deficits. As we will discuss, somatodyspraxia is often associated with *both* tactile and proprioceptive processing deficits, and with deficits in *both* anticipatory projected action sequences as well as deficits in responsive, input-dependent, segmental actions (see Table 4–1; see also Chapter 10).

What we are saying is that individuals with somatodyspraxia may display all of the motor planning deficits we see in individuals with bilateral integration and sequencing disorders. The distinction is that, for those with somatodyspraxia, the motor planning deficits may be more severe. With the addition of deficits in tactile perception, we hypothesize that feedback-dependent motor planning deficits may be *superimposed* on the feedforward-dependent deficits seen in bilateral integration and sequencing disorders.

Finally, we must acknowledge that much of what we hypothesize about both somatodyspraxia and bilateral integration and sequencing deficits is based on a tradition of research spanning more than three decades that heretofore has (a) not *fully* recognized the important contributions of proprioception to motor planning, (b) attributed many of the important contributions of proprioception *solely* to tactile perception (e.g., body scheme), and (c) distinguished between tactile- or somatosensory-based deficits in motor planning and vestibular-based deficits in bilateral motor control. That is, children identified as having vestibular bilateral integration disorders *were not previously viewed as having dyspraxia* (Ayres 1972a, 1979).

Therefore, the purpose of this section is to expand on the important concepts pertaining to the role of tactile and proprioceptive (and possibly vestibular) information we discussed in Chapters 4 and 5, and to apply them to the client who has the *combined* deficits associated with somatodyspraxia.

## Role of Somatosensation

Ayres (1972a, 1979, 1989) suggested that, rather than actual brain damage, somatodyspraxia is due to an impairment in perception of sensory, especially tactile, information. Based on a series of factor-analytic studies (Ayres, 1965, 1966, 1969, 1977), in which an association repeatedly was found between motor planning and tactile discrimination, Ayres (1972a, 1979) proposed that a close relationship exists between problems in perception of tactile information, problems in body scheme, and motor planning problems.

Ayres' most recent factor analyses of SIPT scores resulted in the identification of a factor characterized by poor motor planning (low praxis test scores). Although she labeled this factor somatopraxis, the only somatosensory test that consistently loaded on this factor was Graphesthesia, a low test score that also is commonly associated with bilateral integration and sequencing deficits (see Chapter 4). The other somatosensory tests tended to load on factors she labeled as being associated with somatosensory processing (Ayres, 1989) (see also Chapter 8). Based on the analysis of actual case profiles which revealed that children with low scores on the praxis tests also often had low scores on the somatosensory tests (A. J. Ayres, personal communication, February 20, 1988), and her historical perspective that motor planning deficits commonly are associated with poor tactile discrimination, she labeled this practic disorder somatodyspraxia. Thus, Ayres viewed dysfunction in the perception of tactile information as a critical link in the problem of somatodyspraxia.

The distinction here is subtle, but very important. Children with bilateral integration and sequencing deficits also have low scores on the praxis tests that loaded on the factor Ayres labeled as somatopraxis. As we stated earlier, children with somatodyspraxia differ from those with bilateral integration and sequencing deficits in that they have low scores on the tests that loaded on *both* the factor labeled *somatopraxis* and the factor labeled *somatosensory processing* (see Table 1–4). Thus, the label for the somatopraxis factor might more appropriately have been simply *praxis* (or some other, more "neutral" term).

## Body Scheme as a Basis for Praxis

As we discussed in detail in Chapter 4, "body scheme" refers to an internal model of the body in action. It is largely unconscious and built from sensations and previous responses to external stimuli, especially proprioceptive information associated with corollary discharge (see Chapter 4).

As we stated earlier, Ayres (1972a, 1979, 1985) may have overemphasized the role of tactile discrimination in the development of the body scheme. For example, she said motor planning involves the development of a semiconscious motor scheme that begins with the development of tactile sensory awareness (Ayres, 1972a). She elaborated on this hypothesis by stating that "sensory input from the skin and joints, but especially from the skin, helps develop, in the brain, the model or internal scheme of the body's design as a motor instrument" (p. 168). The relationship between sensation and adaptive motor behavior in the development of an adequate body scheme is highlighted by her statement that

> the somatomotor system is constantly in a state of change in pattern, with the somatic changes arising from movement, leaving in the brain some memory by which to guide a similar or more complicated movement the next time it is needed. The use of the body determines the concept or scheme of the body through the result of action and the stimuli resulting from the action. (pp. 169–170)

Ayres (1972a) suggested that "if the information which the body receives from its somatosensory receptors is not precise, the brain has a poor basis on which to build its scheme of the body" (p. 170).

Ayres (1972a, 1975, 1979, 1985) consistently hypothesized that the body scheme (termed *body percept* in 1985) is critical to the ability to motor plan, and that processing of tactile as well as proprioceptive information is of critical importance in the development of an adequate body scheme. Other investigators (e.g., Schilder, 1935) also have emphasized the importance of an adequate body scheme and suggested that processing and integration of tactile, vestibular-proprioceptive, and visual information contributes to its development. Recent evidence suggests that proprioception, derived from active participation in adaptive sensorimotor behavior, is of primary importance in the development of body scheme (see Chapter 4). Like Ayres, Piaget (1952) emphasized sensorimotor experiences and adaptive motor behavior (active participation) as important to the development of an internal model of the body.

## Research on Somatosensory Systems

Because Ayres' (1965, 1966, 1969, 1971, 1972b, 1977) factor-analytic studies identified a close and repeated relationship between motor planning and somatosensory processing, it is important to examine more fully the role of the tactile system and its relationship to motor planning. The traditional view of the tactile system was reviewed in Chapter 5. Essentially, the dorsal column medial lemniscal system has been viewed as being primarily responsible for the discrimination of the spatial and temporal characteristics of stimuli, whereas the anterolateral system has been viewed as serving the more general aspects of sensation, including pain and temperature (Mountcastle, 1980).

Based on experimental research with monkeys, cats, and rats, as well as on clinical observation of humans with spinal cord damage, new roles have emerged for the dorsal column (Vierck, 1978; Wall, 1970). That is, research has indicated that the dorsal column medial lemniscal system has a role in more than just discrimination of tactile information. Wall (1970) identified two classes of deficits that resulted from dorsal column lesions, those that pertain to motor performance, and those that pertain to attention, orientation, and anticipation. These behaviors, summarized in Table 6–2, are hypothesized to be critical to motor planning. As we discussed, many of these behaviors also are seen in the client the bilateral integration and sequencing deficits. Thus, we must question whether some or all of these behaviors are proprioceptive- as well as tactually-dependent. As we proceed to discuss the specific characteristics of the deficits within each class of behaviors, we will attempt to compare the deficits noted in animals to the behaviors we often see in clients with somatodyspraxia. However, in so doing, we recognize that such extrapolation is highly theoretical and speculative, and *must be interpreted with caution.*

**TABLE 6–2. NEWER VIEWS ON THE ROLE OF THE DORSAL COLUMN MEDIAL LEMNISCAL SYSTEM**

| *Motor* |
| --- |
| Initiation of voluntary movements |
| Performance of complex movement sequences and refined manual dexterity |
| Handling objects in space |
| Flexion of joints |

| *Selective Attention, Orientation, and Anticipation* |
| --- |
| Unraveling competing stimuli |
| Initiating and controlling internal search |
| Anticipatory components of sequential behavior patterns |

## MOTOR DEFICITS

Following dorsal column lesions, monkeys tended not to initiate voluntary movement and did not actively explore their environments. Among the most speculative of our extrapolations is to suggest that this may be similar to the behavior seen in clients with somatodyspraxia who, like Keisha, often prefer sedentary activities. The monkeys also evidenced particular problems in complex movement sequences and in refined manual dexterity; both (a) the ability to make adjustments to subtle changes in response to moving objects or contour of objects, and (b) thumb-to-finger opposition were impaired (Vierck, 1978; Wall, 1970). This latter finding, since it is not commonly associated with bilateral integration and sequencing deficits, makes us wonder whether Keisha's poor tactile discrimination may be related more to her poor manipulation and fine motor planning abilities than to her gross motor planning deficits. Vierck (1978) suggested that "the dorsal column relay to the motor cortex occurs quickly and appears to specify the direction of fine distal movements rather than the reaction of the entire limb" (p. 144). The possibility of a dissociation between fine and gross motor planning emphasizes the need to differentially examine both aspects of developmental dyspraxia in clients. Unfortunately, the SIPT visuomotor tests (Design Copying and Motor Accuracy) are limited in their ability to differentiate between fine motor planning deficits and poor visuomotor skill.

The third, and related, motor aspect noted was a clumsiness in handling objects in space. Hand and finger movements were slow and inept when reaching for food even though fine delicate movements occurred with personal grooming. Mountcastle and colleagues (Mountcastle, Lynch, Georgopoulos, Sakata, & Acuna, 1975) presented findings on the complex interaction of tactile, proprioceptive, and visual information in the areas of the parietal lobe, particularly areas 5 and 7, that may help us to understand this distinction between personal and extrapersonal space. In research with monkeys, Mountcastle and colleagues found cells in area 7 that responded only if the monkey was reaching for something in extrapersonal space. Using regional cerebral blood flow studies, researchers also have found that different areas of the brain are activated as a function of personal vs. extrapersonal space (Roland, Skinhoj, Lassen, & Larsen, 1980).

In Keisha's case, we observed that she had problems with buttoning (personal space), as well as with manipulating puzzles (extrapersonal space). We have no way of knowing if one is more impaired than the other. Therefore, a fruitful area of research would be an examination of praxis for actions performed on the body vs. away from the body. Certain investigators have begun to explore this in children (Conrad, Cermak, & Drake, 1983; Kaplan, 1968; Overton & Jackson, 1973).

Finally, there is evidence that the dorsal column medial lemniscal system may be more involved in flexion than extension. Lesions of the dorsal column produced flexion hypotonia in monkeys. It is interesting for us to speculate as to whether this finding relates to the observation that clients, like Keisha, with somatodyspraxia have particular problems in supine flexion (Ayres, 1979). We also feel that it is important to differentiate between the poor total body flexion seen in clients with somatodyspraxia, and the difficulty in *righting the head* from the supine position seen in clients with vestibular-proprioceptive processing disorders (see Chapter 4). In total body flexion, the tactile component *may be* particularly important.

## ATTENTION, ORIENTATION, AND ANTICIPATION

Wall (1970) reported a case in which a patient had sustained a lesion of the dorsal column 10 years prior to testing and who, at the time of testing, had normal cutaneous threshold and two-point discrimination. However, when the patient was distracted by having to read aloud, he demonstrated deficits in detecting tactile stimuli. This indicated that the dorsal column might play some role in organization by sorting out information, since when the patient was attending to one stimulus (reading), he could not simultaneously direct his *attention* to the tactile stimulus.

In a study of rats with dorsal column lesions, stimulation of the hind leg resulted in the animal's withdrawing its leg, but did not result in the animal's turning its head to locate the stimulus, as would normally be expected. This may indicate that the dorsal column is involved in those movements that bring in more sensory information (viz. orientation).

This research suggests that the dorsal column medial lemniscal system is involved in *initiating and controlling internal search* that is then followed by active exploration or external search in *anticipation* of gathering more sensory information. That is, in early *orientation*, the stimulus (e.g., touch to leg) triggers a motor response in which the animal (or person) directs its sense organs (*attention*) to the location of the stimulus. "This motor response has the effect of collecting more afferent information about the circumstances surrounding a stimulus detected by the somatosensory system" (Wall, 1970, p. 518). Research has indicated that when the dorsal columns are lesioned, "this type of exploration occurs at a very low rate" (p. 518).

Thus, signals arriving over the dorsal column medial lemniscal system trigger exploratory behavior and may serve to guide movement to gather sensation by contributing to the programming of motor responses that will help generate further sensation. In other words, the dorsal columns are involved in orientation, initiation of action, and exploratory movements.

Imagine being handed an object and asked to identify what it is without looking at it. As you turn it over in your hand and run your fingers along the contours or edges, somehow the search is organized into a logical, anticipatory motor manipulation sequence that contributes to the organized gathering of sensory information about the object. We might speculate that the same organizing process occurs when we hand a young child a small toy, even when the child simultaneously can gather information through both the visual and tactile sensory channels. Perhaps Keisha's poor tactile discrimination abilities impaired her ability to organize, and benefit from, object manipulation.

Another study further supports the hypothesis that the dorsal column medial lemniscal system is necessary for the *anticipatory components of projected action sequences*, which are impaired in clients with *both* bilateral integration and sequencing disorders and somatopraxis. In this study, cats with lesions of the dorsal column were unable to jump over barriers while being carried on a moving conveyor belt even though they could see the barrier (Melzack & Southmayd, 1974). They needed the tactile stimulus of their paws making contact with the bar before they would jump. That is, their impairments pertained to feedforward more than feedback motor control. When proprioceptive control of projected action sequences is impaired, there is increased reliance on tactile inputs (See Chapter 4). An important difference between the client with somatodyspraxia and the client with bilateral integration and sequencing deficits *may be* that the client with somatodyspraxia also is limited in his or her ability to benefit from the provision of tactile information.

Two examples of clients who have difficulty with anticipatory components of behavior come to mind. While both of these boys happened to have somatodyspraxia, clients with bilateral integration and sequencing deficits are likely to demonstrate similar behaviors. In one instance, Scott, one of the boys, stood on a platform and was asked to swing on a trapeze across a set of pillows, to return, and then on the second pass, to let go and drop down directly onto the pillows. Scott was unable to anticipate at what point to let go in order to land on the pillows. Even when his feet scraped the surface of the pillows, he would swing to the far end and return, passing over the pillows again and landing on the platform. The second example comes from a report of the mother of an 11-year-old boy. She said that as she watched her son, Ralph, pull his sled back up the hill, she saw another boy on a sled coming down the hill directly toward Ralph. She did not yell because she was sure Ralph had seen the other sled and that he would get out of the way. However, Ralph kept pulling his sled up the hill and the other boy ran into him. When his mother later asked Ralph if he had seen the other sled, Ralph replied that he had seen it, but he had not realized that it would hit him.

In summary, the dorsal column medial lemniscal system seems to be involved not only in tactile and proprioceptive discrimination, but also in complex movement sequences and refined manual dexterity; manipulation in space; selective attention, orientation, and anticipation; and programming of complex movement sequences. Comparison of the client with somatodyspraxia and the client with bilateral integration and sequencing deficits suggests that the tactile (or polymodal) contributions pertain especially to manual dexterity and manipulation (see also Chapter 5), and to selective attention and orientation. Future research may further clarify the relative contributions of the tactile and vestibular-proprioceptive systems.

## Summary of Neuroanatomical Base

Adult-onset apraxia most frequently occurs following brain damage to the left hemisphere, particularly the parietal and frontal lobes. However, damage to other structures also has been associated with apraxia. Developmental dyspraxia is not specifically associated with any particular type of brain damage (Knuckey, Apsimon, & Gubbay, 1983; Nass, 1983). Rather, the integrity of many different neural structures appears to be important. The contributions of the processing of tactile and proprioceptive sensory information to the development of praxis have been highlighted. Wherever possible, the unique contributions of the tactile system to somatodyspraxia have been clarified. It is interesting that the role of sensory processing has been only minimally discussed with regards to adult-onset apraxia. It may be that sensory integration is more critical to the developing child than it is to the adult. Yet, it remains unfortunate that there is such limited research on the possible differences in somatosensory contributions to motor planning abilities that develop across the age span.

## CONCEPTUAL FACTORS IN DYSPRAXIA

Although Ayres (1972a, 1979) early work on dyspraxia emphasized the role of the tactile system in motor planning, Ayres also stressed the cortical role in praxis. In 1972, she stated that "as movement assumes meaning, the child learns to motor plan or *how to cortically direct his movements* [italics added]" (1972a, p. 170), and that "the major substrate of praxis is believed to be diencephalic and cortical" (p. 171). Her more current views have expanded and elaborated on the cortical contributions to praxis. In a seminal piece in 1985, Ayres, stated that

> the brain must have various kinds of information to enable it to motor plan. First, it must have the idea of the purposeful act. It must be able to conceptualize the action and its goal. Then it must be able to know how the body is designed and

how it functions as a mechanical being. That information comes from the tactile, kinesthetic, other proprioceptive, and vestibular systems. Vision also helps. (p. 24)

In recent factor and cluster analyses of SIPT scores, Ayres (1989) identified a group of children whose SIPT scores were associated with visual-perceptual as well as motor planning deficits. She called this cluster group visuo- and somatodyspraxia because of a hypothesized common conceptual link between praxis and visual perception. That is, Ayres (1989) noted that there is evidence to suggest visual perception and praxis are closely aligned and suggested that "a conceptual system common to praxis also appears to serve visual perception" (p. 199) (see also Chapter 8).

## ASSESSMENT OF SOMATODYSPRAXIA

### Differential Identification of Practic Disorders

As we have stressed throughout this chapter, the identification of somatodyspraxia requires assessment of both tactile and vestibular-proprioceptive sensory processing as well as motor planning. The specific tests of the SIPT and related clinical observations of neuromotor behavior helpful in identifying somatodyspraxia are listed in Table 6–1. As with any sensory integrative disorder, identification is based on a meaningful cluster of test scores indicative of a deficit, in this case, in tactile discrimination (with or without concurrent deficits in vestibular-proprioceptive processing), and a meaningful cluster of scores indicative of poor motor planning.

As we have pointed out on numerous occasions, the child who has a meaningful cluster of scores indicative of dyspraxia and a meaningful cluster of scores indicative of vestibular-proprioceptive processing deficits, but *normal* tactile discrimination abilities would most likely be identified as having a bilateral integration and sequencing disorder (rather than somatodyspraxia). (Low scores on Graphesthesia are expected in children with bilateral integration and sequencing deficits as well as in those with somatodyspraxia.) A client with poor motor coordination who does not show difficulty in the processing of tactile or vestibular-proprioceptive information, and who does not have a history of difficulty processing information in these domains, would *not* be considered to have a sensory integrative disorder and would not likely be a client for whom sensory integration procedures are appropriate. This includes the client who has low scores on Praxis on Verbal Command in the *absence* of a sensory processing disorder.

### History Taking and Interview Techniques

Careful interview of parents and teachers, combined with the use of a sensory history questionnaire (Larson, 1982) can be very helpful in clarifying the presenting problem and the sequelae to the practic disorder. For example, a report that the child achieved motor milestones such as sitting and crawling at an appropriate age, but is now having difficulty with more complex tasks such as buttoning and fastening zippers, would alert a therapist to the need to evaluate for a possible motor planning problem. In Table 6–3 we have presented a motor development checklist for young children. Other commonly associated behaviors are noted in Table 6–1. We want to stress, however, that behavioral problems and motor delays are not necessarily

TABLE 6-3. MOTOR DEVELOPMENT CHECKLIST FOR PRESCHOOLERS*

| Task | Age Achieved |
|---|---|
| Bangs two sticks together after demonstration | 18 months |
| Uses spoon, spilling little | 2 years |
| Uses fork to pierce food | 2 years |
| Can climb out of large low box | 2 years |
| Rides a tricycle | 3 years |
| Uses scissors to snip | 3 years |
| Buttons small buttons | 4 years |
| Pumps self on swing | 4 years |
| Can neatly cut out a circle | 5 years |
| Skips reciprocally | 5-6 years |
| Ties shoelaces | 6 years |
| Rides a two-wheeled bicycle without training wheels | 6-7 years |

*Adapted from Ayres (1979).

indicative of a practic disorder. Rather, we feel it is more appropriate to think that developmental delays may be one result of a practic disorder. The results of both the referral information and history taking with the child's parents and teachers should guide the therapist's selection of formal assessment tools and clinical observation methods (Dunn, 1990).

## Standardized Assessments

The most comprehensive tests of praxis for children are the SIPT (Ayres, 1989). As we have already discussed, they assess a variety of aspects of praxis. Somatodyspraxia is a disorder of praxis that is coupled with a disorder of tactile and, possibly, vestibular-proprioceptive processing. Therefore, poor performance on tests of praxis must occur concomitantly with low scores on the tactile tests. Vestibular-proprioceptive test scores also may be low, and poor vestibular-proprioceptive processing can contribute to somatodyspraxia. The tactile tests are described in Chapter 5 and the assessment of vestibular-proprioceptive processing is discussed in Chapter 4.

Although the SIPT are excellent tests, they are standardized only for children from 4 years to 8 years, 11 months of age. Thus, therapists must consider other tests for clients on either side of this age range. Table 6-4 presents a list of standardized tests that assess various aspects of motor planning and visuomotor skill, and which may provide alternatives to the SIPT. These tests also have limitations. For example, the Miller Assessment for Preschoolers (Miller, 1988), a well-standardized test that assesses some aspects of sensory integration, is a screening tool and is not designed specifically to examine different types of disorders in sensory integration and praxis. Similarly, the Bruininks-Oseretsky Test of Motor Proficiency (Bruininks, 1978) is a well-standardized test of motor function and covers a broad age range (5 to 14 years), but it does not assess sensory processing.

The Luria Nebraska Neuropsychological Battery: Children's Revision (Golden, 1987) is a 149-item multidimensional battery designed to diagnose general and specific cognitive deficits. This test, which is standardized for children from 8 to 12 years of age, includes 11 scales and takes about $2\frac{1}{2}$ hours to administer. Two scales assess functions that are similar to those assessed in the SIPT. The first is the Motor Function Scale, a 34-item subtest which includes items that involve copying positions assumed by the examiner, sequencing, oral praxis, and visuomotor skill. The second scale, the Tactile Scale, includes 16 items that assess localization of tactile stimuli, graphesthesia, and stereognosis. In contrast to the SIPT, the Luria Nebraska Neuro-

**TABLE 6–4. OTHER STANDARDIZED TESTS THAT ASSESS ASPECTS OF MOTOR PLANNING AND VISUOMOTOR SKILL**

| Test | Age (years) |
|------|-------------|
| Bruininks-Oseretsky Test of Motor Proficiency (Bruininks, 1978) | $4\frac{1}{2}$–$14\frac{1}{2}$ |
| Purdue Perceptual Motor Survey (Roach & Kephart, 1966) | 6–10 |
| Test of Motor Impairment (Stott, Moyes, & Henderson, 1984) | 5–13 |
| Frostig Movement Skills Battery (Orpet, 1972) | 6–12 |
| Quick Neurological Screening Test (Mutti, Sterling, & Spaulding, 1978) | 5–15 |
| Test of Motor Proficiency (Gubbay, 1975) | 8–12 |
| Meeting Street School Screening Test (Hainesworth & Siqueland, 1969) | $4$–$7\frac{1}{2}$ |
| Bender Gestalt Test (Koppitz, 1963) | 5–17 |
| Developmental Test of Visual Motor Integration–Revised (Beery, 1989) | 2–15 |
| Developmental Test of Visual Perception (Frostig, Lefever, & Whittlesey, 1963, 1966) | 4–8 |
| Miller Assessment for Preschoolers (Miller, 1988) | 2–5 |
| Pediatric Examination of Education Readiness (PEER) (Levine, 1982) | 4–6 |
| Pediatric Early Elementary Examination (PEEX) (Levine, 1983) | 7–9 |
| Pediatric Examination of Educational Readiness at Middle Childhood (PEERAMID) (Levine, 1985) | 9–15 |
| Luria Nebraska Neuropsychological Battery: Children's Revision (Golden, 1987) | 8–12 |

psychological Battery: Children's Revision only provides total scores for each domain of function (e.g., tactile, motor). As with the SIPT, advanced specialized training is needed to administer and interpret this test.

Additionally, because of the cognitive aspects of praxis, it is helpful to obtain from a psychologist an assessment of the client's intelligence. As we discussed earlier, a client whose poor-for-chronological-age practic abilities are *consistent* with his or her lower overall cognitive abilities would not be considered to be dyspraxic.

## Skilled Clinical Observation

### HAPTIC EXPLORATION

As we discussed in Chapter 5, a stereognosis task in which the client is asked to identify an object through the sense of touch can provide information about both his or her tactile discrimination abilities and his or her motor (manipulative) abilities. In this chapter, we will focus on the motor components, although the separation of the two is somewhat artificial.

As part of our clinical observations, we can observe how the client initiates active, exploratory manipulation. Research also has demonstrated a developmental progression in the acquisition of haptic manipulation strategies, with the accuracy of object identification being related to the level of sophistication of the haptic manipulation strategies used by the client during the testing (Abravanel, 1972a, 1972b; Hoop, 1971a, 1971b, Jennings, 1974; Kleinman, 1979; Wolff, 1972; Zaporozhets, 1965, 1969). Contour following (moving the fingers around the edge of the object) was found to be the optimum strategy for use in identifying shapes (Lederman & Klatsky, 1987). A description of the developmental progression for haptic manipulation strategies of common objects and shapes based on a summary of the work of Piaget and Inhelder (1948) and Zaporozhets (1965, 1969) follows.

$2\frac{1}{2}$ to 4 years:   Children may play with the object (e.g., push) but there is no active manual exploration. Grasping or touching of the object is seen, but the palm remains still when making contact with the object.

4 to 5 years:    Beginning of crude exploration is observed. Grasping of the object with the palm and middle of the fingers is seen; exploration remains passive. By 4 years, 6 months, exploration is done in a global, haphazard manner that includes probing for distinctive features.

5 to 6 years:    Systematic use of both hands (palms and fingers) begins. Isolated analysis of distinctive features, without studying the whole form, can be observed.

6 to 7 years:    Use of a systematic method of exploration can be seen. Contour following is used.

## MOTOR PERFORMANCE

Observing the client performing a variety of tasks and interacting with objects in the physical environment can provide the occupational therapist with invaluable information about how the client's practic abilities may be impacting on the client's gross and fine motor abilities. The therapist can observe the child in the classroom as he or she colors, uses scissors, or writes. This also may provide an opportunity to observe the child's ability to manage zippers, snaps, and buttons in preparation for recess or toileting activities. Observing the child in gym class provides the therapist with information about the child's gross motor skills.

Other clinical observations that frequently are associated with somatodyspraxia include the ability to assume the supine flexion position, sequential finger touching, and ability to perform rapid alternating movements. Finally, because somatodyspraxia is most evident when the client is performing novel or unfamiliar tasks, the therapist may find it helpful to observe the child in structured play situations that involve the use of sensory integration treatment equipment. For example, Parham (1987) described a child who wanted to ride on a scooter board and "instead of going through the motions that would bring her into a prone position on the board, . . . simply stood next to it, stepping in place repeatedly" (p. 31).

The performance disorder of the client with somatodyspraxia often is relatively subtle. Usually, the client with somatodyspraxia is not "totally unable" to perform tasks. Rather, he or she exhibits more trial and error, more effort, and poorer quality of performance. It is therefore critical for the therapist to have an experiential knowledge of normal development and the qualitative aspects of movement. This requires more than just a "textbook knowledge" of developmental milestones. The therapist must know and have a "feeling for" both *what* clients at different ages can do and *how* they do it. Evaluation of the *quality* of performance is essential.

# THEORETICAL ISSUES FOR THE INTERVENTION OF SOMATODYSPRAXIA

As we consider issues for intervention, let us return to Keisha. When we evaluated Keisha, we found that she had poor tactile perception and vestibular-proprioceptive processing. She also had marked difficulty on tests requiring motor planning and visuomotor coordination. We concluded that she had somatodyspraxia involving both gross and fine motor planning. We felt that her poor visuomotor coordination was an end product of her motor planning difficulties. This affected her handwriting, her self-care skills, and her play behavior.

As we began to think about planning an occupational therapy intervention program for Keisha based on the theory of sensory integration, we recalled that we wanted to provide her with enhanced opportunities to take in tactile, vestibular-proprioceptive, and visual (polymodal) sensory information within the context of her planning and producing meaningful adaptive behavior. Because she had problems with both gross and fine motor planning, we wanted to guide her in the choice of activities that involved both components. As we proceeded, we also wanted to consider certain theoretical issues related to the intervention for somatodyspraxia that reflect continuing or changing views on the nature of dyspraxia.

## Cognitive Processes

The first of these issues pertains to the utilization of an approach to intervention that incorporates "cognitive processes," including *visual direction of body action* and *verbal mediation and monitoring.* The provision of visual direction involves (a) reminding the client to look at what he or she is doing and where he or she is going, and (b) demonstrating the activity so as to provide the client with a visual model of how the activity is performed. Verbal mediation and monitoring include requesting the client to verbalize what is to be done and what has been done.

It should be emphasized that the focus in treatment remains on the goal, or intention, of the action rather than on specific movements. For example, if Keisha wanted to climb to the top of a playground jungle gym, we might ask her to look up at the top of the gym, or we might show her how we "climb to the top." Keisha's intention would not be to reciprocally flex and extend her legs in a certain manner, or to place her hand on one bar of the jungle gym and her foot on the next bar. Rather, her goal would be to reach the top of the jungle gym. Thus, we would focus her attention on, and demonstrate, the intention. Moreover, if we asked Keisha to describe what she wanted to do, she would formulate a representation that relates to the cognitive aspect of the action of climbing to the top (Jeannerod, 1988).

We hypothesize that, because Keisha has difficulty processing and integrating polymodal sensory information, she has difficulty planning both feedforward-dependent projected action sequences and responsive, feedback-dependent, segmental motor actions. Therefore, our goal is to *provide enhanced polymodal information* that she can use to conceptualize and plan adaptive motor behavior. We believe that the inclusion of these cognitive components (visual direction and verbal mediation), when combined with the provision of enhanced tactile, vestibular-proprioceptive, and visual information, can further augment the available information Keisha needs to plan and produce motor action sequences. That is, she can combine the sensory information needed to plan an action with the cognitive processes that enhance her ability to plan "what to do" and "how to do it" (Brooks, 1986).

## Application of Principles of Transfer of Learning to Praxis

As we discussed earlier, one of the problems that clients like Keisha face is difficulty in developing *schemas or neuronal models of action* that can be generalized (Ayres, 1985; Brooks, 1986; Schmidt, 1988). That is, since their abilities to develop schemas are deficient, practiced skills remain highly specific to the particular task they have practiced and do not generalize to other similar activities. In most instances, however, learning involves variations and elements of, or similarities to, previous learning tasks or circumstances. Lindner (1986) emphasized that "this influence on the learning of a given task from practicing or learning other tasks should be one of the most important factors in learning" (p. 65). Therefore, it is important that we consider very carefully what skills to work on during our intervention. While our goal is that Keisha will develop an enhanced ability to develop schemas or neuronal models that can be generalized, it also is important that we focus our intervention on those skills that are most relevant to her daily life task performance needs.

In Keisha's case, we might want to implement an integrated intervention program, which combines the use of sensory integrative treatment procedures with behavioral skills training (see Chapter 13), and to emphasize the manipulative and visuomotor skills that she needs for dressing, handwriting, and play. In so doing, it will be important to determine whether teaching Keisha to attend to specific perceptual or conceptual features of tasks will transfer to other self-care, classroom, or play tasks.

The literature on transfer of training may yield useful intervention-related information to consider in an integrated approach (Marteniuk, 1976; Schmidt, 1975, 1988). The schema theory of motor learning may be particularly useful to explore since it predicts that a schema is strengthened through variability of practice (Shapiro & Schmidt, 1982; Schmidt, 1988). This view is consistent with Ayres' (1972a) view of the importance of varying the task in order to achieve generalizability.

## Action Systems Theory and the Importance of Context

A recent approach to understanding behavior has focused on the idea that spatial knowledge of the external world is derived from the experiences of movement associated with visual experiences and memories. Thus, recent theories of motor control have begun to examine the perceptual control of action (Reed, 1988). This view, known as *action systems theory*, focuses on the functional specificity and meaning of actions, and emphasizes the need to study actions within natural contexts. This view is consistent with the spiral process of self-actualization presented in Chapter 1.

> Further, active participation in a meaningful activity, and the planning and production of an adaptive behavior, are central to this conceptual model [of the spiral process of self-actualization]. *Meaningful* is defined as having significance, value, or purpose, when viewed from the perspective of the client; the term connotes the requirement of active interpretation of sensory information. In order for an activity to be meaningful, the client must be in control of, and be able to make sense of or interpret, the sensory experience. Therefore, whether or not an activity is meaningful depends on what the client experiences. (Fisher & Murray, this volume, p. 20)

This view also is consistent with the centrality to occupational therapy of participation in meaningful and purposeful behavior (see Chapter 1). Fidler and Fidler (1978) asserted that purposeful activity provides the action-learning experience essential for skill acquisition. Gliner (1985) emphasized the interaction between the individual and the environment (object and task), and not the movement itself, and suggested that the environment provides meaning and support to the person performing the action. King (1978) also maintained that adaptive behavior can be organized best through active involvement in doing an activity. She stated that, in purposeful activity, attention is directed toward the object, or the goal, rather than toward the movement, and that this pattern of attention is typical of the natural processes of motor skill development.

Praxis is the ability that enables us to interact effectively with the physical environment (Ayres, 1985). However, it must also be recognized that the environment guides praxis (Ayres, 1985; Gibson, 1988; Jeannerod, 1988). Ayres (1972a, 1979, 1985) consistently emphasized that it is the therapist's role to set up an environment to appropriately challenge the client. She recognized, as do many other researchers, that "skills are always jointly determined by the organism, the task, and the precise environment in which the actions take place" (Connolly & Dalgleish, 1989, p. 894). The environment has consequences for skilled performance; as the environmental context changes, so do the consequences of the client's actions.

For example, we can imagine that after we have worked with Keisha for several weeks, she might select the activity of swinging on a trapeze and letting go so that she will land in a pile of pillows. We feel that this would be an excellent activity for Keisha, as she will need to work on planning and executing projected action sequences. As we think ahead about implementing this activity, we realize that we can set up the situation so that she starts from the top of a set of three steps positioned 10 feet away from the pillows, or we can structure the situation so that she starts from the top of a small stool 6 feet away from the pillows. In either case, the goal will be the same, landing on the pillows. If we offer Keisha the opportunity to try both variations of the activity, and if she reaches the intended goal, her overall action plan will have to be flexible so that it can be readjusted as required by the implemented changes in the environmental context.

We are aware, however, that Keisha, like other clients with dyspraxia, lacks this flexibility. She can learn an action (skill) in one context (environment), but has difficulty adjusting it to fit a slightly different situation. Therefore, we view the sensory integration treatment environment as an ideal situation for allowing Keisha to experiment with multiple variations of an activity where the goal remains the same. We will accomplish this by modifying the environmental context. Consistent with action systems theory, the emphasis will be on the outcome as it relates to anticipated results. How the action is produced is of relatively less importance in action systems theory (Lindner, 1986). This is, in many ways, similar to sensory integration theory, which emphasizes the importance of sensory processing rather than motor output per se.

The relevance and importance of action systems theory for remediation of dyspraxia has not yet been fully articulated. We feel, however, that its potential impact may be multifaceted. The theory recognizes that objects do provide guides for action. Ayres (1972a, 1985) always emphasized the importance of the therapist designing the environment in order to provide the client with the "just right" challenge. Viewed from the perspective of action systems theory, sensory integrative treatment equipment provides "affordances" that enable the client to (a) perceive the meaning of the situation (what to do with the therapy equipment) and (b) act on it. The client's actions are guided, in part, by the nature of the equipment and its perceptual characteristics.

## SUMMARY AND CONCLUSIONS

Somatodyspraxia is a developmental disorder of motor planning. It can be characterized as a "disorder of doing," which is believed to be the result of difficulty in processing certain types of sensory information, most notably tactile, proprioceptive, and sometimes vestibular information. Somatodyspraxia impacts on the client's performance of activities of daily living and on his or her interactions within the environment. Clients with somatodyspraxia have particular difficulty in learning to perform new motor tasks. Clinical observations of the client's motor performance, standardized testing, and parent and teacher interviews all contribute to identification of the clinical picture. With the development of the Sensory Integration and Praxis Tests (SIPT) (Ayres, 1989), the nature of a motor planning disorder can be more fully explored. Treatment of the disorder involves a multifaceted approach that includes providing opportunities to take in enhanced tactile, vestibular-proprioceptive, and visual (polymodal) sensory information within the context of planning and producing meaningful adaptive behavior. The client's active participation and the environmental context are vital elements in the intervention for somatodyspraxia.

# REFERENCES

Abravanel, E. (1972a). How children combine vision and touch when perceiving the shape of objects. *Perception and Psychophysics, 12*, 171–175.

Abravanel, E. (1972b). Short-term memory for shape information processed intra- and intermodally at three ages. *Perceptual and Motor Skills, 35*, 419–425.

Agostoni, E., Coletti, A., Orlando, G., & Tredici, G. (1983). Apraxia in deep cerebral lesions. *Journal of Neurology, Neurosurgery, and Psychiatry, 46*, 804–808.

Ayres, A. J. (1965). Pattern of perceptual-motor dysfunction in children: A factor analysis study. *Perceptual and Motor Skills, 20*, 335–368.

Ayres, A. J. (1966). Interrelationships among perceptual-motor functions in children. *American Journal of Occupational Therapy, 20*, 68–71.

Ayres, A. J. (1969). Deficits in sensory integration in educationally handicapped children. *Journal of Learning Disabilities, 2*, 160–168.

Ayres, A. J. (1971). Characteristics of types of sensory integrative dysfunction. *American Journal of Occupational Therapy, 25*, 329–334.

Ayres, A. J. (1972a). *Sensory integration and learning disorders.* Los Angeles: Western Psychological Services.

Ayres, A. J. (1972b). Types of sensory integrative dysfunction among disabled learners. *American Journal of Occupational Therapy, 26*, 13–18.

Ayres, A. J. (1975). Sensorimotor foundations of academic ability. In W. M. Cruickshank & D. P. Hallahan (Eds.), *Perceptual and learning disabilities in children. Vol. 2: Research and theory,* (pp. 301–358). New York: Syracuse University.

Ayres, A. J. (1976). *The effect of sensory integrative therapy on learning disabled children: The final report of a research project.* Pasadena, CA: Center for the Study of Sensory Integrative Dysfunction.

Ayres, A. J. (1977). Cluster analyses of measures of sensory integration. *American Journal of Occupational Therapy, 31*, 362–366.

Ayres, A. J. (1979). *Sensory integration and the child.* Los Angeles: Western Psychological Services.

Ayres, A. J. (1985). *Developmental dyspraxia and adult onset apraxia.* Torrance, CA: Sensory Integration International.

Ayres, A. J. (1989). *Sensory Integration and Praxis Tests.* Los Angeles: Western Psychological Services.

Ayres, A. J., Mailloux, Z., & Wendler, C. L. (1987). Developmental dyspraxia: Is it a unitary function? *Occupational Therapy Journal of Research, 7*, 93–110.

Ayres, L. P. (1920). *A scale for measuring the quality of handwriting in children.* New York: Russell Sage Foundation.

Basso, A., Capitani, E., Laiacona, M., & Zanobio, M. E. (1985). Crossed aphasia: One or more syndromes. *Cortex, 21*, 25–45.

Basso, A., Capitani, E., Sala, S., Laiacona, M., & Spinnler, H. (1987). Ideomotor apraxia: A study of initial severity. *Acta Neurology of Scandinavia, 76*, 142–146.

Basso, A., Luzzatti, C., & Spinnler, H. (1980). Is ideomotor apraxia the outcome of damage to well-defined regions of the left hemisphere? *Journal of Neurology, Neurosurgery, and Psychiatry, 43*, 118–126.

Beery, E. (1989). *The Developmental Test of Visual-Motor Integration* (3rd rev.). Cleveland, OH: Modern Curriculum.

Benbow, M. (1990). *Loops and other groups: A kinesthetic writing system.* Tucson, AZ: Therapy Skill Builders.

Benbow, M. D. (1987). *Sensory and motor measurements of dynamic tripod skill.* Unpublished master's thesis, Boston University.

Bezzi, R. (1962). A standardized manuscript scale for grades 1, 2, and 3. *Journal of Education Research, 25*, 339–340.

Brinkman, C., & Porter, R. (1979). Supplemental motor area of the monkey: Activity of neurons during performance of a learned motor task. *Journal of Neurophysiology, 42*, 681–709.

Brookhart, J. M., & Mountcastle, V. B. (1984). *Sensory processes.* Bethesda, MD: American Physiological Society.

Brooks, V. B. (1986). How does the limbic system assist motor learning? A limbic comparator hypothesis. *Brain Behavior Evolution, 29,* 29–53.

Bruininks, R. H. (1978). *Bruininks-Oseretsky Test of Motor Proficiency.* Circle Pines, MN: American Guidance Service.

Cermak, S. (1985). Developmental dyspraxia. In E. A. Roy (Ed.), *Neuropsychological studies of apraxia and related disorders,* (pp. 225–248). New York: North-Holland.

Connolly, K. & Dalgleish, M. (1989). The emergence of a tool using skill in infancy. *Developmental Psychology, 25,* 894–912.

Conrad, K. E., Cermak, S. A., & Drake, C. (1983). Differentiation of praxis among children. *American Journal of Occupational Therapy, 37,* 466–473.

Dawdy, S. C. (1981). Pediatric neuropsychology: Caring for the developmentally dyspraxic child. *Clinical Neuropsychology, 3,* 30–37.

DeRenzi, E., Faglioni, P., Sorgato, P. (1982). Modality-specific and supramodal mechanisms of apraxia. *Brain, 105,* 301–312.

DeRenzi, E., Motti, F., & Nichelli, P. (1980). Imitating gestures. A quantitative approach to ideomotor apraxia. *Archives of Neurology, 37,* 6–10.

Dunn, W. (1990). *Pediatric occupational therapy: Facilitating effective service provision.* Thorofare, NJ: C. B. Slack.

Faglioni, P., & Basso, A. (1985). Historical perspectives on neuroanatomical correlates of limb apraxia. In E. A. Roy (Ed.), *Neuropsychological studies of apraxia and related disorders* (pp. 3–44). New York: North-Holland.

Fidler, G. S., & Fidler, J. W. (1978). Doing and becoming: Purposeful action and self-actualization. *American Journal of Occupational Therapy, 32,* 305–310.

Freeman, F. N. (1915). An analytical scale for judging handwriting. *Elementary School Journal, 15,* 432–441.

Frostig, M., Lefever, W., & Whittlesey, R. B. (1963). *The Marianne Frostig Developmental Test of Visual Perception (1963 standardization).* Palo Alto, CA: Consulting Psychologists.

Frostig, M., Lefever, W., & Whittlesey, R. B. (1966). *Scoring Manual for the Marianne Frostig Developmental Test of Visual Perception.* Palo Alto, CA: Consulting Psychologists.

Geschwind, N. (1975). The apraxias: Neural mechanisms of disorders of learned movement. *American Scientist, 63,* 188–195.

Geschwind, N., & Galaburda, A. M. (1985). Cerebral lateralization: Biological mechanisms, associations, and pathology: I. A hypothesis and a program for research. *Archives of Neurology, 42,* 428–459.

Gibson, E. J. (1988). Exploratory behavior in the development of perceiving, acting and the acquiring of knowledge. *Annual Review of Psychology, 39,* 1–41.

Gliner, J. A. (1985). Purposeful activity in motor learning theory: An event approach to motor skill acquisition. *American Journal of Occupational Therapy, 39,* 28–34.

Goldberg, G. (1985). Response and projection: A reinterpretation of the premotor concept. In E. A. Roy (Ed.), *Neuropsychological studies of apraxia and related disorders* (pp. 251–266). New York: North-Holland.

Golden, J. (1987). *Luria-Nebraska Neuropsychological Battery: Children's Revision.* Los Angeles: Western Psychological Services.

Gonzalez-Rothi, L. J., Mack, L., Heilman, K. M. (1986). Pantomime agnosia. *Journal of Neurology, Neurosurgery and Psychiatry, 49,* 451–454.

Gordon, N., & McKinlay, I. (Eds.) (1980). *Helping clumsy children.* New York: Churchill-Livingstone.

Gubbay, S. S. (1975). *The clumsy child.* Philadelphia W. B. Saunders.

Gubbay, S. S. (1978). The management of developmental dyspraxia. *Developmental Medicine and Child Neurology, 20,* 643–646.

Gubbay, S. S. (1979). The clumsy child. In F. C. Rose (Ed.), *Pediatric neurology* (pp. 145–160). London: Blackwell.

Gubbay, S. S. (1985). Clumsiness. In P. J. Vinken, G. W. Bruyn, & H. L. Klawans (Eds.), *Handbook of clinical neurology* (rev. series) (pp. 159–167). New York: Elsevier.

Hainesworth, K., & Siqueland, L. (1969). *Early identification of children with learning disabilities: The Meeting Street School Screening Test.* Providence, RI: Crippled Children and Adults of Rhode Island.

Hoop, N. H. (1971a). Haptic perception in preschool children, part I: Object recognition. *American Journal of Occupational Therapy, 25,* 340–344.

Hoop, N. H. (1971b). Haptic perception in preschool children, part II: Object manipulation. *American Journal of Occupational Therapy, 25,* 415–419.

Jeannerod, M. (1988). *The neural and behavioral organization of goal-directed movements: Oxford psychology series.* Oxford: Clarendon.

Jennings, P. A. (1974). Haptic perception and form reproduction by kindergarten children. *American Journal of Occupational Therapy, 28,* 274–280.

Kaplan, E. (1968). *The development of gesture.* Unpublished doctoral dissertation, Clark University, Worcester, MA.

King, L. J. (1978). Toward a science of adaptive responses. *American Journal of Occupational Therapy, 32,* 429–437.

Kleinman, J. J. (1979). Developmental changes in haptic exploration and matching accuracy. *Developmental Psychology, 15*, 480-481.

Knuckey, N., Apsimon, T., & Gubbay, S. S. (1983). Computerized axial tomography in clumsy children with developmental apraxia and agnosia. *Brain and Development, 5*, 14-19.

Knuckey, N., & Gubbay, S. S. (1983). Clumsy children: A prognostic study. *Australian Pediatric Journal, 19*, 9-13.

Kolb, B., & Whishaw, I. Q. (1985). Can the study of praxis in animals aid in the study of apraxia in humans? In E. A. Roy (Ed.), *Neuropsychological studies of apraxia and related disorders* (pp. 203-224). New York: North-Holland.

Koppitz, M. (1963). *Bender Gestalt Test for young children*. New York: Grune & Stratton.

Larson, K. A. (1982). The sensory history of developmentally delayed children with and without tactile defensiveness. *American Journal of Occupational Therapy, 36*, 590-596.

Lederman, S. J., & Klatzky, R. L. (1987). Hand movements: A window into haptic object recognition. *Cognitive Psychology, 19*, 342-368.

Levine, M. D. (1982). *Pediatric Examination of Educational Readiness (PEER)*. Cambridge, MA: Educators Publishing Service.

Levine, M. D. (1983). *Pediatric Early Elementary Examination (PEEX)*. Cambridge, MA: Educators Publishing Service.

Levine, M. D. (1984). Cumulative neurodevelopmental debts: Their impact on productivity in late middle childhood. In M. D. Levine and P. Satz (Eds.), *Middle childhood: Development and dysfunction*. Baltimore, MD: University Park.

Levine, M. D. (1985). *Pediatric Examination of Educational Readiness at Middle Childhood (Peeramid)*. Cambridge, MA: Educators Publishing Service.

Levine, M. D. (1987). Motor implementation. In M. D. Levine (Ed.), *Developmental variation and learning disorders* (pp. 208-240). Cambridge, MA: Educators Publishing Service.

Levine, M. D., Oberklaid, F., & Meltzer, L. (1981). Developmental output failure: A study of low productivity in school aged children. *Pediatrics, 67*, 18-25.

Lezak, M. D. (1983). *Neuropsychological assessment* (2nd ed.). New York: Oxford University.

Lindner, K. J. (1986). Transfer to motor learning: From formal discipline to action systems theory. In L. D. Zaichkowsky & C. Z. Fuchs (Eds.), *The psychology of motor behavior: Development, control, learning and performance* (pp. 65-87). Ithaca, NY: Mouvement Publications.

Luria, A. R. (1963). *Restoration of function after brain injury*. New York: Pergamon.

Luria, A. R. (1980). *Higher cortical functions in man*. New York: Basic Books.

Marteniuk, R. G. (1976). *Information processing in motor skills*. New York: Holt, Rinehart & Winston.

McHale, K. (1987). *Integrating children with fine motor difficulties into regular classrooms: An approach to identifying and solving problems*. Unpublished master's thesis. Rhode Island College, Providence, RI.

Melzack, R., & Southmayd, J. E. (1974). Dorsal column contributions to anticipatory motor behavior. *Experimental Neurology, 42*, 274-281.

Miller, L. J. (1988). *Miller Assessment for Preschoolers*. San Antonio, TX: Psychological Corporation.

Mountcastle, V. B., Lynch, J. C., Georgopoulos, A., Sakata, H., & Acuna, C. (1975). Posterior parietal association cortex of the monkey: Command functions for operations within extra-personal space. *Journal of Neurophysiology, 38*, 871-908.

Mutti, M., Sterling, H. M., & Spaulding, N. V. (1978). *Quick Neurological Screening Test* (rev. ed.). Novato, CA: Academic Therapy Publications.

Nass, R. (1983). Ontogenesis of hemispheric specializations: Apraxia with congenital left hemisphere lesions. *Perceptual and motor skills, 57*, 775-782.

Orpet, R. E. (1972). *Frostig Movement Skills Test Battery*. Palo Alto, CA: Consulting Psychologists.

Overton, W., & Jackson, J. (1973). The representation of imagined objects in action sequences: A developmental study. *Child Development, 44*, 309-314.

Paillard, J. (1982). Apraxia and the neurophysiology of motor control. *Philosophical Transactions Royal Society of London, B298*, 111-134.

Parham, D. (1987). Evaluation of praxis in preschoolers. In Z. Mailloux (Ed.), *Sensory integrative approaches in occupatinal therapy*, (pp. 23-26). New York: Haworth.

Piaget, J., & Inhelder, B. (1948). *The child's conception of space*. New York: Norton.

Piaget, J. (1952). *The origins of intelligence in children*. New York: International Universities.

Poeck, K. (1982). Two types of motor apraxia. *Archives Italiennes de Biologie, 120*, 361-369.

Rapcsak, S. Z., Gonzalez-Rothi, L. J., & Heilman, K. M. (1987). Apraxia in a patient with atypical cerebral dominance. *Brain and Cognition, 6*, 450-463.

Reed, E. (1988). From the motor theory of perception to the perceptual control of action. In E. S. Reed (Ed.), *James J. Gibson and the psychology of perception*. New Haven, CT: Yale University.

Roach, C., & Kephart, C. (1966). *The Purdue Perceptual-Motor Survey*. San Antonio, TX: Psychological Corporation.

Roland, P. E., Larsen, B., Lassen, N. A., & Skinhoj, E. (1980). Supplementary motor area and other cortical areas in organization of voluntary movements in man. *Journal of Neurophysiology, 43*, 118-136.

Roland, P. E., Skinhoj, E., Lassen, N. A., & Larsen, B. (1980). Different cortical areas in man in organization of voluntary movements in extrapersonal space. *Journal of Neurophysiology, 43*, 137-150.

Royeen, C. B., & Fortune, J. C. (1990). TIE: Touch inventory for school aged children. *American Journal of Occupational Therapy, 44,* 155–160.

Safire, W. (1989, June 11). Rethinking reclama. *The New York Times Magazine,* p. 20.

Schilder, P. (1935). *The image and appearance of the human body.* London: Routledge & Kegan Paul.

Schmidt, R. A. (1975). A schema theory to discrete motor skill learning. *Psychological Review, 82,* 225–260.

Schmidt, R. A. (1988). *Motor control and learning: A behavioral analysis* (2nd ed.). Champaign, IL: Human Kinetics.

Schneck, C. M. (1988). *Developmental changes in the use of writing tools in normal 3.0 to 6.11 year old children.* Unpublished doctoral dissertation, Boston University.

Shapiro, D. C., & Schmidt, R. A. (1982). The schema theory: Recent evidence and developmental implications. In J. A. S. Kelso & J. E. Clark (Eds.), *The development of motor control and co-ordination,* (pp. 113–150). New York: John Wiley & Sons.

Shaw, L., Levine, M., & Belfer, M. (1982). Developmental double jeopardy: A study of clumsiness and self-esteem in children with learning problems. *Journal of Developmental Behavior Pediatrics, 3,* 191–196.

Siegel, L. S., & Feldman, W. (1983). Nondyslexic children with combined writing and arithmetic learning disabilities. *Journal of Clinical Pediatrics, 22,* 241–244.

Stott, D. H., Moyes, F. A., & Henderson, S. E. (1984). *The Test of Motor Impairment* (Henderson rev.) San Antonio, TX: The Psychological Corporation.

Thorndike, E. L. (1910). American handwriting scale. *Teacher's College Record, 11,* 83–175.

Vierck, C. J. (1978). Interpretations of the sensory and motor consequences of dorsal column lesions. In G. Gordon (Ed.), *Active touch: The mechanisms of recognition of objects by manipulation: A multidisciplinary approach,* (pp. 139–160). Oxford: Pergamon.

Wachs, H., & Vaughn, L. (1977). *Wachs analysis of cognitive structures.* Los Angeles: Western Psychological Services.

Wall, P. D. (1970). Sensory role of impulses traveling in the dorsal columns. *Brain, 93,* 505–524.

Walton, J. N., Ellis, E., & Court, S. D. M. (1963). Clumsy children: A study of developmental apraxia and agnosia. *Brain, 85,* 603–613.

Watson, R. T., Fleet, W. S., Gonzalez-Rothi, L., Heilman, K. M. (1986). Apraxia and the supplemental motor area. *Archives of Neurology, 43,* 787–792.

Wolff, P. (1972). The role of stimulus-correlated activity in children's recognition of nonsense forms. *Journal of Experimental Child Psychology, 24,* 427–441.

Zaporozhets, A. V. (1965). The development of perception in the preschool child. *Monographs of the Society for Research in Child Development, 30,* 82–101.

Zaporozhets, A. V. (1969). Some of the psychological problems of sensory training in early childhood and the preshcool period. In A.R. Leont'ev & A.R. Luria (Eds.), *A handbook of contemporary soviet psychology* (pp. 86–120). New York: Basic Books.

# APPENDIX 6–A

# Fine Motor Functions and Handwriting

Clinical observations have indicated that while many children have difficulty with both total body and fine motor planning, there are some children whose deficits are primarily in one realm. Impairment in fine motor function is significant because it can interfere with a child's ability to do manipulative tasks. Educationally, its impact is seen clearly in handwriting. In this section, we will discuss the importance of handwriting, characteristic problems seen in clients who have poor handwriting, and strategies for remediating these problems.

Handwriting is important because it may be a graphic symptom of a learning disability (Levine, 1985). Problems in handwriting have been associated with arithmetic deficits, organization and short-term memory deficits (Siegel & Feldman, 1983), and sensory integrative dysfunction (Ayres, 1979). Fine motor demands are great within the academic environment. McHale (1987) observed 11 second, fourth, and sixth grade classrooms and recorded the frequency of time spent in tasks demanding fine motor functions. She found that, depending on the classroom, 20 to 60 percent of the classroom activities required fine motor function.

Levine, Oberkland, and Meltzer (1981) emphasized that around fourth grade there is a marked increase in the academic demand for written output, which continues to increase as the child gets older. Handwriting problems often interfere with a child's ability to communicate and to "show what he or she knows." The child with fine motor and handwriting problems often cannot finish assignments on time; because writing is difficult, the child may try to complete a written assignment in as few words as possible. If a child has to focus on the mechanical aspects of writing, he or she is not able to fully attend to the content of information. Thus, there is a "tradeoff" with other functions. One child we treated said, "Whenever I write, I lose my memory. I can either write or think but I can't do both." Another child reported that when he had to take extensive notes in class, he could not understand what the teacher was saying.

## WHAT IS POOR HANDWRITING?

Problems in handwriting may be characterized by a number of different features. However, of utmost importance is legibility and speed. Characteristic problems may include the following:

1. Poor quality of the stroke, including tight, jagged, or squeezed strokes

**166**

2. Improper spacing, including difficulty with alignment of words, spacing between words, spacing of letters, or letter formation
3. Inappropriate uphill or downhill slant
4. Disorganized and nonuniform lettering, including letters that are too small or too large and mixed letter types (cursive and printed, upper and lower case)
5. Inability to sustain legibility of writing

Problems with handwriting may be due to problems with form and space perception; motor planning and motor memory; sequencing; and somatosensory processing, or visuomotor coordination. Levine (1985) emphasized the need to differentiate problems with the mechanical aspects of handwriting from problems with the language component that affects word finding, sentence formulation, and punctuation. For example, the child whose handwriting problems are primarily characterized by letter reversals, although producing poor writing, is probably experiencing primarily language deficits (Levine, 1985).

We have found that a problem in handwriting is one of the most frequent reasons that school-aged children are referred to occupational therapy. While there are a number of tests to identify problems in handwriting (Ayres, 1920; Bezzi, 1962; Freeman, 1915; Stott, Moyes, & Henderson, 1985; Thorndike, 1910), perhaps the best measure is the teacher's assessment of the writing product (Schneck, 1988). The teacher has a classroom of children against which to compare a particular child's handwriting, years of experience to draw upon, and multiple samples of the child's work. For a one-time assessment (especially if the child is aware that his or her handwriting is being evaluated), the child may put forth exceptional conscious effort and produce a good product. However, this same child may not be able to sustain that level over time or to produce the same quality of writing while he or she is attending simultaneously to the content of the assignment.

Once a determination has been made that a child has a problem in handwriting, it is critical to determine why the child has the problem in order that remediation strategies can be implemented to best meet the needs of the child. While practice in handwriting is certainly one strategy, it may be more effective when paired with teaching techniques that capitalize on the child's strengths, with remediation programs that deal with developing foundational skills, and with compensation methods. Analysis of handwriting problems will be addressed first, followed by a discussion of different remediation strategies.

Levine (1985) identified a number of different types of problems that may result in handwriting deficits. These are evaluated in the fine motor section of the Pediatric Examination of Educational Readiness at Middle Childhood, a test for children aged 9 to 15. Results of the SIPT assessment also can serve to clarify the nature of the problem. That is, using the SIPT, we can determine whether the problem reflects somatosensory processing difficulty resulting in "motor memory" problems or whether the problem is one of visual form and space analysis. The Wachs Analysis of Cognitive Structures (WACS) (Wachs & Vaughan, 1977), standardized for preschool- and early-school-aged children, also can provide a basis for task analysis.

To give the reader an idea of the types of problems that commonly occur, we will address a few of the areas identified by Levine (1985). Some children who have poor handwriting have inadequate somatosensory perception. This may be manifested by problems in finger identification, or in knowing the precise position of his or her arms and hands. The child who does not adequately process somatosensory information must rely heavily on vision. That child may position his or her head close to the paper in order to visually monitor what his or her hand is doing. In order to try to increase somatosensory feedback, the child may develop poor pencil grasp characterized by stabilization of distal joints. While this may be adequate for small amounts of writing, it is very fatiguing (Levine, 1985).

An example of the ways in which poor pencil grasp can result in problems is demonstrated by John, who tends to hold his pencil too close to the tip. Because the circumference is smaller at the tip, he must exert more pressure to maintain control. This prolonged grip of a smaller object is tiring for John. In addition, his thumb tends to get in the way so that John cannot see what he is writing. He compensates by leaning to the side and tilting his head. This results in John using his other arm to support his body weight so that he doesn't lose his balance and fall out of his chair. Unfortunately, this also means that his other arm is no longer available for stabilizing his paper.

Another type of problem may relate to deficits in motor planning or motor memory. The movements needed for writing are not automatic; the child must think about them all the time. A child with a problem of this nature seems to have difficulty forming and retrieving the proprioceptive-dependent neuronal models or engrams of the letters. As a result, the child may make the same letter three or four different ways.

In examining the motor planning and motor memory contributions to handwriting, it is important to examine both copying and spontaneous writing. Spontaneous writing involves feedforward control of the written output, and is dependent on the ability to utilize neuronal models or memories. Conversely, copying is feedback-dependent. Thus, we might speculate that a child with bilateral integration and sequencing deficits would be able to copy, but would have more difficulty with spontaneous writing. A child with somatodyspraxia, however, who has problems with both feedback and feedforward motor control, is more likely to be impaired in both copying and spontaneous writing.

Problems in handwriting may be compounded by a number of factors, including poor muscle tone and poor shoulder stability. Poor muscle tone and stability can lead to poor posture, fatigue, decreased speed, laborious writing, and poor pencil grasp. Inadequate strength of the finger muscles or an imbalance between flexor and extensor muscle strength also may contribute to poor pencil grasp and problems with handwriting (Benbow, 1987).

## REMEDIATION

Three approaches to remediation will be discussed: demystification, bypass strategies, and direct intervention strategies. These are by no means mutually exclusive, but rather are compatible approaches. *Demystification* involves "taking the mystery out of the situation" by explaining the nature of the problem to the child, his teachers, and his parents. This will help the individuals involved to understand that the problem is not laziness or "stupidity." This process is discussed in detail in Chapter 11, where we refer to it as "reframing."

*Bypass strategies* involve "circumventing the problem." This may mean starting the child on a typewriter or on a word processing system. While these certainly may help, it is usually a slow process until the child is able to produce at a rate that is worthwhile to the child.

We believe that it is preferable to start the child with keyboarding instruction immediately; the hunt-and-peck method should be avoided because the child may be extremely resistant to giving up this method later in order to learn proper keyboarding. In our experience, children are ready to begin keyboarding by the third grade. While some children may be ready sooner, the child must be able to isolate individual finger movements and this often is delayed in children who have motor coordination problems. Benbow (M.D. Benbow, personal communication, March 15, 1988) has suggested that it may be preferable to begin keyboarding instruction with a typewriter rather than a word processor, because with a typewriter the child gets more feedback. Also, if the child's finger lingers on the keys of a computer keyboard, the computer will produce multiple copies of the same letter.

Another bypass strategy is to alter expectations for the child. An example is to prioritize simultaneous demands in an assignment. For example, if the child is asked to write a composition on Abraham Lincoln, and if the goal of the assignment is for the child to show the teacher what he or she knows about Lincoln, then spelling, punctuation, capitalization, and good handwriting can be "sacrificed." Another example is to reduce the volume of work to be completed, for example, to ask the child to complete 5 carefully selected math problems instead of 15.

A final example of the bypass approach to treatment involves environmental manipulations that may make it easier for the child to perform. Specific examples of this include placing a device on the pencil that facilitates proper pencil grasp, using graph paper to aid the child's spatial organization, or providing the child with adapted writing utensils and slanted surfaces on which to write. The implementation of bypass strategies are effected through the consultation process discussed in Chapter 11.

The third approach to the remediation of handwriting deficits is the *direct intervention approach*. Since the ultimate goal is for a child's writing to become fluid and automatic, the child should not always have to think about letter formation and should be able to produce volume without fatigue. Thus, practice with letter formation certainly is needed. Repeated practice in the deficient skill (writing letters) is one approach to intervention. An alternate approach involves analysis of the child's motor skills and sensory processing abilities that contribute to, and underlie, the handwriting problem. It also is necessary to analyze the child's learning style in order to determine how to match the child's learning style with the teacher's strategies for teaching. For example, one would want to examine the child's ability to benefit from verbal mediation in an effort to facilitate letter formation. When the child draws an M, does telling the child to start at the "bottom" and "go up and down and up and down" in order to "draw two mountains" help the child? Is a proprioceptive approach, such as moving the child's arm and hand, or having the child practice the motions in the air, helpful to the child?

Intervention involves utilizing the child's strengths and remediating his or her deficits. Benbow's (1990) handwriting program *Loops and Other Groups* is an example of a program that utilizes both verbal mediation and proprioceptive input in the teaching of cursive writing.

In addition to intervention that focuses on the handwriting itself, we also might select an approach to intervention that would emphasize the remediation of underlying problems. For example, if the child fatigues easily because of low muscle tone, then we might choose to intervene by improving muscle tone (see Chapter 4). However, if the underlying problem is difficulty with form and space perception or construction, the approach to intervention would be quite different (see Chapter 13). If the primary problem is a more general motor planning problem with an underlying somatosensory base, we might intervene by using a sensory integration approach.

Finally, while various approaches to remediation of handwriting problems have been identified, we view them as compatible. We feel that the best intervention strategy for any child usually reflects a combination of several of these approaches.

# CHAPTER 7

# Hemispheric Specialization

**Elizabeth A. Murray, ScD, OTR**

*The right hemisphere synthesizes over space. The left hemisphere analyzes over time.*

*Levy, 1974, p. 167*

Ayres (1972, 1976, 1979, 1989), through the development of sensory integration theory, has been a pioneer in addressing the contributions of subcortical structures to normal development and in noting possible indicators of subcortical dysfunction in some children who have learning disabilities. We should understand, however, that learning disabilities are considered by most psychologists (e.g., Rourke & Strang, 1983) and educators (e.g., Davidson, 1983) to be reflective of dysfunction primarily of higher cortical processes.

Although sensory integrative dysfunction may exist along with, and may even contribute to, cortical dysfunction, probably the actual problems these learning-disabled children experience in academic learning ultimately result from problems in cortical function. As occupational therapists, we may use sensory integration treatment procedures designed to improve function at subcortical levels, but we need to be aware of the child's total picture of strengths and weaknesses, not just those in one specific area. Ayres herself noted patterns that appeared to reflect left and right hemisphere function in several of her factor-analytic studies (Ayres, 1969, 1976).

## PURPOSE AND SCOPE

The purpose of this chapter is to provide the occupational therapist with a basic understanding of the concepts of hemispheric specialization and lateralization of function in the cerebral cortex. Additionally, this chapter will include discussion of the research base of hemispheric specialization and the application of these findings both to the normal population and to those with learning disabilities.

In order to place research in its proper perspective, we will begin our discussion with two children who have difficulties associated with hemispheric dysfunction. Next, terminology will be defined; a review of the various research methods that have been used to assess aspects of hemispheric specialization will be presented, along with variables that may affect these findings.

An understanding of the contributions of each hemisphere to behavior in the normal population is needed before we can discuss fully the deficits in children with learning disabilities. Researchers (e.g., Eccles, 1973) have described the behaviors associated with each hemisphere. The research describing these behaviors will be critiqued, and behaviors typically associated with each hemisphere will be reviewed.

Next, we will summarize the findings of research with subjects with learning disabilities, along with hypotheses on the mechanisms of dysfunction. Behaviors typical of children with left and right hemisphere dysfunctions will be described. Most of this research is from the fields of neurology, psychology, and education. We need to be aware that *there is no existing research on hemisphere function in children with sensory integrative dysfunction.*

Finally, we will consider the evaluation and intervention for children with hypothesized hemisphere dysfunction. Tests from the Sensory Integration and Praxis Tests (SIPT) (Ayres, 1989) that may give indications of left or right hemisphere dysfunction will be discussed, along with observations that may be made with other assessments. We will end with a discussion of intervention, including the role of sensory integration procedures in the intervention of children with hemisphere dysfunction.

## CLINICAL PICTURE OF HEMISPHERE DYSFUNCTION

We begin with descriptions of two boys, Jimmy and Ross. Both have been diagnosed as learning-disabled. Both have been receiving special education services for several years. While both Jimmy and Ross have been identified as having learning disabilities, they present two very different pictures and require two different approaches to remediation. Jimmy is typical of a young man with what is described as left hemisphere dysfunction, while Ross' profile is similar to that of children who are thought to have a deficit in the right hemisphere. However, in both of these cases (and in the cases of most individuals for whom these diagnoses are made), there is no actual evidence of any frank pathology in the brain.

### Jimmy: A Case Study of an Adolescent with Left Hemisphere Dysfunction

Jimmy, 14 years old, is quiet and somewhat shy. He tends to speak in relatively short sentences and does not elaborate on what he has said. Jimmy's parents were concerned about his speech development early on. He did not talk until much later than his siblings, preferring to point and gesture to communicate. When he could not make himself understood, Jimmy frequently had temper tantrums. His nursery school teacher also was concerned about Jimmy's delayed speech and recommended a language evaluation. Jimmy was diagnosed as having a deficit in both receptive and expressive language.

Jimmy has had problems in school from kindergarten onward. Learning to read was especially difficult; he had trouble attaching sounds to letters, so it was hard for him to "sound out" or decode words. Reading aloud was painfully slow. Jimmy's ability to read remains well below his grade level. He has trouble in subjects such as history and English, which require much reading and long written assignments.

Jimmy also has difficulty understanding what is said to him, particularly when the information is lengthy or complex. As a young boy, he was thought by his parents and teachers to have an attention deficit, as he frequently appeared not to be listening and did not always follow directions.

Jimmy has a good sense of numbers. His shop teacher finds that he has an excellent sense of size and proportion and is easily able to estimate. Jimmy also has good mechanical abilities; he made his own bicycle out of parts that he found in a local junkyard.

## Ross: A Case Study of an Adolescent with Right Hemisphere Dysfunction

Ross is a very verbal teenager. His ambition is to be a sports announcer. Ross' parents did not have any major concerns about him as a young boy. They did note that he had more trouble learning to dress himself than did his older brother, and that he always seemed to be disheveled. However, he learned to talk at an early age, and many of their friends commented on how verbal he was. Ross' nursery school teacher observed that he was poor at drawing and avoided puzzles, but she felt these were the result of immaturity and was not concerned.

Ross had no difficulty with reading in the primary grades. Problems arose later, however, when he needed to summarize or synthesize what he read. It was at this point, when he was 8 years old, that Ross was evaluated, and special education services were provided.

Math was always particularly difficult for Ross. Although he was able to memorize his number facts, he had trouble applying these to everyday situations. He also was delayed in learning to tell time and in money skills.

Ross enjoys being in the company of his peers, but he has few friends. He is poor at reading nonverbal cues and consequently acts inappropriately in many social situations. He is a frequent target of practical jokes.

Ross' teachers note that he has problems organizing his work. Although he is good at remembering details, he is poor at making inferences and answering "why" questions.

These portraits of Jimmy and Ross illustrate the skills associated with each hemisphere. In order to understand how their skills were identified, we will review the research procedures and findings.

## RESEARCH IN HEMISPHERIC SPECIALIZATION

In 1861, Broca presented the results of autopsies on the brains of two patients who had developed disturbances in speaking. In both cases, lesions were found in the posterior frontal lobe of the left hemisphere. A decade later, Wernicke described a case of a patient who had lost the ability to comprehend speech. Postmortem autopsy revealed a lesion in the left temporal lobe. These and similar findings, combined with the observation that massive damage to the right hemisphere did not result in any noticeable impairment in language, led to the hypothesis that language abilities were localized in the left hemisphere. Because it was known that the left hemisphere controls the right hand, which is the preferred hand for the majority of the population, the assumption was made that the left hemisphere was dominant or superior to the right. The term *cerebral dominance* was used to refer to this control (Harris, 1988; Joynt & Goldstein, 1975; Luria, 1980).

Although there were reports of problems with spatial perception and orientation in patients with right hemisphere lesions, and it was suggested that the right hemisphere may have a dominant role in nonverbal skills, most studies of brain-injured patients throughout the late 1800s and early 1900s emphasized the role of the left hemisphere in language (Luria, 1980). It was not until the latter half of this century that particular attention was paid to the special functions of the right hemisphere.

Because it has now become increasingly apparent that each hemisphere is specialized for different functional abilities, the term *hemispheric specialization* has come to be preferred to cerebral dominance. Hemispheric specialization implies that each hemisphere has a specialized role, rather than that the one hemisphere is more important than, or dominant over, the other. *Lateralization* refers to the process whereby hemispheres become specialized for a particular function; that is, a functional ability is said to be lateralized to one hemisphere or the other. Language is lateralized to the left hemisphere in most right-handed people. An ability may be *strongly lateralized*, meaning one hemisphere has the major control, or it may be *weakly lateralized*, indicating more sharing of the ability between the two hemispheres (Hiscock & Kinsbourne, 1982). In this section, we will present a summary of the methods used to assess hemispheric specialization. The following section will demonstrate how the findings from this body of research have been used to describe the functions of the two hemispheres.

## Research on Subjects with Neurological Impairment

As can be seen from the previous discussion, interest in hemispheric specialization stemmed from observations of loss of skills in patients with unilateral lesions. Researchers (cf. Aram & Whitaker, 1988; Jason, 1986) continue to study these patients. In addition, subjects who have undergone specific surgical procedures, such as severing of the corpus callosum or removal of one hemisphere, have enabled researchers (e.g., Gazzaniga, 1975; Ogden, 1989) to study the functions of the two hemispheres. In Table 7–1, we present a listing of these patients, together with a description of the diagnoses and the ways in which they have been assessed to study hemispheric specialization. The reader is referred to Dennis (1980), Eccles (1973), Gazzaniga (1975), Luria (1980), and Ogden (1989) for more specific information about these procedures.

**TABLE 7–1. TYPES OF NEUROLOGICALLY-IMPAIRED SUBJECTS USED TO STUDY HEMISPHERIC SPECIALIZATION**

| *Type of Patient* | *Description of Lesion* | *How Assessed* |
|---|---|---|
| Unilateral brain injury | Lesion of only one hemisphere, generally due to cerebrovascular accident or traumatic injury | Compare sequelae to damage in left hemisphere to sequelae to damage in right hemisphere |
| Commissurotomy | Surgical procedure in which the corpus callosum and anterior commissure (fibers that transmit information between the two hemispheres) are severed; generally performed for intractable seizures | Present stimuli to one hemisphere in isolation |
| Hemispherectomy | Surgical removal of one hemisphere, generally because of tumor, disease, or seizures | Assess skills of remaining hemisphere |

A major drawback to studies that include brain-injured and surgical patients as subjects is that the studies are on abnormal subjects, such as those with known brain disease or lesions, or severe epilepsy. In many studies of brain-injured subjects, we do not know the precise location of the injury, and there is often the possibility of some bilateral involvement. Further, while we can assess the loss of function, we do not know how those skills were organized in that individual's brain before the injury. For example, in patients who have undergone severing of the corpus callosum (referred to as commissurotomy, or "split-brain" patients), abnormalities in the brain were present during early development, resulting in severe epilepsy. We would expect some reorganization of function to have occurred in many of these instances to compensate for the abnormalities; thus, what is true of these subjects with regard to hemispheric specialization may not be true of the general population.

A loss of skill stemming from a brain lesion does not necessarily indicate that the skill itself was controlled by the specific area of damage. It is possible, for example, that damage to connecting fibers interferes with the transmission of information that is important to another area of the brain, resulting in depressed performance of skills controlled by the second area. We must be particularly careful in making assumptions about loss of skills in children who have suffered early unilateral brain lesions. Whereas it is known that plasticity of the brain, or its ability to functionally reorganize following damage, continues throughout life, the younger nervous system is thought to be more plastic than the older nervous system, as many cells have not yet matured or myelinated. Thus there is greater potential in the young child for other areas of the brain, as they mature, to take on skills normally performed by those in the lesioned area (Liederman, 1988).

These studies, then, do not tell us how the normal brain functions; rather, they provide us with some information about how the brain functions after a lesion or brain surgery. In order to provide a more complete picture of hemispheric specialization in the normal brain, we need ways to study specialization in normal subjects.

## Measures Used to Study Normal Subjects

While early researchers of hemispheric specialization studied patients with brain injuries, a variety of new techniques have been developed that enable researchers to study hemispheric specialization in normal subjects. These include morphological studies, measures of laterality, and physiological measures. Although there are limitations to each of these procedures, they have provided us with a better picture of hemispheric specialization in the normal brain.

### MORPHOLOGICAL STUDIES

Up until the 1960s, the hemispheres of the brain were thought to be anatomically similar. However, Geschwind and Levitsky (1968) found, on postmortem studies, that an area of the temporal cortex called the *planum temporale* was generally larger in the left hemisphere than in the right. The planum temporale includes the auditory association area (Wernicke's area) that is related to the comprehension of language. Galaburda and his associates (Galaburda, 1984; Galaburda, LeMay, Kemper, & Geschwind, 1978) confirmed the findings of Geschwind and Levitsky through subsequent postmortem studies. These asymmetries also have been found in the brains of infants (Witelson & Pallie, 1973) and fetuses (Chi, Dooling, & Gilles, 1977; LeMay, 1984; LeMay & Geschwind, 1978; Wada, Clarke, & Hamm, 1975).

The development of computerized tomography (CT) scanning has provided a method of observing the anatomy of the brain in living subjects. The CT scan is a computerized x-ray of the brain that can be used to determine if any structural abnormalities exist. Morphological asymmetries, based on CT scans, have been reported by LeMay and her associates (LeMay 1976, 1984; LeMay & Geschwind, 1978; LeMay & Kido, 1978). These have included a relatively larger area in the right frontal lobe and a larger area in the left occipital lobe. More recently, a technique called magnetic resonance imaging (MRI) has provided even more precise images of the structure of the brain. Currently, however, both CT scans and MRI are used mainly for diagnostic purposes in persons with suspected lesions. The procedures also are expensive, which has limited their general use in studying brain morphology in normal subjects.

In summary, evidence exists that there are structural differences between the two hemispheres. However, these findings do not answer the question of whether or not there are parallel functional differences.

## MEASURES OF LATERALITY

*Laterality* refers to *the degree to which* either sensory reception or motor output on one side of the body is superior to the reception or output on the other side. As the primary reception of most sensory input and the control of some motor output are regulated by the contralateral hemisphere, measures of laterality are thought to reflect degree of *lateralization* (specialization) of function within each hemisphere. It is important to understand the difference between these two terms. Laterality refers to a *measured* superiority of function (e.g., hand preference). Because laterality is based on tests, we can only *infer* the degree of lateralization within the central nervous system.

Perceptual-motor theorists have traditionally assessed laterality in terms of handedness and eye preference, as well as foot preference. Their assumption, based on the early concept of cerebral dominance, is that hand, eye, and foot preference should all be consistent. That is, if a person is right-handed, he or she would show a preference for the right eye and right foot. Any variation was referred to as inconsistent laterality or crossed dominance and was felt to indicate inadequate lateralization of function in the hemispheres (Delacato, 1966; Kephart, 1960; Orton, 1937). This concept of laterality is no longer accepted for several reasons. First, motor control of most movements is bilateral, meaning that both ipsilateral and contralateral pathways control movements (Hiscock & Kinsbourne, 1982). The major exception to this rule is refined finger movements, which are under the control of the contralateral hemisphere (Lawrence & Kuypers, 1968). Thus, whereas writing and drawing with the right hand would indicate primarily left hemisphere control, throwing a ball (another task often used to asses lateral dominance) would not. Further, the foot used to kick a ball would be under the control of both hemispheres. [It has been observed that children who are born without arms, and who use their feet for the manipulation of objects, demonstrate an evenly distributed right vs. left foot preference for writing (A.G. Fisher, personal communication, March 23, 1990)]. Similarly, there is no evidence that the eye used for sighting a target is an indication of preference of one hemisphere. Rather, regardless of which eye is preferred, information seen through that eye goes to both hemispheres, with stimuli from the right visual field going to the left hemisphere and vice-versa (Hiscock & Kinsbourne, 1982). Finally, research has shown that there is little correlation between eye and hand preference in the normal population (Porac & Coren, 1981), indicating that crossed dominance is not reflective of dysfunction.

While some traditional measures of laterality are no longer thought to be valid, there are newer measures that are more accepted. Specific test paradigms used to assess laterality for sensory inputs, referred to as tests of *perceptual asymmetry*, have been developed that involve the auditory, visual, and tactile modalities. Stimuli presented to sensory receptors for these senses on one side of the body are thought to be processed initially either exclusively or predominantly by the contralateral hemisphere. For example, what we see in our left visual field is initially processed in the right visual cortex. Further, although both the auditory and tactile systems are strongly represented both ipsilaterally and contralaterally, the crossed primary sensory pathways are functionally superior to the uncrossed pathways. Thus, if one side of the body is more efficient at responding appropriately to a particular sensory presentation, it is hypothesized that the opposite hemisphere is specialized for that particular task. For example, if a group of subjects were able to read more words correctly when they were presented to the right visual half-field than the left visual half-field, we might conclude that written words are more efficiently processed by the left hemisphere.

Table 7–2 provides a review of tests of perceptual asymmetry. The reader is referred to Hiscock (1988) for an excellent review of these measures.

Tests of perceptual asymmetry have been criticised, despite their widespread use. The tasks themselves generally are not motivating; thus, attention to the tasks may not be optimal (Bradshaw, Burden, & Nettleton, 1986; Hiscock, 1988). Behavioral measures of asymmetry also have low test-retest reliability, with up to one third of subjects showing a different pattern of response on retesting (Bradshaw et al. 1986; Koomar & Cermak, 1981). Although these tests may give a picture of patterns of hemispheric specialization within a group of people, they are less helpful in assess-

## TABLE 7–2. MEASURES OF PERCEPTUAL ASYMMETRY

| *Sensory Modality* | *Test* | *Procedure* | *Examples of Stimuli* |
| --- | --- | --- | --- |
| Auditory | Dichotic listening | Paired auditory stimuli are presented to each ear simultaneously through earphones<br>Subject identifies stimuli verbally | Syllables, words, environmental sounds |
| Visual | Tachistoscope | Visual stimuli are presented to left or right visual half-field for very brief durations (<200 msec) in order to prevent scanning, which would move the stimulus into the other visual half-field<br>Subject identifies stimuli either verbally or by matching | Written words, numerals, dots, pictures of objects or faces |
| Tactile | Haptic, dichhaptic | Stimuli are manipulated by either one hand (haptic) or both hands simultaneously (dichhaptic)<br>Subject identifies stimulus by naming or matching | Letters, shapes |

ing individuals. Additionally, correlations between different measures of perceptual asymmetry generally are low (Boles, 1989; Hiscock, Antoniuk, Prisciak, & von Hessert, 1985). It also is important to remember that, in tests of perceptual asymmetry, *both* hemispheres are able to perform the task. The studies indicate *only* that one hemisphere is more efficient (faster or more accurate) than the other hemisphere.

Many of the hypotheses of differences between the two hemispheres have been based on research using tests of perceptual asymmetry. These tests provide a picture of only a very small slice of behavior in an artificial situation. For example, tachistoscopic presentation requires that a stimulus be shown for only milliseconds, so that the subject cannot scan it visually. In daily life, scanning is automatic, and both visual half-fields receive and process whatever is seen. Further, while a left hemisphere advantage may occur for processing of syllables, we cannot generalize from this observation that all language is thus a function of the left hemisphere. Available research does document the existence of asymmetries of sensory processing in the human brain, but it provides no qualitative information on actual differences in functional abilities in daily life.

## PHYSIOLOGICAL MEASURES

Other measures have been used to allow us to study the function of the brain during activity by indicating areas of the brain that are activated when the subject is engaged in a specific task. These measures have been used to provide evidence of lateralization. Table 7–3 provides a summary of these measures. The reader is referred to Brandeis and Lehman (1989); Ciecielski (1989); Deutsch, Bourbon, Papanicolou, and Eisenberg (1988); Duffy, Denckla, and Sandini (1980); Heiss, Herholz, Pawlik, Wagner, and Weinhard (1986); and Risberg (1986) for more specific information about these procedures.

There are limitations to these physiological measures. All brains are not activated identically, so that the pictures obtained will vary from subject to subject.

**TABLE 7–3. PHYSIOLOGICAL MEASURES USED TO ASSESS HEMISPHERIC SPECIALIZATION**

| Test | What Is Measured | Procedure |
| --- | --- | --- |
| Electroencephalogram (EEG) | Electrical activity of brain | Electrodes attached to skull; specific output at each site is recorded graphically |
| Event-related potentials (ERP) | Electrical activity of brain | As above, but activity is in response to specific sensory input (e.g., sound, light) |
| Brain electrical activity mapping (BEAM) | Electrical activity of brain | Provides computerized picture of areas of relative activation of the brain, at rest or during activity |
| Regional cerebral blood flow (rCBF) | Blood flow through brain (increased blood flow indicates increased activation in that region) | Subject inhales, or is injected with, a gas with very low-level radioactivity. Gas enters bloodstream, and areas of increased blood flow are charted. Can be used at rest or during activity |
| Positron emission tomography (PET) | Similar to above | Similar to above |

Further, these measures all require technical expertise both to administer and to interpret the results. They also require expensive, sophisticated equipment. Even though no two subjects show identical patterns of activation, these measures do demonstrate that there is variability among individuals, while still allowing us to look for trends.

# NEURAL ORGANIZATION OF THE HEMISPHERES

Semmes (1968) has proposed differences in the neural organization of the two hemispheres that may parallel the functional differences found with the preceding measures. In studies of tactile perception with adults who were brain-injured, she and her associates found that, whereas deficits in the right hand were attributable specifically to lesions of the sensorimotor cortex, tactile deficits in the left hand occurred when there were lesions either within or outside the sensorimotor cortex of the right hemisphere. Similar findings were observed when hand strength was analyzed, with right-hand strength impaired as a result of left sensorimotor lesions, but strength in the left hand impaired as a result of lesions either outside or within the sensorimotor cortex of the right hemisphere. Semmes' conclusion was that the left hemisphere has a more focal, or precise organization, with similar functional units located near each other. She suggested that this organization may facilitate precise coding needed for speaking. The right hemisphere, however, is more diffusely organized, with convergence of dissimilar functional units. Thus, the right hemisphere has an advantage in synthesizing unlike inputs. Semmes proposed that this organization may give the right hemisphere an advantage in performing spatial tasks.

Rourke (1988) also described the right hemisphere as more intermodal and integrating than the left. He hypothesized that the right hemisphere is dependent on connecting fibers for both learning and maintaining skills, noting that the skills for which the right hemisphere is specialized generally demand more complex inputs from a variety of sources. These connecting fibers, on which the right hemisphere depends, include the corpus callosum (connecting the two hemispheres), association fibers (connecting the anterior and posterior regions of the cortex), and projection fibers (connecting the hemispheres with the brainstem).

Rourke (1988) indicated that, like the right hemisphere, the left hemisphere is dependent on connecting fibers for the learning of skills. Once learned, however, the skills for which the left hemisphere is specialized become more localized and less dependent on multiple inputs. Thus, the left hemisphere, according to Rourke (1988), is less dependent than the right on these connections, particularly the callosal and projection fibers, for skill maintenance.

# HEMISPHERIC SPECIALIZATION AND BEHAVIOR

There are many significant limitations on the usefulness of the above methods in studying hemispheric specialization. Results from studies also are not consistent. Further, some studies have shown differences between men and women (Harris, 1978; Inglis & Lawson, 1981; McGlone, 1978) and between right-handed and left-handed subjects (Harris & Carlson, 1988; Hugdahl & Anderson, 1989). Other studies have suggested that differences in hemispheric specialization are related to rate of physical maturation (Vrbancic & Mosley, 1988; Waber, 1976, 1977). However, some

TABLE 7–4. BEHAVIORS ATTRIBUTED TO THE LEFT AND RIGHT HEMISPHERES

| Behavior | Left Hemisphere | Right Hemisphere |
|---|---|---|
| Cognitive style | Processing information in a sequential, linear manner<br>Observing and analyzing details | Processing information in a simultaneous, holistic, or gestalt manner<br>Grasping overall organization or pattern |
| Perception/cognition | Processing and producing language | Processing non-verbal stimuli (environmental sounds, speech intonation, complex shapes and designs)<br>Visual-spatial perception<br>Drawing inferences, synthesizing information |
| Academic skills | Reading: sound-symbol relationships, word recognition, reading comprehension<br>Performing mathematical calculations | Mathematical reasoning and judgment<br>Alignment of numerals in calculations |
| Motor | Sequencing movements<br>Performing movements and gestures to command | Sustaining a movement or posture |
| Emotions | Expression of positive emotions | Expression of negative emotions<br>Perception of emotion |

overall trends are apparent. Specific patterns of thinking and behavior have been attributed to each hemisphere. Table 7–4 presents a brief summary of these patterns. We will discuss some of these patterns here, asking that the reader keep in mind that this is a simplified presentation of the volumes of research that have been done on this topic.

## Cognitive Style

Perhaps the most important difference between the left and right hemispheres is the style or approach that each is thought to use in processing information. The left hemisphere is hypothesized to process information in a *sequential, linear* manner. It also is thought to be superior at observing and analyzing details (Kumar, 1973). Evidence to support these hypotheses comes from several sources. Patients with left hemisphere lesions have been found to have difficulty with performing sequences of motor movements and with remembering sequences of colored lights and sounds (Carmon & Nachson, 1971). Using dichotic listening tests, researchers (cf. Krashen, 1975) have found the right ear to be more efficient (called a right ear advantage) at remembering Morse code messages (in which short and long sounds are presented sequentially) and sequences of pitches. Subjects also have been found to be superior both at remembering the sequence in which fingers of their right hands were touched (Nachshon & Carmon, 1975) and at performing sequences of movements with their right hands when right-hand and left-hand performance were compared (Kimura & Archibald, 1974). The left hemisphere also has been found to be superior at remembering sequences of stimuli presented tachistoscopically (Tomlinson-Keasey & Kelly, 1979). This is commonly referred to as a left visual-field advantage.

In contrast, the right hemisphere has been described as superior at *simultaneous processing* and *holistic* (gestalt) thinking, that is, thinking in terms of complex wholes, rather than parts (Kumar, 1973). The right hemisphere is thought to use a more intuitive approach to problem solving, considering several alternatives at one time. Both adults and children who have right hemisphere lesions have particular difficulty with copying complex designs. Their designs tend to be full of details, but they show impairment of overall organization (Lezak, 1983; Stiles-Davis, Janowsky, Engel, & Nass, 1988). Experiments with individuals following commissurotomy have demonstrated that the left hand (right hemisphere) is superior to the right hand (left hemisphere) at sorting shapes when two attributes (height and width) had to be considered at the same time (Kumar, 1973). Subjects can more readily recall which fingers on their left hands have been touched when several fingers are touched simultaneously (Nachshon & Carmon, 1975).

Subjects with brain injuries to either the right or left hemisphere have difficulty copying and drawing representational designs in both two and three dimensions (Lezak, 1983). However, there are qualitative differences between the drawings of these two groups that appear to reflect differences in hemispheric processing style. Patients with left hemisphere lesions tend to oversimplify, maintaining a general sense of the design, but leaving out the internal details. By contrast, the designs of subjects with right hemisphere lesions are full of details, but lack overall organization (Kirk & Kertesz, 1989; Lezak, 1983). The problem usually is more severe in individuals with right hemisphere lesions. Further, the drawing ability of patients with right hemisphere lesions does not improve over time (Lezak, 1983; Villa, Gainotti, & DeBonis, 1986).

Although a deficit in reproducing designs originally was called constructional apraxia, it is now more commonly referred to as a deficit in *constructional abilities*, as it is felt to be reflective of a spatial, rather than motor, deficit (Cermak, 1984; Lezak, 1983). It should be noted that deficits in constructional abilities are found more commonly in patients with right hemisphere damage, including young children with early right hemisphere lesions (Stiles-Davis et al., 1988). Further studies using EEGs have demonstrated increased right hemisphere activity during constructional tasks (Dawson, Warrenburg, & Fuller, 1985).

## Perception and Cognition

The major aspect of cognition that has been attributed to the left hemisphere is language, both expressive and receptive. Studies of patients with brain injuries have historically focused on the receptive and expressive aphasia found frequently in patients with left hemisphere lesions. Patients who have had commissurotomies, although able to recognize some simple words presented to the right hemisphere, are able to use language to describe only what has been presented to the left hemisphere (Gazzaniga, 1975). Children with early lesions of the left hemisphere have been found to have particular difficulty with the syntax of language (Aram & Whitaker, 1988). Further, studies of perceptual asymmetry consistently have demonstrated a left hemisphere advantage for linguistic stimuli. Studies using dichotic listening with children as young as $2\frac{1}{2}$ years of age have demonstrated a right ear advantage for linguistic stimuli (Bever, 1971; Kamptner, Kraft, & Harper, 1984), and a right ear advantage has been found consistently in children aged 3 years and older (Kinsbourne & Hiscock, 1977; Eling, Marshall, & van Galen, 1981). Similarly, tachistoscopic studies with children who were presented with linguistic stimuli (numerals, letters, and words) generally have found a right visual field advantage in these children (Davidoff & Done, 1984; Ellis & Young, 1981; Yeni-Komshian, Isenberg, & Goldberg, 1975).

The right hemisphere has been postulated to be more efficient than the left when processing nonverbal stimuli. Studies of adults with brain injuries have demonstrated that those adults have difficulty perceiving and remembering complex stimuli that are hard to label or describe (Lezak, 1983). Some (although not all) studies using dichotic listening have demonstrated a left ear advantage for music and environmental sounds (Bryden & Allard, 1982; Knox & Kimura, 1970; Piazza, 1977). In studies involving dichhaptic presentation of shapes that could not be verbally encoded, the left hand has been found to be superior (Hiscock, 1988). Nonverbal stimuli used with children in tachistoscopic studies have included facial recognition, dot enumeration, and color recognition. Results have tended to show a left visual field advantage (Turkewitz & Ross-Kossak, 1984; Young & Bion, 1979), although this result has not been consistent (Jones & Anuza, 1982; Saxby & Bryden, 1985).

The most notable ability attributed to the right hemisphere is its superiority with tasks involving spatial perception. Patients with injuries to the right hemisphere have been found to perform particularly poorly on tasks of visual-spatial ability, including copying block designs (constructional abilities) and completing puzzles (Lezak, 1983; Luria, 1980). Following commissurotomy, patients are able to complete geometric puzzles more efficiently with the left than the right hand, further suggesting right hemisphere superiority (Gazzaniga, 1975). Studies using tachistoscopic presentation and regional cerebral blood flow have shown the right hemisphere to be more active during various visual-spatial tasks, including spatial location and mental rotation (Deutch, et al., 1988; Risberg, Halsey, Wills, & Wilson, 1975). Problems with perception of their own bodies in space also can be seen in the tendency of patients with right hemisphere injuries to neglect the left side of space (Lin, 1989), and in the difficulty that many of these patients have in dressing (dressing "apraxia") (Poeck, 1986).

While patients with right hemisphere lesions seldom develop aphasia, many do demonstrate a monotonic (lacking intonation and rhythm) pattern to their speech. Although these patients may be quite talkative, they frequently have little depth or organization to the content of their speech (Lezak, 1983). Some patients also have had difficulty understanding complex stories and humorous material (Rivers & Love, 1980; Wapner, Hamby, & Gardner, 1981). Wapner and associates (Wapner et al., 1981) also noted that, when asked to explain a story, patients with right hemisphere lesions often repeated verbatim what had been told to them, rather than providing a summary of the story. These patients had difficulty drawing any inferences and, at times, added material that was irrelevant to the story (Wapner, Hamby, & Gardner, 1981).

## Academic Skills

### READING

The contributions of the two hemispheres to academic performance is not well documented, perhaps because of the complexity of academic tasks. While deficits in reading and in written language have been associated with left hemisphere lesions in adults (Lezak, 1983; Luria, 1980), children with lesions to either hemisphere have been found to have deficits in reading when compared with normal peers (Aram & Whitaker, 1988). This may indicate that both hemispheres contribute to learning reading. Left hemisphere lesions in children appear to cause more significant deficits in reading, especially comprehension, than right hemisphere lesions (Aram & Whitaker, 1988). Studies using tachistoscopes have demonstrated that letter and word recognition both are performed more efficiently by the left hemisphere (Hiscock, 1988). However, the recognition or decoding of words is only a small part of the skill of reading.

## MATHEMATICS

Studies of hemispheric specialization related to mathematics have concentrated on the ability of subjects to perform calculations. In adults, loss of the ability to perform mental and written calculations (acalculia) has been associated with lesions of the left hemisphere (Luria, 1980; Rosselli & Ardila, 1989). Lesions of the right hemisphere also may result in errors in written calculations. However, in this case, the errors are due to problems in aligning the numerals, rather than inability to perform the calculations (Benson & Weir, 1972; Rosselli & Ardila, 1989). Patients with right hemisphere lesions also have been found to be poor at mathematical reasoning and judgment (Rosselli & Ardila, 1989).

There are little data on mathematical disabilities in children with brain injuries. Hecaen (1983) reported acalculia to be associated with left hemisphere lesions, while Kiessling, Denckla, and Carlton (1983) indicated that children with lesions of the right hemisphere performed more poorly on written computations than did children with left hemisphere lesions. Voeller's (1986) study of children with right hemisphere deficits indicated that they had relatively more difficulty with computation skills than with reading single words.

While most of these studies have concentrated on subjects' abilities to perform calculations, mathematics is more complex than mere computational skills. Some mathematics educators have hypothesized that the right hemisphere has an important role in understanding and applying mathematical concepts (Davidson, 1983; Wheatley, 1983). This hypothesis is based on associations found between visual-spatial abilities and the understanding of mathematical concepts (Harris, 1978; Murray, 1988; Piemonte, 1982). Thus, in mathematical ability, as in reading, both hemispheres make important contributions.

## Motor Skills

One deficit associated with left hemisphere lesions in adults is *apraxia*, in which patients have been noted to have difficulty with performing (a) *previously learned* movements, (b) gestures to commands, and (c) sequences of movements. The left hemisphere's superiority at sequencing movements has been further demonstrated by Kimura (1977; Kimura & Archibald, 1974). In her experiments with both normal subjects and subjects with brain injuries, the right hand was found to be superior to the left in imitating sequences of movements. However, Canavan and his associates (Canavan, Passingham, Marsden, Quinn, Wyke, & Polkey, 1989) noted decreased motor sequencing in patients with right temporal lobectomies, but not in those with lobectomies of the left temporal lobe. Further, Jason (1986) found that frontal lesions of either hemisphere affected the subjects' abilities to perform rapid motor sequences. Stockmeyer (1980) has hypothesized that the right hemisphere is specialized for "holding" postures. This hypothesis is consistent with the finding of motor impersistence, or the inability to sustain a movement or posture, in patients with right lesions (Kertesz, Nicholson, Chancelliere, Kassa, & Black, 1985).

## Emotions

As with motor and academic skills, the two hemispheres have been hypothesized to have different specialized roles in the perception and expression of emotion. Patients with lesions of the left hemisphere have been described as negative, anxious, and depressed, while those with right hemisphere lesions often are categorized as indifferent or sometimes euphoric (Gainotti, 1972; Robinson & Price, 1982; Sackheim, Greenberg, Weiman, Gur, Hungerbuhler, & Geschwind, 1982). Thus, the left hemisphere is believed to have a major role in positive emotions, while negative emotions are more closely linked to the right hemisphere. Some studies of normal adults, using tachistoscopic presentation, have provided support for these hypotheses. These studies have demonstrated a left hemisphere advantage for perception of faces that have a happy expression and a right hemisphere advantage when the faces presented are sad (Davidson, Schaffer, & Saron, 1985; Reuter-Lorenz, Givis, & Moscovitch, 1983). Schiff and Lamon (1989) have demonstrated this same difference between the two hemispheres in the expression of emotions.

Other studies have demonstrated that the right hemisphere is specialized for the perception of emotion, regardless of content. Patients with right hemisphere lesions have been found more impaired at recognizing the emotional tone of facial expressions than patients with left hemisphere lesions (Cicone, Wapner, & Gardner, 1980; Benowitz, Bear, Rosenthal, Mesulam, Zaidel, & Sperry, 1983). Children with known or suspected right hemisphere lesions have been reported by Voeller (1986) to have difficulty interpreting social cues and expressing their own feelings. Several researchers have found normal subjects to have a left ear advantage on dichotic listening tests when recognizing the emotional tone of a sentence, regardless of the emotion presented (Ley & Bryden, 1982; Saxby & Bryden, 1984).

These disparate findings may be related to differences between perceiving and expressing emotions. Kinsbourne and Bemporad (1984) hypothesized that the parietal lobes are more involved with the analysis of input (perception), while the frontal lobes are more important in the control of action, which could include expression of emotions.

Fox and Davidson (1988) have presented evidence to support the hypothesis of Kinsbourne and Bemporad (1985). Using electroencephalographic (EEG) studies, they found increased activation of (a) the left frontal lobe during activities that elicit positive emotional expressions, and (b) the right frontal lobe during activities that elicit negative emotional responses. They further found that the right parietal lobe is active regardless of the type of emotions elicited. Based on these findings, Fox and Davidson (1988) hypothesized that the perception of emotion is a function of the right parietal lobe, whereas emotional expression may be controlled by both hemispheres. They further hypothesized that the right hemisphere plays a stronger role in expressing negative behaviors while the left is more involved with the expression of positive emotion.

## LIMITATIONS OF THE LEFT-RIGHT DICHOTOMY

Hemispheric specialization has become a popular subject in many professional fields and in the popular press. Individuals have become interested in discovering their *hemisphericity*, or preferred hemisphere for problem solving (Kinsbourne, 1982). A linear, analytical approach to solving problems is said to reflect left hemisphere preference, while an approach that is integrative and holistic is indicative of a preference for the right hemisphere. Consultants in management are developing "left brain" and "right brain" styles of organization. Educators, in particular, have adopted this concept of "left-brain" vs. "right-brain" thinking (Gray, 1980). The current educational system has been described as too left-brain oriented, and some educational literature has begun to emphasize the importance of teaching to the more creative right hemisphere (Harris, 1988; Prince, 1978). While this concept is intuitively appealing, it is oversimplified, and there are many limitations to this conceptualization of the difference in function of the two hemispheres.

The strict left hemisphere–right hemisphere dichotomy in the application of hemispheric specialization does not take into consideration other aspects of the functional organization of the brain. Cortical functions also differ between anterior and posterior regions (Luria, 1980). The frontal lobes have been described as having an executive function; they are thought to be responsible for developing and organizing a plan for the attainment of a goal. As such, they have been described as being responsible for future-oriented behavior (Walsh & Pennington, 1988). Posterior areas of the brain play a major role in the reception, association, and integration of both sensory inputs and motor outputs.

Any model of brain function also must take into account the effects of the subcortical structures on the cortex and vice-versa. For example, studies have indicated that specific areas of the thalamus project to language areas of the cortex, and that damage to this area of the thalamus can result in language impairment. Subcortical areas are essential to the organization and initiation of movement (see also Chapters 4 and 6). Kinsbourne (1982) also has emphasized the importance of the brainstem in cortical functions. He has stated that ascending activation from the brainstem to the cortex is essential for cortical functions.

Finally, and most importantly, existing tests of hemispheric specialization, both those assessing broad skills such as language, and those assessing very specific perceptual asymmetries, cannot reflect the complexity of functioning of the brain in everyday life. We are at all times attending to complex stimuli from a variety of sources. While we may be engaged in one specific task, our central nervous systems are responding to many inputs. Further, one task may require many different types of thinking and processing.

For example, Sally is preparing a new recipe for a party she is giving. She needs to be able to read and understand the recipe, follow a sequence of directions, measure out the ingredients, and determine when these ingredients have been appropriately mixed. At the same time, Sally is watching an interview on the television. She is listening to what is being said and comparing the ideas expressed with her own ideas. When the doorbell rings, she stops what she is doing and opens the door for her first guest. She returns to the kitchen, remembering where she left off in the recipe, and, by listening to the interview, making assumptions about the part of the interview she did not hear. At the same time, Sally is estimating whether the meal will be prepared by 6 o'clock. In addition, Sally is using her arms and hands for the food preparation and walking both in the kitchen and to the front door. When she drops something on the floor, she bends down to pick it up.

It is obvious from this example that it is impossible to attribute the multitude of functions in everyday life to any one specific part of the brain. While some parts of the central nervous system may be more active than others, there is activity at all levels at all times, and cooperation throughout the brain is the sine qua non of the central nervous system (Jeeves & Baumgartner, 1986).

# HEMISPHERIC SPECIALIZATION AND SENSORY INTEGRATION THEORY

In her earlier work, Ayres suggested that sensorimotor processes, such as bilateral integration and postural responses, fostered the lateralization of cerebral function (Ayres, 1975). Sensory integration theory has postulated that bilateral integration, or the ability to use the two sides of the body in a coordinated manner, is a necessary basis for the development of hand preference (Berk & DeGangi, 1983). Poor bilateral integration and weak hand preference have been thought, in turn, to reflect weak or inadequate lateralization of function in the two hemispheres, and the implication has been made that there is a delay in lateralization. Further, Ayres (1976) found an association between indicators of central vestibular system dysfunction and poor bilateral integration. Based on this finding, she hypothesized that vestibular dysfunction may contribute to deficits in bilateral integration and to inadequate lateralization (Ayres, 1979). Treatment that provided opportunities for intake of enhanced vestibular information, then, was thought to improve lateralization of the hemispheres.

Recent evidence of functional asymmetry in infants, combined with the anatomical asymmetries found in fetal and infant brains, have prompted the conclusion that the degree to which each hemisphere will be lateralized for different functions, including hand preference, is present at birth (Crowell, Jones, Kapunial, & Nakagawa, 1973; Molfese & Betz, 1988). Further, researchers using dichotic listening generally have found no increase in strength of ear advantage as children get older; this suggests that the degree of lateralization is innate (Obrzut, 1988; Obrzut & Boliek, 1986). Thus, poor bilateral integration and weak hand preference do not reflect a delay in lateralization.

Although lateralization may not develop, the central nervous system does; the relative specialization of each hemisphere for certain skills becomes more apparent as a child matures. When we see an increase in hand preference and the development of more complex language, we have, in the past, assumed that this behavior reflects an increase in lateralization. However, these observations are in fact more likely to reflect a maturing of functional abilities in a brain that already is lateralized (Molfese & Segalowitz, 1988). Thus, while sensory integration may enhance brain function (including cortical function) it most likely does not actually affect lateralization.

We also need to remember that *weak* lateralization, or a lack of hemispheric asymmetry, is not synonymous with *inadequate* lateralization. Weak lateralization does not, in and of itself, indicate dysfunction, nor is it suggestive of immaturity. While it does suggest more sharing of skills between the two hemispheres, there is to date no empirical support to suggest that a lack of asymmetry results in inefficiency. In fact, weak lateralization is a finding typical of left-handed subjects who have no disability (Kinsbourne, 1988).

Sensory integration theory emphasizes improved sensory processing at a subcortical level. However, the brain communicates at all levels. In Chapter 4, we discussed the notion that cortical projections of vestibular-proprioceptive inputs are related to planning and executing bilateral and sequenced movements. In Chapter 6, we indicated that praxis in children may be related both to cortical function and to somatosensory processing. Thus, we have indications of a relationship between sensory processing and cortical function (although not to the specific function of one hemisphere). Therefore, in certain instances, improved sensory processing could be expected to have a positive effect on other aspects of cortical functioning.

If sensory processing is intact, however, there is no indication of sensory integrative dysfunction. Therefore, there is no reason to suggest that therapy using sensory integration treatment procedures will result in improved function of either hemisphere. Based on her research, Ayres (1979) appropriately expressed concern that children with hemisphere dysfunction, without indications of deficits of sensory integration, might not benefit from intervention programs *using a sensory integration approach*, although occupational therapy intervention based on other approaches may be beneficial. However, when there are indications of dysfunction in both sensory processing *and* hemisphere function, we might speculate that there is some relationship between the two, particularly if the dysfunction is associated with the right hemisphere. Recall that Rourke (1988) hypothesized that cortical-subcortical connections were of particular importance in *maintaining* the specialized skills of the right hemisphere. In making this speculation, we need to keep in mind that currently there is little experimental evidence that improved sensory integration results in an improvement of function in the specialized abilities of either hemisphere.

## HEMISPHERIC SPECIALIZATION AND LEARNING DISABILITIES

Hemispheric specialization has long been used to provide a model to explain learning disabilities. The concept that reading disabilities (dyslexia) were the result of weak or abnormal lateralization was popularized in the 1930s by Orton (1937). While Orton's model is not generally accepted today, the concept that learning disabilities are related to left or right hemisphere dysfunction has become increasingly popular, and research support for this conceptualization has grown substantially (Harris, 1988).

Research findings based on measures of perceptual asymmetry, as well as morphological and physiological studies, are inconsistent, but they do suggest that at least some children with learning disabilities show patterns of cerebral organization that differ from those of most normal children. One reason for the inconsistency in results from these studies may be due to variability in the definitions, and selection, of subjects with learning disabilities (Bryden, 1988; Obrzut, 1988). In fact, children with learning disabilities do not form a homogeneous group. Rather, there appear to be subtypes of classifications within the broad diagnostic category of learning disabilities characterized by different patterns of strengths and weaknesses (Mattis, French, & Rapin, 1975; Strang & Rourke, 1985).

### Inferential Measures of Hemisphere Dysfunction

In addition to the research methods described earlier, hemispheric specialization in children with learning disabilities has been studied using what might be called inferential measures. Because these measures also are frequently used in clinical assessments, the use of inferential measures will be described in more detail.

The concept of hemispheric specialization has been used as one method of categorizing children with learning disabilities. Clinically, this categorization is done by giving a child a battery of both verbal and nonverbal tests. If the child performs significantly more poorly on the verbal tests than on the nonverbal ones, a left hemisphere deficit is inferred. Similarly, if the performance is poorer on the nonverbal tests, a deficit is inferred to exist in the right hemisphere (Gordon, 1988; Rourke, 1988; Strang & Rourke, 1985). These hypotheses are based, in part, on the performances on verbal and non-verbal tests of patients with unilateral brain injuries.

Probably the test most frequently used in assessing verbal vs. non-verbal skills in children is the Wechsler Intelligence Scale for Children – Revised (WISC – R) (Wechsler, 1974). This standardized intelligence test consists of 10 subtests, 5 of which measure verbal skills and 5 of which measure non-verbal, or performance, skills. In addition to the overall IQ score, separate IQ scores are obtained for the verbal and performance subtests. Some studies of patients with unilateral brain injuries, using the adult version of this test, have indicated that those with left hemisphere lesions perform more poorly on the verbal tests than the performance tests, whereas the opposite pattern is found for patients with lesions of the right hemisphere (Black, 1980; Warrington, James, Maciejewski, 1986). Based on these findings, it is often assumed that significant discrepancies of 15 points or more (Wechsler, 1974) between the verbal and performance IQ scores on the WISC – R are reflective of inefficiency of one hemisphere (e.g., Strang & Rourke, 1985). Thus, if a child had a verbal IQ of 100 and a performance IQ of 84, we might infer a right hemisphere dysfunction. Significant discrepancies between verbal and performance IQs are found in many, but not all, children with learning disabilities (Rourke & Strang, 1983; Strang & Rourke, 1985).

Kaufman (1979) has pointed out that styles of processing (sequential vs. simultaneous) may be a more important distinction between the two hemispheres than any differences in the content processed. Kaufman and Kaufman (1983) have developed an intelligence test for children that provides separate scores for sequential processing and simultaneous processing. They describe their test, the Kaufman Assessment Battery for Children (K – ABC), as being based on cerebral specialization research. A relatively lower score (generally 12 to 15 points lower) on the sequential-processing subscale would indicate a left hemisphere deficit, whereas, if the simultaneous-processing subscale is lower, an inefficiency of the right hemisphere might be hypothesized. Some support for this hypothesis has been provided by Obrzut and his associates (Obrzut, Obrzut, Bryden, & Bartels, 1985), who found an association between a right ear advantage for syllables on dichotic listening tests and the sequential-processing subscale in learning-disabled and normal children.

Another method of assessment that may be used to make inferences about hemisphere function has been developed by Waber and Holmes (1985) using the Rey-Osterrieth Complex Figure (Lezak, 1983). The ability to copy this complex figure is a measure of two-dimensional constructional ability. As we discussed earlier, although lesions of either hemisphere can result in deficits in construction, there are qualitative differences in these deficits. Those with left hemisphere lesions tend to maintain the overall configuration of the figure to be copied, while losing the details. Lesions of the right hemisphere, by contrast, tend to result in a loss of the overall design, resulting in a collection of details.

Using this knowledge of differences in approach, Waber and Holmes (1985) have devised a scoring system to be used with children that categorizes their replications as part-oriented, configurational, or intermediate (a combination of the two approaches). For example, a part-oriented approach in a design that is relatively well drawn may reflect a preference for this style when approaching complex tasks.

However, if the design is poorly drawn and lacking in overall configuration, we might conclude that there is an inefficiency of the right hemisphere.

Waber and Holmes (1985, 1986) have noted these different styles in children with learning disabilities and have found them to be even more pronounced when the child is asked to draw the figure from memory shortly after copying it. Weintraub and Mesulam (1983) used the Rey-Osterrieth Complex Figure with adolescent and adult patients who had suspected right hemisphere dysfunction. Although no major problems were noted when copying the design, their subjects showed major impairment when asked to draw the design from memory immediately after copying it. Their reproductions were notable for distortions and omissions, and they lacked a sense of the overall configuration of the design.

While we may use measures such as those above to make inferences about hemispheric specialization, it is important to remember that poor performance in one area is not proof of hemisphere inefficiency. Moreover, good language skills do not necessarily indicate a strong left hemisphere; children who have had their left hemispheres removed at a young age show few, if any, significant problems with language (Witelson, 1977), and there are indications that these children may have more long-term problems with complex visual-spatial tasks (Ogden, 1989).

A few studies of children and adults with learning disabilities have linked sensory or motor asymmetry with specific areas of deficit, supporting an association of these deficits with hemisphere dysfunction. Rourke and his associates (Rourke, 1988; Rourke, Young, & Leenaars, 1989) have noted an association between nonverbal deficits and both poor tactile perception and psychomotor incoordination, particularly on the left side. Similarly, in a review of case histories of 14 patients with what were described as "nondyslexic learning disabilities," Weintraub and Mesulam (1983) noted left-sided motor asymmetries (posturing or slowed rapid movements) in all cases. Research by Ayres (1976) indicated an association between a right ear advantage on dichotic listening tests and measures of auditory-language abilities. However, Hynd, Obrzut, and Obrzut (1981) found no association between ear preference on a dichotic listening test and verbal-performance discrepancies on the WISC-R.

Thus, it is not clear that measures such as the WISC-R are indicative of hemisphere function. They are valuable, however, in determining patterns of strengths and weaknesses for learning within subtypes of children with learning disabilities, and in providing information needed to develop a remedial program for an individual child.

## Clinical Picture of Hemisphere Dysfunction

Researchers and clinicians who have described the clinical picture of left and right hemisphere dysfunction have relied, to a great extent, on the inferential measures described above, as well as on observations of individuals in daily activities. The following sections will present descriptions of the characteristics commonly associated with left and right hemisphere dysfunction in children with learning disabilities. Because the vast majority of this research is conducted by psychologists and educators, the emphasis has been on the cognitive and academic profile that can be obtained. However, there are some aspects of the research that relate closely to the immediate concerns of occupational therapists.

## LEFT HEMISPHERE DYSFUNCTION

Left hemisphere dysfunction is strongly associated with language deficits and reading disabilities. Typically, children with hypothesized left hemisphere dysfunction have trouble early on associating the letters of the alphabet with their specific sounds in order to "decode" words. Language deficits also make reading comprehension difficult (Rourke & Fiske, 1988). Remembering details and the sequence of steps in an activity also can be a problem. This problem often is reflected in difficulty with complex mathematical calculations (Davidson, 1983).

Other problems associated with left hemisphere dysfunction are more relevant to occupational therapy. Although apraxia in the adult is associated with lesions of the left hemisphere, and dyspraxia in children has not been associated with a specific hemisphere, we have observed that some children with hypothesized left hemisphere dysfunction may have trouble performing sequences of motor skills. This problem could affect skills requiring fine motor sequencing, such as handwriting, buttoning, and shoe-tying, as well as gross motor activities that involve projected action sequences, such as some competitive sports and dances (see also Chapter 6).

Children with poor language skills may frequently feel socially isolated, owing to their difficulty in communicating with others. At times this problem may lead to inappropriate behaviors, such as acting out, in order to gain the attention of others (Brumback & Staton, 1982). Recognizing this as a potential problem can be helpful when working with children who appear to have left hemisphere dysfunction.

Jimmy's profile is reflective of a pattern hypothesized to be due to left hemisphere inefficiency. His language disability, noted at an early age, is considered a hallmark of this dysfunction, as is his difficulty with reading. Jimmy has trouble remembering details and sequences of events, which can make subjects such as history quite difficult for him. His problems with sequencing also can be seen when he does mathematics. Jimmy has trouble remembering the steps used to complete multidigit multiplication and long-division problems. In contrast, Jimmy's good spatial skills give him an intuitive understanding of mechanical devices and machinery. He has an excellent sense of size and proportion, and, when building furniture in his woodworking class, he prefers to estimate lengths rather than go through the tedious process of measuring exactly.

## RIGHT HEMISPHERE DYSFUNCTION

Rourke (1988, 1989) has described right hemisphere dysfunction as a non-verbal learning disability. While the outstanding characteristic of left hemisphere dysfunction is the language disability, there is no one major impairment that suggests poor right hemisphere function (Brumback & Staton, 1982). Rather, we look for a cluster of symptoms.

One problem commonly found in children with right hemisphere dysfunction is difficulty in organizing and synthesizing information. It may be hard for such children to understand the main idea of a lesson or to make inferences and generate new ideas (Rourke, 1988, 1989). Furthermore, understanding mathematical concepts often does not come easily. Particular problems commonly seen include difficulty with time, money, and measurement concepts (Brumback & Staton, 1982; Davidson, 1983).

Some children with hypothesized right hemisphere dysfunction have trouble in the initial stages of reading. Letter recognition can be difficult, and the initial emphasis on sight words, which requires recognition of a visual configuration, increases the early demand on visual-perception skills in reading (Bakker, 1983). It has been noted, however, that most children with intact language skills are able to master the use of phonics to decode words and are often relatively successful in reading (Bakker, 1983; Strang & Rourke, 1985; Weintraub & Mesulam, 1983).

Many children with non-verbal learning disabilities are very talkative, with extensive vocabularies and no obvious problems with the syntax of language. However, analysis of the content of their speech often reveals a tendency to be tangential and a strong reliance on jargon and clichés (Rourke, 1988; Strang & Rourke, 1985).

Psychosocial or emotional problems also are frequently observed in children with hypothesized right hemisphere dysfunction. They seem unable to attend to non-verbal aspects of communication, such as gestures and voice intonation, as well as other children do, and they often miss inferences or "hidden meanings" in what is said to them. Many also display less emotion, through voice and gestures, than their peers (Brumback, 1988; Brumback & Staton, 1982; Ozols & Rourke, 1985; Weintraub & Mesulam, 1983). Further, they may have problems when presented with novel social situations. It can be difficult for them to "read" the situation and come up with an appropriate strategy or "game plan." Consequently many of these children have a real dislike of new situations. Depression also has been noted to be more common in children and adults with non-verbal learning disabilities than in those whose problems are more language-based (Brumback, 1988: Brumback & Staton, 1982; Fletcher, 1989; Rourke et al., 1989; Weintraub & Mesulam, 1983). Problems with attention also have been noted to be prevalent in children with indicators of right hemisphere dysfunction (Brumback, 1988; Brumback & Staton, 1982; Rourke, 1988).

Children with hypothesized right hemisphere dysfunction, or non-verbal learning disabilities, have several problems that are commonly addressed by occupational therapy. They generally have difficulty with constructional tasks and other activities involving visual-spatial skills, such as drawing and completing puzzles.

Problems with handwriting also are typically seen, particularly when these children are initially learning to write. Letters are poorly formed, and the size of letters is not consistent. Spacing between words also is variable (Brumback & Staton, 1982; Rourke, 1989). Problems with handwriting can interfere with written calculations. Just as in the case of adults with brain injuries, these children often have problems with alignment of numerals when writing mathematics problems (Rourke & Strang, 1983).

Clumsiness frequently is mentioned when describing children with suggested right hemisphere dysfunction; it is especially noticeable in games and sports that require making judgments about movement of the body or an object through space (Brumback & Staton, 1982). Gubbay (1975) noted that the performance IQ was often lower than the verbal IQ in children with developmental dyspraxia (see Chapter 6). A poor sense of body scheme may interfere with learning dressing skills.

Ross' pattern of strengths and weaknesses is typical of an adolescent with hypothesized dysfunction of the right hemisphere. He has major difficulties with aspects of learning that involve organizing and synthesizing information. Although he is able to recall specific details in stories he has read, he is unable to relate the main idea and has trouble answering inferential questions. Similarly, in history class, he is noted for his ability to remember names and dates, but it is difficult for him to explain how events are related.

Ross' great difficulty with mathematics is considered to be reflective of his deficits in visual-spatial abilities. Although he has been able to memorize his number facts, it is hard for him to apply these facts in day-to-day situations, which suggests that he has difficulty understanding mathematical concepts and applications.

Ross also has been described as clumsy. He has particular difficulty with skills that require spatial judgments, such as playing ball games. His clumsiness, combined with his difficulties with social skills, have resulted in his being avoided by his peers.

## Evaluation of Hemisphere Dysfunction in Learning Disabilities

When evaluating children with suspected sensory integration dysfunction, we frequently include assessments that also may allow us to *hypothesize* about hemisphere functioning. One reason for doing this is that it provides a more complete picture of possible neurological dysfunction. Another reason for attempting to determine if a child's problems may be related to hemisphere dysfunction is that this information can guide us in determining appropriate interventions. Although a sensory integrative approach may be beneficial in improving dysfunction that is thought to be due to subcortical disorders, as discussed earlier, it is not the approach of choice with children whose problems appear to be solely cortically based.

We will discuss tests from the SIPT (Ayres, 1989), as well as other types of tests and observations that would be useful in assessing hypothesized functions of the left and right hemispheres. The SIPT were *not* designed to assess dysfunction within the cerebral hemispheres. However, there are several tests of the SIPT that may prove helpful in postulating dysfunction within one of the hemispheres. In the following sections, we will discuss the use of the SIPT and other assessment tools that can be helpful when making a judgment about hypothesized hemisphere dysfunction. We need to keep in mind that, like the WISC–R, the measures described here are inferential. As always, we are looking for a *meaningful cluster* of low scores or poor performances, rather than isolated instances of deficit.

### THE SENSORY INTEGRATION AND PRAXIS TESTS

Possible left hemisphere dysfunction may be indicated by a low score on Praxis on Verbal Command. Praxis on Verbal Command is a test that requires the child to assume a position when given a verbal direction (e.g., "Put your elbows together"). Factor analysis indicated a relationship between low scores on this test, which has an obvious language component, and increased duration of nystagmus after rotation on the Postrotary Nystagmus Test (Ayres, 1989). Ayres (1976, 1979) suggested that increased postrotary nystagmus may be reflective of a lack of cortical inhibition and, based on her research, hypothesized that it was particularly related to dysfunction of the left hemisphere. Thus, a low score on Praxis on Verbal Command and increased postrotary nystagmus, *in combination*, may reflect dysfunction within the left hemisphere (Ayres, 1989). Additionally, as sequencing has been associated with left hemisphere function, those tests of the SIPT that involve sequencing of movement (i.e., Sequencing Praxis, Oral Praxis, Bilateral Motor Coordination, and, possibly, Standing and Walking Balance) could also be used when making assumptions about the integrity of the left hemisphere. In fact, research using the SIPT indicated that a low score on Praxis on Verbal Command is associated with poor performance on the tests that involve motor sequencing (Ayres, 1989). The pattern of *increased* postrotary nystagmus, along with *depressed scores* on Praxis on Verbal Command, Sequencing Praxis, Oral Praxis, Bilateral Motor Coordination, and Standing and Walking Balance, *in the absence of indicators of vestibular-proprioceptive dysfunction*, suggests left hemisphere dysfunction rather than sensory integrative dysfunction. Note, however, that when deficits in planning bilateral projected action sequences are associated with left hemisphere dysfunction, the disorder is *not referred to as a deficit in bilateral integration and sequencing* (see Chapters 4 and 6).

As the perception of form and space, as well as constructional abilities, are associated with the *right hemisphere*, low scores on tests of these areas may suggest dysfunction in that hemisphere. Tests of form and space perception on the SIPT include Space Visualization, which requires shape discrimination as well as mental rotation of shapes, and Figure-Ground Perception, in which a child must recognize a figure either among overlapping figures or embedded in a rival background. The SIPT also include two tests of constructional abilities, Design Copying and Constructional Praxis. Design Copying is a test of two-dimensional construction that requires the child to copy increasingly complex shapes. The Constructional Praxis test, in which the child copies two different block constructions, is a test of three-dimensional construction. Low scores on these tests, as well as on the form and space tests, might contribute to a picture suggestive of right hemisphere dysfunction. We should note that Ayres has labelled Design Copying and Constructional Praxis as tests of visuopraxis (Ayres, 1989). However, as discussed earlier, tests that involve construction are more commonly (and appropriately) referred to as tests of constructional abilities (see also Chapter 8).

Another test that may be associated with right hemisphere function is Manual Form Perception, in which shapes are recognized by touching and manipulating them (haptic perception). As mentioned earlier, some studies have indicated that haptic perception of shapes, particularly those that cannot be verbally encoded, is performed more efficiently by the right hemisphere.

Several tests of the SIPT provide separate scores for the left and right sides of the body. However, given the low test-retest reliability of these scores, *it is not recommended* that they be used to support an assessment of possible hemisphere dysfunction (Ayres, 1989).

## OTHER METHODS OF EVALUATION

Given that the primary deficit in children with hypothesized *left hemisphere* dysfunction is in language, scores on assessments of expressive and receptive language are essential predictors. Additionally, in older children, a significant delay in reading also may be an indicator of dysfunction. These two primary areas of assessment, then, are the domain of disciplines other than occupational therapy (e.g., speech and language pathology and special education). When delays are suspected, a referral is indicated.

Occupational therapy assessment may find indications of problems with motor sequencing on items from tests of motor skills such as the Bruininks-Oseretsky Test of Motor Proficiency (Bruininks, 1978), or through informal observation of motor activities. Additionally, indications of motor asymmetry, with the right side of the body performing more poorly than the left, would suggest possible left hemisphere dysfunction.

Occupational therapy testing may be more helpful when assessing right, rather than left, hemisphere dysfunction. Tests of visual perception, such as the Test of Visual-Perceptual Skills (Non-Motor) (Gardner, 1982) and assessments of visuomotor or constructional abilities, such as the Developmental Test of Visual-Motor Integration (Beery, 1989), are commonly given by occupational therapists to provide information about a child's ability to perform tasks associated with the right hemisphere. Additionally, we often observe a child performing activities such as moving his or her body through space, copying block designs, or completing puzzles. We need to keep in mind, however, that right hemisphere dysfunction is not the *only* reason for poor performances on any of these tests or activities. Again, indications of motor asymmetry, with the left side of the body performing more poorly than the right, should be noted.

Tests such as the Rey-Osterrieth Complex Figure (Lezak, 1983; Waber & Holmes, 1985), which allows us to watch a child's approach to a task, as well as to analyze the final product, also can provide valuable information. For example, a child may copy a design using a more segmented or piecemeal approach, suggesting a left hemisphere style. Conversely, the approach may be more holistic, representative of a right hemisphere style.

Additionally, it is generally helpful to have the results of a psychological evaluation, using either the K–ABC to assess simultaneous vs. sequential processing, or the WISC–R, which provides a sample of verbal vs. non-verbal functions. Naturally, these evaluations should be administered by a psychologist.

## Intervention for Hemisphere Dysfunction

When a child's problems are felt to be due solely to dysfunction in either the left or right hemisphere, intervention *based on sensory integration theory* would not be appropriate. This does not mean that occupational therapy is not indicated. However, it is well beyond the scope of this book to provide a detailed discussion of intervention approaches that could be used for these children. The following sections will provide only a brief discussion of the intervention for hemisphere dysfunction, including when sensory integration procedures may be appropriate.

### INTERVENTION FOR LEFT HEMISPHERE DYSFUNCTION

Language deficits are the major problem in children with left hemisphere dysfunction, so it is essential to have a child evaluated by a speech and language pathologist if such a dysfunction is suspected. Intervening with a child who has a language disability requires the expertise of a speech and language pathologist; a carefully designed educational program also is essential. Occupational therapists do not have the necessary training to treat language deficits.

Occupational therapy may be helpful in improving difficulties with motor sequencing, which can affect skills such as handwriting, managing fasteners, and mastering the sequence of steps necessary to ride a bicycle. Depending on the problems and the needs of the child, the therapist could help the child to practice a specific skill (e.g., fastening a button) or could provide activities that allow the child to practice sequencing alone. Additionally, if motor asymmetries are found, intervention could be aimed at improving right-sided function.

### INTERVENTION FOR RIGHT HEMISPHERE DYSFUNCTION

Many of the deficits seen in children with hypothesized right hemisphere dysfunction are those that may be addressed by occupational therapy. Visual-perceptual problems are a common area that is frequently treated. Additionally, clumsiness and difficulties with moving through space would be appropriate areas for occupational therapy intervention. If we had been able to treat Ross as a young boy, we would have wanted to address his problems with dressing and handwriting, his general clumsiness, and his overall difficulty in organizing himself and his life. Because occupational therapists also are trained in psychosocial dysfunction, it may be appropriate at some point for a therapist to help Ross with his difficulty in both expressing and understanding emotions. Another important role with Ross would be in consulting with his parents and his teachers to help them understand how his disability affects his daily life and what they can do to help Ross achieve independence. (For some excellent suggestions that could be used when consulting for children with hypothesized right hemisphere dysfunction, see Strang & Rourke, 1985.)

## USE OF SENSORY INTEGRATIVE PROCEDURES FOR CHILDREN WITH HEMISPHERE DYSFUNCTION

It is possible for a child with hemisphere dysfunction also to show subcortical deficits. As many researchers have noted, ascending activation from subcortical mechanisms plays an important role in hemisphere function. Thus, in some children who appear to have inefficiency in one or both hemispheres, we would not be surprised to find indicators of subcortical dysfunction, such as poor tactile perception, or indicators of poor processing of vestibular-proprioceptive information. For example, in addition to indicators of right hemisphere dysfunction, Ross may have low muscle tone and problems with balance, both possible indicators of vestibular-proprioceptive dysfunction. While a portion of his occupational therapy intervention program would emphasize improving his ability to organize himself and his world, it also would be appropriate to use sensory integrative procedures designed to enhance vestibular-proprioceptive function. We need to be aware, however, that these procedures are expected to affect subcortical function, improving Ross' muscle tone and balance and, in this way, to result in improved motor skills. It should not be assumed that they will improve his hemisphere deficit. Although Rourke (1988) hypothesized that subcortical-cortical connections may be of particular importance to the right hemisphere, any specific link at this point between sensory integration procedures and improved cortical function is tenuous.

Many sensory integration treatment procedures include activities that would address the specific motor problems that may occur with right or left hemisphere dysfunction. For example, some activities used require a child to perform a sequence of movements, a problem for some children with left hemisphere dysfunction. Similarly, many activities, particularly those using suspended equipment, are designed, in part, to improve a child's sense of his or her body in space; body scheme often is an area of deficit for children with dysfunction of the right hemisphere. It would be appropriate, then, when designing an intervention program, to combine some treatment procedures that are based on sensory integrative principles with other types remedial activities aimed more directly at teaching specific skills. Let it be understood that, in this situation, we are using these activities in order to improve these specific skills. We are *not* treating a sensory integration problem.

# CONCLUSION

In this chapter, we have presented a summary of research in hemispheric specialization, along with clinical pictures of *hypothesized* left and right hemisphere dysfunction. Although we may observe the behaviors that have been associated with disorders of the left or right hemisphere, occupational therapists *do not diagnose* hemisphere dysfunction. We do, however, address many of the described behaviors during intervention, and concepts from hemispheric specialization may provide a framework for understanding these behaviors.

Just as some, but not all, persons with learning disabilities may have sensory integrative dysfunction, some but not all, persons with sensory integrative dysfunction may have deficits of the left or right hemisphere. Although sensory integration theory does not directly address the specialization of the two hemispheres, it is a theory of brain function. Recognizing problems at *all levels* of brain function is essential for a full understanding of the difficulties encountered by the clients that we serve.

# REFERENCES

Aram, D. M., & Whitaker, H. A. (1988). Cognitive sequelae of unilateral lesions acquired in early childhood. In D. L. Molfese & S. J. Segalowitz (Eds.), *Brain lateralization in children: Developmental implications* (pp. 417–436). New York: Guilford.

Ayres, A. J. (1969). Deficits in sensory integration in educationally-handicapped children. *Journal of Learning Disabilities, 2*, 44–51.

Ayres, A. J. (1972). *Sensory integration and learning disorders.* Los Angeles: Western Psychological Services.

Ayres, A. J. (1975). Sensorimotor foundations of academic ability. In W. M. Cruickshank & D. P. Hallahan (Eds.), *Perceptual and learning disabilities in children, Vol 2: Research and theory* (pp 301–358). Syracuse, NY: Syracuse University.

Ayres, A. J. (1976). *The effect of sensory integrative therapy on learning disabled children: The final report of a research project.* Los Angeles: University of Southern California.

Ayres, A. J. (1979). *Sensory integration and the child.* Los Angeles: Western Psychological Services.

Ayres, A. J. (1989). *Sensory Integration and Praxis Tests.* Los Angeles: Western Psychological Services.

Bakker, D. J. (1983). Hemispheric specialization and specific reading retardation. In M. Rutter (Ed.), *Developmental neuropsychiatry* (pp. 498–506). New York: Guilford.

Beery, K. (1989). *The VMI: Developmental Test of Visual-Motor Integration.* Cleveland, OH: Modern Curriculum.

Benowitz, L. I., Bear, D. M., Rosenthal, R., Mesulam, M. M., Zaidel, E., & Sperry, R. (1983). Hemispheric specialization in nonverbal communication. *Cortex, 19*, 5–11.

Benson, D. F., & Weir, W. F. (1972). Acalculia: Acquired anarithmetia. *Cortex, 8*, 465–472.

Bever, T. G. (1971). The nature of cerebral dominance in speech behavior of the child and adult. In R. Huxley & E. Ingram (Eds.), *Language acquisition: Models and methods* (pp. 231–261). London: Academic.

Black, F. W. (1980). WAIS verbal-performance discrepancies as predictors of lateralization in patients with discrete brain lesions. *Perceptual and Motor Skills, 51*, 213–214.

Boles, D. B. (1989). Do visual field asymmetries intercorrelate? *Neuropsychologia, 27*, 697–704.

Bradshaw, J. L., Burden, V., & Nettleton, N. C. (1986). Dichotic and dichhaptic techniques. *Neuropsychologia, 24*, 79–91.

Brandeis, D., & Lehmann, D. (1986). Event-related potentials of the brain and cognitive processes: Approaches and applications. *Neuropsychologia, 24*, 150–159.

Bruininks, R. (1978). *Bruininks-Oseretsky Test of Motor Proficiency.* Circle Pines, MN: American Guidance Service.

Brumback, R. A. (1988). Childhood depression and medically treatable learning disability. In D. L. Molfese & S. J. Segalowitz (Eds.), *Brain lateralization in children: Developmental implications* (pp. 463–506). New York: Guilford.

Brumback, R. A., & Staton, R. D. (1982). An hypothesis regarding the commonality of right hemisphere involvement in learning disability, attentional disorder, and childhood major depressive disorder. *Perceptual and Motor Skills, 50*, 1163–1167.

Bryden, M. P. (1988). Does laterality make any difference? Thoughts on the relation between cerebral asymmetry and reading. In D. L. Molfese & S. J. Segalowitz (Eds.), *Brain lateralization in children: Developmental implications* (pp. 509–526). New York: Guilford.

Bryden, M. P., & Allard, F. A. (1981). Do auditory perceptual asymmetries develop? *Cortex, 17*, 313–318.

Canavan, A. G. M., Passingham, R. E., Marsden, C. D., Quinn, N., Wyke, M., & Polkey, C. E. (1989). Sequencing ability in parkinsonians, patients with frontal lobe lesions and patients who have undergone unilateral temporal lobectomies. *Neuropsychologia, 27*,d 787–798.

Carmon, A., & Nachshon, I. (1971). Effect of unilateral brain damage on perception of temporal order. *Cortex, 7*, 410–418.

Cermak, S. A. (1984). Constructional Apraxia. *Sensory Integration Special Interest Section Newsletter, 7*(3), 1–4.

Chi, F. G., Dooling, E. C., & Gilles, F. H. (1977). Left-right asymmetries of the temporal speech areas of the human fetus. *Archives of Neurology, 34*, 346–348.

Cicone, M., Wapner, W., & Gardner, H. (1980). Sensitivity to emotional expressions and situations in organic patients. *Cortex, 16*, 145–158.

Ciesielski, K. T. (1989). Event-related potentials in children with specific visual cognitive disability. *Neuropsychologia, 27,* 303–313.

Crowell, D. H., Jones, R. H., Kapuniai, L. E., & Nakagawa, J. K. (1973). Unilateral cortical activity in newborn infants: An early index of cerebral dominance? *Science, 180,* 205–208.

Davidson, R. J. & Fox, N. A. (1988). Cerebral asymmetry and emotion: Developmental and individual differences. In D. L. Molfese & S. J. Segalowitz (Eds.), *Brain lateralizatiion in children: Developmental implications* (pp. 191–206). New York: Guilford.

Davidoff, J. B., & Done, D. J. (1984). A longitudinal study of the development of visual field advantage for letter matching. *Neuropsychologia, 22,* 311–318.

Dawson, G., Warrenberg, S., & Fuller, P. (1985). Left hemisphere specialization for facial and manual imitation. *Psychophysiology, 22,* 237–243.

Delacato, C. (1966). *Neurological organization in reading.* Springfield, IL: Charles C. Thomas.

Dennis, M. (1980). Capacity and strategy for syntactic comprehension after left or right hemidecortication. *Brain and Language, 10,* 287–307.

Deutsch, G., Bourbon, W. T., Papanicoluou, A. C., & Eisenberg, H. M. (1988). Visuospatial tasks compared via activation of regional cerebral blood flow. *Neuropsychologia, 26,* 445–452.

Duffy, F. H., Denckla, M. B., Bartels, P. H., & Sandini, G. (1980). Dyslexia: Regional differences in brain electrical activity by topographic mapping. *Annals of Neurology, 7,* 412–420.

Eccles, J. C. (1973). *The understanding of the brain.* New York: McGraw-Hill.

Eling, P., Marshall, J. C., & Van Galen, G. (1981). The development of language lateralization as measured by dichotic listening. *Neuropsychologia, 19,* 767–773.

Ellis, A. W., & Young, A. W. (1981). Visual hemifield asymmetry for naming concrete nouns and verbs in children between seven and eleven years of age. *Cortex, 17,* 617–624.

Fletcher, J. M. (1989). Nonverbal learning disabilities and suicide: Classification leads to prevention. *Journal of Learning Disabilities, 22,* 176–179.

Gainotti, G. (1972). Emotional behavior and hemispheric side of lesion. *Cortex, 8,* 41–55.

Galaburda, A. M. (1984). Anatomical asymmetries. In N. Geschwind & A. M. Galaburda (Eds.), *Cerebral dominance: The biological foundations* (pp. 11–25). Cambridge, MA: Harvard University.

Galaburda, A. M., & Kemper, T. L. (1979). Cytoarchitctonic abnormalities in developmental dyslexia: A case study. *Annals of Neurology, 6,* 94–100.

Galaburda, A. M., LeMay, M., Kemper, T. L., & Geschwind, N. (1978). Right-left asymmetries in the brain. *Science, 199,* 852–856.

Gardner, M. F. (1982). *Test of Visual-Perceptual Skill (Non-Motor).* Seattle, WA: Special Child.

Gazzaniga, M. S. (1975). Review of the split brain. *UCLA Educator, 17*(2), 9–16.

Geschwind, N., & Levitsky, W. (1968). Human brain: Left-right asymmetries in temporal speech region. *Science, 161,* 186–187.

Gordon, H. W. (1988). The effect of "right brain/left brain" cognitive profiles on school achievement. In D. L. Molfese & S. J. Segalowitz (Eds.), *Brain lateralization in children: Developmental implications* (pp. 237–256). New York: Guilford.

Gray, E. C. (1980). Brain hemispheres and thinking styles. *The Clearing House, 54,* 127–131.

Gubbay, S. S. (1975). *The clumsy child.* Philadelphia: W.B. Saunders.

Harris, L. J. (1988). Right-brain training: Some reflections on the application of research on cerebral hemispheric specialization to education. In D. L. Molfese & S. J. Segalowitz (Eds.), *Brain lateralization in children: Developmental implications* (pp. 207–236). New York: Guilford.

Harris, L. J. (1978). Sex differences in spatial ability: Possible environmental, genetic, and neurological factors. In M. Kinsbourne (Ed.), *Asymmetrical function of the brain* (pp. 405–521). Cambridge: Cambridge University.

Harris, L. J., & Carlson, D.F. (1988). Pathological left-handedness: An analysis of theories and evidence. In D. L. Molfese & S. J. Segalowitz (Eds.), *Brain lateralization in children: Developmental implications* (pp. 289–372). New York: Guilford.

Hecaen, H. (1983). Acquired aphasia in children: Revisited. *Neuropsychologia, 21,* 581–587.

Heiss, W-D., Herholz, K., Pawlik, G., Wagner, R., & Weinhard, K. (1986). Positron emission tomography in neuropsychology. *Neuropsychologia, 24,* 141–149.

Hiscock, M. (1988). Behavioral asymmeries in normal children. In D. L. Molfese & S. J. Segalowitz (Eds.), *Brain lateralization in children: Developmental implications* (pp. 85–169). New York: Guilford.

Hiscock, M., Antoniuk, D., Prisciak, K., & von Hessert, D. (1985). Generalized and lateralized interference between concurrent tasks performed by children. Effecs of age, sex, and skill. *Developmental Psychology, 1,* 29–48.

Hiscock, M., & Kinsbourne, M. (1982). Laterality and dyslexia: A critical review. *Annals of Dyslexia, 32,* 177–227.

Hugdahl, K., & Andersson, B. (1989). Dichotic listening in 126 left-handed childen: Ear advantages, familial sinistrality and sex differences. *Neuropsychologia, 27,* 999–1006.

Hynd, G. W., Obrzut, J. E., & Obrzut, A. (1981). Are lateral and perceptual asymmetries related to WISC–R and achievement test performance in normal and learning-disabled children? *Journal of Consulting and Clinical Psychology, 49,* 977–979.

Inglis, J., & Lawson, J. S. (1981). Sex differences in the effects of unilateral brain damage on intelligence. *Science, 212,* 693–695.

Jason, G. W. (1986). Performance of manual copying tasks after focal cortical lesions. *Neuropsychologia, 24,* 181–191.

Jeeves, M. A., & Baumgartner, G. (1986). Methods of investigation in neuropsychology. *Neuropsychologia, 24,* 1–4.

Jones, B., & Anuza, T. (1982). Sex differences in cerebral lateralization in 3- and 4-year-old children. *Neuropsychologia, 20,* 347–350.

Kamptner, L., Kraft, R. H., & Harper, L. V. (1984). Lateral specialization and social-verbal development in preschool children. *Brain and Cognition, 3,* 42–50.

Kaufman, A. S. (1979). Cerebral specialization and intelligence testing. *Journal of Research and Development in Education, 12,* 96–107.

Kaufman, A. S., & Kaufman, N. L. (1983). *Kaufman Assessment Battery for Children.* Circle Pines, MN: American Guidance Service.

Kephart, N. (1960). *The slow learner in the classroom.* Columbus, OH: Charles Merrill.

Kertesz, A., Nicholson, I., Chanceliere, A., Kassa, K., & Black, S. E. (1985). Motor impersistence: A right-hemisphere syndrome. *Neurology, 35,* 662–666.

Kiessling, L. S., Denckla, M. B., & Carlton, M. (1983). Evidence for differential hemispheric function in children with hemiplegia cerebral palsy. *Developmental Medicine and Child Neurology, 25,* 727–734.

Kimura, D. (1977). Acquisition of a motor skill after left-hemisphere damage. *Brain, 100,* 527–542.

Kimura, D. & Archibald, Y. (1974). Motor functions of the left hemisphere. *Brain, 97,* 337–350.

Kinsbourne, M. (1982). Hemispheric specialization and the growth of human understanding. *American Psychologist, 37,* 411–420.

Kinsbourne, M. (1988). Sinistrality, brain organization, and cognitive deficits. In D. L. Molfese & S. J. Segalowitz (Eds.), *Brain lateralization in children: Developmental implications* (pp. 259–280). New York: Guilford.

Kinsbourne, M., & Bemporad, B. (1984). Lateralization of emotion: A model and the evidence. In N. A. Fox & R. J. Davidson (Eds.), *The psychobiology of affective development* (pp. 259–291). Hillsdale, NJ: Lawrence Erlbaum Associates.

Kinsbourne, M., & Hiscock, M. (1977). Does cerebral dominance develop? In S. J. Segalowitz & F. A. Gruber (Eds.), *Language development and neurological theory* (pp. 171–191). New York: Academic.

Kirk, A., & Kertesz, A. (1989). Hemispheric contributions to drawing. *Neuropsychologia, 27,* 881–886.

Knox, C., & Kimura, D. (1970). Cerebral processing of nonverbal sounds in boys and girls. *Neuropsychologia, 8,* 227–237.

Koomar, J. A., & Cermak, S. A. (1981). Reliability of dichotic listening using two stimulus formats with normal and learning-disabled children. *American Journal of Occupational Therapy, 35,* 456–463.

Kumar, S. (1973). The right and left of being internally different. *Impact of Science on Society, 23,* 53–64.

Lawrence, D., & Kuypers, H. (1968). The functional organization of the motor system in the monkey. *Brain, 91,* 1–14.

LeMay, M. (1976). Morphological cerebral asymmetries of modern man, fossil man, and nonhuman primate. *Annals of the New York Academy of Science, 280,* 349–366.

LeMay, M. (1984). Radiological, developmental, and fossil asymmetries. In N. Geschwind & A. M. Galaburda (Eds.), *Cerebral dominance: The biological foundations* (pp. 26–42). Cambridge, MA: Harvard University.

LeMay, M. & Geschwind, N. (1978). Asymmetries of the human cerebral hemispheres. In A. Caramazza & E. B. Zurif (Eds.), *Language acquisition and language breakdown* (pp. 311–328). Baltimore, MD: Johns Hopkins.

LeMay, M., & Kido, D. K. (1978). Asymmetries of the cerebal hemispheres on computed tomograms. *Journal of Computer-Assisted Tomography, 2,* 471–476.

Levy, J. (1974). Psychobiological implications of brain asymmetry. In S. J. Dimond & J. C. Beaumont (Eds.), *Hemisphere function in the human brain* (pp. 121–182). New York: John Wiley & Sons.

Ley, R. G., & Bryden, M. P. (1982). A dissociation of right and left hemispheric effects for recognizing emotional tone and verbal content. *Brain and Cognition, 1,* 3–9.

Lezak, M. D. (1983). *Neuropsychological assessment* (2nd ed). New York: Oxford University.

Leiderman, J. (1988). Misconceptions and new conceptions about early brain damage, functional asymmetry, and behavioral outcome. In D. L. Molfese & S. J. Segalowitz (Eds.), *Brain lateralization in children: Developmental implications* (pp. 375–400). New York: Guilford.

Lin, K-C., (1989). *A meta-analysis of the efficacy of cognitive and peceptual retaining on unilateral neglect in pos-CVA patients.* Unpublished master's thesis, Boston University.

Luria, A. R. (1980). *Higher cortical functions in man* (2nd ed.). New York: Basic Books.

Mattis, S., French, J. H., & Rapin, I. (1975). Dyslexia in children and young adults: Three independent neuropsychological syndromes. *Developmental Medicine and Child Neurology, 17,* 150–163.

McGlone, J. (1978). Sex differences in functional brain asymmetry. *Cortex, 14,* 122–128.

Molfese, D. L., & Betz, J. C. (1988). Electrophysiological indices of the early development of lateralization for language and cognition, and their implications for predicting later development. In D. L. Molfese & S. J. Segalowitz (Eds.), *Brain lateralization in childen: Developmental implications* (pp. 171–190). New York: Guilford.

Molfese, D. L., & Segalowitz, S. J. (Eds.). (1988). *Brain lateralization in children: Developmental implications.* New York: Guilford.

Murray, E. A. (1988). The relationship between visual-spatial abilities and mathematics achievement in normal and learning-disabled boys (Doctoral dissertation, Boston University, 1987). *Dissertation Abstracts International, 48*A, 2011.

Nachshon, I., & Carmon, A. (1975). Hand preference in sequential and spatial discrimination tasks. *Cortex, 11,* 123–131.

Obrzut, J. E. (1988). Deficient lateralization in learning-disabled children: Developmental lag or abnormal cerebral organization? In D. L. Molfese & S. J. Segalowitz (Eds.), *Brain lateralization in children: Developmental implications* (pp. 567–590). New York: Guilford.

Obrzut, J. E., & Boliek, C. A. (1986). Lateralization characteristics in learning disabled children. *Journal of Learning Disabilities, 19,* 308–314.

Obrzut, J. E., Obrzut, A., Bryden, M. p., & Bartels, S. G. (1985). Information processing and speech lateralization in learning-disabled children. *Brain and Language, 25,* 87–101.

Ogden, J. A., (1989). Visuospatial and other "right-hemispheric" functions after long recovery periods in left-hemispherectomized subjects. *Neuropsychologica, 27,* 765–776.

Orton, S. T. (1937). *Reading, writing, and speech problems in children.* New York: Norton.

Ozols, E. J., & Rourke, B. P. (1985). Dimensions of social sensitivity in two types of learning-disabled children. In B. P. Rourke (Ed.), *Neuropsychology of learning disabilities: Essentials of subtype analysis* (pp. 281–301). New York: Guilford.

Piazza, D. M. (1977). Cerebral lateralization in young childen as measured by dichotic listening and finger tapping tasks. *Neuropsychologia, 15,* 417–425.

Poeck, K. (1986). The clinical examination of motor apraxia. *Neuropsychologia, 24,* 129–134.

Porac, C., & Coren, S. (1981). *Lateral preferences and human behavior.* New York: Springer-Verlag.

Prince, G. (1978, November). Putting the other half of your brain to work. *Training,* 57–61.

Risberg, J. (1986). Regional cerebral blood flow in neuropsychology. *Neuropsychologia, 24,* 135–140.

Risberg, J., Halsey, J. H., Wills, E. L., & Wilson, E. M. (1975). Hemispheric specialization in normal man studied by bilateral measurements of the regional cerebral blood flow. *Brain, 98,* 511–524.

Rivers, D. L., & Love, R. J. (1980). Language performance on visual processing tasks in right hemisphere lesion cases. *Brain and Language, 10,* 348–366.

Robinson, R. G., & Price, T. R. (1982). Post-stroke depressive disorders: A follow-up study of 103 patients. *Stroke, 13,* 623–628.

Rosselli, M., & Ardila, A. (1989). Calculation deficits in patients with right and left hemisphere damage. *Neuropsychologia, 27,* 607–617.

Rourke, B. P. (1988). The syndrome of nonverbal learning disabilities: Developmental manifestations in neurological disease, disorder, and dysfunction. *The Clinical Neuropsychologist, 2,* 293–330.

Rourke, B. P. (1989, April). *Nonverbal learning disabilities.* Paper presented at the Interdisciplinary Doctoral Conference on Verbal and Nonverbal Learning Disabilities, Boston University.

Rourke, B. P., & Fisk, J. L. (1988). Subtypes of learning-disabled childen: Implications for a neurodevelopmental model of differential hemispheric processing. In D. L. Molfese & S. J. Segalowitz (Eds.), *Brain lateralization in children: Developmental implications* (pp. 547–566). New York: Guilford.

Rourke, B. P., & Strang, J. D. (1983). Subtypes of reading and arithmetical disabilities: A neuropsychological analysis. In M. Rutter (Ed.), *Developmental neuropsychiatry* (pp. 473–488). New York: Guilford.

Rourke, B. P., Young, G. C., & Leenaars, A. A. (1989). A childhood learning disability that predisposes those afflicted to adolescent and adult depression and suicide risk. *Journal of Learning Disabilities, 22,* 169–175.

Sackheim, H. A., Greenberg, M. S., Weiman, A. L., Gur, R. C., Hungerbuhler, J. P., & Geschwind, N. 1982. Hemispheric asymmetry in the expression of positive and negative emotions. *Archives of Neurology, 39,* 210–218.

Saxby, L., & Bryden, M. P. (1984). Left-ear superiority in children for processing auditory emotional material. *Developmental Psychology, 21,* 253–261.

Saxby, L., & Bryden, M. P. (1985). Left visual-field advantage in children for processing visual emotional stimuli. *Developmental Psychology, 21,* 253–261.

Schiff, B. B., & Lamon, M. (1989). Inducing emotion by unilateral contraction of facial muscles: A new look at hemispheric specialization and the experience of emotion. *Neuropsychologia, 27,* 923–935.

Semmes, J. (1968). Hemispheric specialization: A possible clue to mechanism. *Neuropsychologia, 6,* 11–26.

Stiles-Davis, J., Janowsky, J., Engel, M., & Nass, R. (1988). Drawing ability in four young children wih congenital unilateral brain lesions. *Neuropsychologia, 26,* 359–371.

Stockmeyer, S. (1980, March). *Hemispheric specialization for motor control.* Paper presented at the Movement Sciences Conference: Neural Basis of Motor Control, Teachers College, Columbia University, New York.

Strang, J. D., & Rourke, B. P. (1985). Adaptive behavior of children who exhibit specific arithmetic disabilities and associated neuropsychological abilities and deficits. In B. P. Rourke (Ed.), *Neuropsychology of learning disabilities: Essentials of subtype analysis* (pp. 302–328). New York: Guilford.

Tomlinson-Keasey, C., & Kelly, R. R. (1979). A task analysis of hemispheric functioning. *Neuropsychologia, 17,* 345–351.

Turkewitz, G., & Ross-Kossak, P. (1984). Multiple modes of right-hemisphere information processing: Age and sex differences in facial recognition. *Developmental Psychology, 20,* 95–103.

Villa, G., Gainotti, G., & DeBonis, C. (1986). Constructive disabilities in focal brain-damaged patients:

Influence of hemispheric side, locus of lesion and coexistent mental deterioration. *Neuropsychologia, 24,* 497–510.

Voeller, K. K. S. (1986). Right-hemisphere deficit syndrome in children. *American Journal of Psychiatry, 43,* 1004–1009.

Vrbancic, M. I., & Mosley, J. L. (1988). Sex-related differences in hemispheric lateralization: A function of physical maturation. *Developmental Neuropsychology, 4,* 151–167.

Waber, D., (1976). Sex differences in cognition: A function of maturation rate. *Science, 192,* 572–574.

Waber, D. (1977). Sex differences in mental abilities, hemisphere lateralization, and rate of physical growth at adolescence. *Developmental Psychology, 13,* 29–38.

Waber, D. P., & Holmes, J. M. (1985). Assessing children's copying productions of the Rey-Osterrieth Complex Figure. *Journal of Clinical and Experimental Neuropsychology, 7,* 264–282.

Waber, D. P., & Holmes, J. M. (1986). Assessing children's memory productions of the Rey-Osterrieth Complex Figure. *Journal of Clinical and Experimental Neuropsychology, 8,* 563–581.

Wada, J. A., Clarke, R., & Hamm, A. (1975). Cerebral hemisphere asymmetry in humans. *Archives of Neurology, 32,* 239–246.

Wapner, W., Hamby, S. & Gardner, H. (1981). The role of the right hemisphere in the apprehension of complex linguisic materials. *Brain and Language, 41,* 15–33.

Warrington, E. K., James, M., & Maciejewski, C. (1986). The WAIS as a lateralizing and localizing diagnostic instrument: A study of 656 patients with unilateral cerebral lesions. *Neuropsychologia, 24,* 223–239.

Wechsler, D. (1974). *Wechsler intelligence Scales for Children–Revised.* New York: Psychological Corporation.

Weintraub, S., & Mesulam, M. M. (1983). Developmental learning disabilities of the right hemisphere: Emotional, interpersonal, and cognitive components. *Archives of Neurology, 40,* 463–468.

Welsh, M. C., & Pennington, B. F. (1988). Assessing frontal lobe functioning in children: Views from developmental psychology. *Developmental Neuropsychology, 4,* 199–230.

Witelson, S. F. (1977). Developmental dyslexia: Two right hemispheres and none left. *Science, 195,* 309–311.

Witelson, S. F., & Pallie, W. (1973). Left hemisphere specialization for language in the newborn: Neuroanatomical evidence of asymmetry. *Brain, 96,* 641–646.

Yeni-Komshian, G. H., Isenberg, D., & Goldberg, H. (1975). Cerebral dominance and reading disability: Left visual field deficit in poor readers. *Neuropsychologia, 13,* 83–94.

Young, A. W., & Bion, P. J. (1979). Hemispheric laterality effects in the enumeration of visually presented collections of dots by children. *Neuropsychologia, 17,* 99–102.

# Part *III*

# EVALUATION AND TREATMENT

# CHAPTER 8

# Sensory Integration and Praxis Tests

**A. Jean Ayres, PhD, OTR**
**Diana B. Marr, PhD**

*Tests yield numbers and numbers can do things that words or ideas cannot do. In occupational and physical therapy, measurement is central to differential diagnosis, gain or loss assessment, establishing client status, predicting response to therapy, building and testing theory, and conveying information across fields. It is difficult to accomplish any of these goals without some form of measurement.*

*Ayres, 1989a, p. xi*

This chapter describes the nature, purpose, development, standardization, validity, reliability, and psychometric basis for the interpretation of the Sensory Integration and Praxis Tests (SIPT) (Ayres, 1989b). This integrated battery of tests was designed to contribute to the clinical understanding of children 4 through 8 years of age with mild to moderate learning, behavioral, or developmental irregularities. The tests that comprise the SIPT are based on a neurobiological model, which primarily addresses the relationships among tactile processing, vestibular-proprioceptive processing, visual perception, and practic ability, all of which are considered essential to organism-environment interaction and the organization of behavior. Therefore, these tests also assess the major *behavioral manifestations of deficits in integration of sensory inputs* from these systems.

## DESCRIPTION OF THE TESTS

Each of the 17 tests in the SIPT is individually administered; the entire test battery generally can be completed in approximately an hour and a half. The tests are computer scored, which ensures precise scoring and allows for complex statistical comparisons between the tested child's pattern of SIPT scores and the typical score patterns observed in six different cluster groups.

The tests included in the SIPT are of the performance type. None of the SIPT requires verbal responses of the child, and only one of the tests is strongly (and intentionally) dependent on auditory-language comprehension. The SIPT are categorized into four *overlapping* groups: (a) measures of tactile and vestibular-proprioceptive sensory processing, (b) tests of form and space perception and visuomotor coordination, (c) tests of practic ability, and (d) measures of bilateral integration and sequencing.

## Tactile and Vestibular-Proprioceptive Sensory Processing Tests

(Kinesthesia, Finger Identification, Graphesthesia, Localization of Tactile Stimuli, Postrotary Nystagmus, Standing and Walking Balance)

These six tests assess integration and interpretation of sensory input from the body. The tactile tests and the *Kinesthesia* (KIN) test together comprise the somatosensory tests. All five somatosensory tests are administered with vision occluded.

In the *Finger Identification* (FI) test, the child points to the finger(s) touched by the examiner. The *Graphesthesia* (GRA) test requires the child to draw the same design on the back of his or her hand that the examiner drew there with a finger. In the *Localization of Tactile Stimuli* (LTS) test, the child touches the spot on his or her hand or arm that was touched by the examiner.

Certain aspects of central nervous system processing of vestibular-proprioceptive sensory input are evaluated by the Kinesthesia test, the *Postrotary Nystagmus* (PRN) test, and by the *Standing and Walking Balance* (SWB) test. The Kinesthesia test measures the conscious perception of position and movement of the arms and hands with vision occluded. Postrotary Nystagmus is identical in design (but not in normative data) to the Southern California Postrotary Nystagmus Test (Ayres, 1975). In administration of Postrotary Nystagmus, the duration of the oculomotor reflex following body rotation is recorded. Both atypically high (prolonged) and atypically low (depressed) scores are considered abnormal. Static and dynamic balance with eyes open and closed are evaluated in Standing and Walking Balance. Body balance is included in the SIPT because of its strong dependence on integration of vestibular-proprioceptive inputs.

## The Form and Space Perception and Visuomotor Coordination Tests

(Space Visualization, Figure-Ground Perception, Manual Form Perception, Motor Accuracy, Design Copying, Constructional Praxis)

The *Space Visualization* (SV) test assesses visual space perception and the ability to mentally manipulate objects in two-dimensional space. In this test, the child is asked to decide which of two blocks will fit into a hole in a formboard. Because motor performance is not required and does not enter into scoring, the test is deliberately one of visual perception, rather than a visuomotor test. Although the child is not required to put the blocks into the formboard, most children do so, providing information about the child's hand preference and the child's tendency to use the contralateral vs. ipsilateral hand in extracorporeal space. Scores derived from these observations are discussed below with the tests of bilateral integration and sequencing.

The *Figure-Ground Perception* (FG) test requires the visual separation of a foreground line drawing from a rival background. This test is motor-free. To eliminate contamination of a strictly visual perception score by motor or practic function, the child indicates his or her answer to each test item by merely pointing to one of six multiple-choice response figures. The child's decision time for each item is recorded, and a time score, separate from the accuracy score, is obtained.

The *Manual Form Perception* (MFP) test evaluates the haptic or stereognostic sense through identification of a plastic form held in the hand. In Part I of this test, the child is asked to point to an equivalent visual stimulus of the form; in Part II, the child is asked to use the other hand to tactually identify an equivalent form.

Visuomotor coordination is assessed by the *Motor Accuracy* (MAc) test. In this test, the child draws a red line over a heavy, curved, printed black line, and the score is based on the extent of error. Separate scores for preferred and nonpreferred hand performance enable comparison of visuomotor coordination of the two hands.

In addition to these four tests of visual and haptic perception and visuomotor coordination, two visuopraxis tests, *Design Copying* (DC) and *Constructional Praxis* (CPr), described later in this chapter, assess visual construction, and include elements of form and space perception. Design Copying also assesses an element of visuomotor coordination.

Based on the results of factor and cluster analysis of SIPT scores, Ayres (1989) labeled this group of tests that tended to be related to one another tests of visuopraxis. The term visuopraxis was used to reflect the common conceptual component between visual perception and motor planning. Visuopraxis does not refer to the *motor* manifestations of a motor planning deficit. Due to confusion in the use of this term, the term visuopraxis should be avoided, and the test scores broken down into the following elements: form and space perception, visual construction, and visuomotor coordination. The individual SIPT associated with each element are summarized in Table 1–1.

## The Praxis Tests

(Design Copying, Constructional Praxis, Postural Praxis, Praxis on Verbal Command, Sequencing Praxis, Oral Praxis)

Practic skill is appraised in six behavioral domains. As mentioned previously, two of these primarily assess visual construction rather than praxis. The Design Copying test evaluates the child's ability to graphically conceptualize, plan, and execute two-dimensional designs. In Part I, the child duplicates a design superimposed on a dot grid. In Part II, the design is copied in a designated blank space. All designs are scored for spatial accuracy; some designs are also scored for atypical drawing approaches such as segmentations, reversals, inversions, and extension of the drawings beyond their designated boundaries (see Ayres, 1989b for more detail). Constructional Praxis uses a block-building task to assess visual construction skill in spatially relating objects to each other in orderly arrangement or systematic assembly. The child's block structures are scored for various errors in block placement, including rotation, reversal, mislocation, and omission.

The major tests of praxis include *Postural Praxis* (PPr), *Praxis on Verbal Command* (PrVC), *Sequencing Praxis* (SPr), and *Oral Praxis* (OPr). Postural Praxis evaluates aptitude in planning and assuming different and unusual body postures. Hand and arm postures are most frequently used, but head, trunk, and finger positions are critical on some of the items. Although Postural Praxis requires visual interpretation of each demonstrated position, no memory of that position is required. Praxis on Verbal Command taps the ability to assume a number of different positions based only on the examiner's verbal command. Sequencing Praxis evaluates competency in perceiving, remembering, and executing a demonstrated sequence of unilateral and bilateral hand and finger positions. In the Oral Praxis test, the child imitates the examiner's movements of the tongue, lips, cheeks, or jaw. Most items consist of a sequence of movements.

## The Bilateral Integration and Sequencing Tests

(Oral Praxis, Sequencing Praxis, Graphesthesia, Standing and Walking Balance, Bilateral Motor Coordination, Space Visualization Contralateral Use, Space Visualization Preferred Hand Use)

Through a series of factor and cluster analyses of SIPT scores, five tests in the SIPT were found to be related to and to assess the domain of bilateral integration and sequencing. Four of these tests, Oral Praxis, Sequencing Praxis, Graphesthesia, Standing and Walking Balance, were described above. The fifth test is *Bilateral Motor Coordination* (BMC). Bilateral Motor Coordination requires the child to imitate smoothly executed movement sequences of hands and feet after they are demonstrated by the examiner. Reciprocal interactions of right and left extremities are stressed to assess integration of function of the two sides of the body.

Two additional scores related to bilateral integration and sequencing, the *Space Visualization Contralateral Use* (SVCU) score and the *Space Visualization Preferred Hand Use* (PHU) score, are derived from the observation of which hand is used to pick up the block placed in the formboard on the Space Visualization test. The Space Visualization Contralateral Use score, a test of crossing midline, is based on the proportion of responses in which the child crosses the midline of the body with the hand to select a block from contralateral space. The Space Visualization Preferred Hand Use score, a measure of hand preference, is based on the proportion of preferred vs. nonpreferred hand use during Space Visualization performance. The preferred hand is defined as the hand the child uses for writing.

## TEST DEVELOPMENT AND STANDARDIZATION

The tests in the SIPT have evolved over several decades. Initially, a number of clinical procedures commonly employed to assess agnosia and apraxia in individuals with adult-onset brain damage were redesigned for use with children with minimal brain dysfunction or learning disabilities. Through statistical analyses (Ayres, 1965, 1969), those procedures that provided the most useful clinical information, and that showed the highest factor loadings and the strongest capacity to discriminate between dysfunctional and normal children, were selected. First appearing as several different individual tests, they were later published in combined form as the Southern California Sensory Integration Tests (SCSIT) (Ayres, 1972a), and as the Southern California Postrotary Nystagmus Test (Ayres, 1975).

The Postrotary Nystagmus test was included in the SIPT, and twelve of the tests in the Southern California Sensory Integration Tests were retained and revised for the SIPT. Decisions as to which of the Southern California Sensory Integration Tests to revise and include in the SIPT were based on the results of a number of factor analyses (Ayres, 1966, 1972b, 1977; Silberzahn, 1975), the ability of the tests to contribute to the understanding of children's problems, and the results of a survey of the faculty of Sensory Integration International. In addition, four new praxis tests were developed for the SIPT.

In developing new tests and revising the tests from the Southern California Sensory Integration Tests, the selection of test items was based on extensive field testing, several pilot studies evaluating each item's capacity to distinguish between dysfunctional and normal children, interrater reliability, and test-retest reliability.

The tests in the SIPT were standardized on a nationwide sample of approximately 2000 children. The children in the SIPT normative sample were chosen to be as representative as possible of the children from 4-0 (4 years, 0 month) to 8-11 (8 years, 11 months) living in the United States. A modified random sampling procedure was used, stratified to reflect the population characteristics from the 1980 US Census. The total number of children tested in each region was based on the number of children between the ages of 4 and 14 reported for each region in the census data; the ethnic composition of the normative sample and the percentage of urban vs. rural children in each region were based on these census figures. Because sensory integration principles are employed throughout Canada, a number of Canadian children also were included in the standardization sample. Table 8–1 shows the geographic distribution of children in the SIPT normative sample.

The normative data analyses for the SIPT were conducted in three stages: (a) preliminary analyses, which examined age- and gender-related differences in SIPT performance, and determined the appropriate scoring and stopping rules for the SIPT tests; (b) computation of means and standard deviations, which included the examination of developmental trends and the normality of the score distribution for each of the 17 tests in the SIPT; and (c) determination of major SIPT scores, based on the extent to which each of the various subscores for each test allowed discrimination between normal and dysfunctional children.

Preliminary analyses indicated significant sex differences on all of the SIPT tests except Manual Form Perception and Postrotary Nystagmus. Therefore, separate norms were developed for boys and girls. There also were significant age effects on all tests except Postrotary Nystagmus. The developmental curves for the tests indicated that the optimal age groupings for the normative data should cover 4-month intervals for children younger than 6 years of age, and 6-month intervals for children aged 6 and older. Therefore, separate norms were developed for boys and girls in each of 12 age groups. For each of these groups, SIPT scores generally fit a normal distribution curve. Means and standard deviations were computed for each normative subgroup, so that each child's score can be reported as an index of the degree to which the child's performance differs from the average performance of children of the same age and gender.

For many of the tests, it was considered desirable to stop testing when the child's performance indicated that he or she was unable to complete any more of the test items. Because items on many tests are administered in order of increasing difficulty, it was possible to determine appropriate stopping rules for 8 of the 17 tests. Stopping rules were added only for those tests in which the predictive validity of the test was not significantly lowered by the use of a stopping rule, and only when the differences were negligible between the scores for the total test and the scores obtained using a stopping rule.

Most of the individual tests in the SIPT yield several different subscores, often including subscores for time and accuracy. For both theoretical and pragmatic reasons, it was expected that children in different diagnostic groups might exhibit different speed-accuracy tradeoffs in test performance. Thus, time-adjusted accuracy scores are important on a number of these tests. Optimal statistical weights for time and accuracy were identified to best discriminate between normal and dysfunctional children within and across the 12 age groups.

## VALIDITY OF THE SIPT

Test validity refers to the ability to draw meaningful inferences from test scores to meet an intended purpose. Three types of validity-related evidence are addressed here: construct-related, content-related, and criterion-related.

TABLE 8–1. NORMATIVE SAMPLE BY AGE, SEX, AND GEOGRAPHIC REGION

| Age Group (yr/mo) | New England | | Mid Atlantic | | South Atlantic | | East No. Central | | East So. Central | | West No. Central | | West So. Central | | Mountain | | Pacific | | Canada | | Total |
|---|---|---|---|---|---|---|---|---|---|---|---|---|---|---|---|---|---|---|---|---|---|---|
| | m | f | m | f | m | f | m | f | m | f | m | f | m | f | m | f | m | f | m | f | |
| 4/0–4/3 | 3 | 2 | 3 | 2 | 2 | 3 | 7 | 5 | 1 | 1 | 2 | 3 | 1 | 1 | 1 | 2 | 4 | 0 | 0 | 1 | 44 |
| 4/4–4/7 | 7 | 3 | 3 | 5 | 5 | 6 | 10 | 9 | 6 | 3 | 6 | 5 | 4 | 6 | 2 | 3 | 3 | 7 | 3 | 3 | 99 |
| 4/8–4/11 | 3 | 5 | 7 | 7 | 7 | 4 | 9 | 7 | 4 | 2 | 4 | 8 | 5 | 4 | 1 | 1 | 9 | 9 | 4 | 4 | 104 |
| 5/0–5/3 | 4 | 6 | 8 | 5 | 6 | 3 | 13 | 17 | 3 | 5 | 2 | 6 | 8 | 7 | 2 | 4 | 6 | 3 | 3 | 0 | 108 |
| 5/4–5/7 | 2 | 6 | 10 | 6 | 16 | 9 | 14 | 17 | 9 | 3 | 6 | 3 | 11 | 12 | 4 | 6 | 7 | 6 | 9 | 3 | 157 |
| 5/8–5/11 | 3 | 3 | 10 | 13 | 16 | 17 | 14 | 20 | 9 | 10 | 5 | 6 | 10 | 9 | 8 | 14 | 7 | 7 | 7 | 4 | 184 |
| 6/0–6/5 | 4 | 3 | 14 | 15 | 21 | 23 | 28 | 24 | 11 | 10 | 8 | 10 | 10 | 14 | 13 | 7 | 12 | 11 | 6 | 8 | 259 |
| 6/6–6/11 | 2 | 2 | 9 | 11 | 22 | 21 | 19 | 18 | 10 | 9 | 6 | 12 | 10 | 11 | 9 | 9 | 10 | 12 | 9 | 7 | 216 |
| 7/0–7/5 | 2 | 2 | 14 | 12 | 17 | 14 | 18 | 19 | 8 | 5 | 11 | 14 | 12 | 12 | 6 | 12 | 10 | 8 | 10 | 9 | 212 |
| 7/6–7/11 | 1 | 4 | 13 | 13 | 15 | 16 | 20 | 25 | 6 | 6 | 8 | 8 | 10 | 12 | 8 | 7 | 12 | 11 | 7 | 9 | 216 |
| 8/0–8/5 | 3 | 2 | 12 | 11 | 14 | 15 | 14 | 20 | 9 | 9 | 10 | 9 | 13 | 6 | 9 | 7 | 6 | 8 | 7 | 7 | 191 |
| 8/6–8/11 | 4 | 5 | 11 | 15 | 22 | 17 | 19 | 25 | 11 | 6 | 5 | 7 | 12 | 8 | 10 | 4 | 6 | 7 | 7 | 6 | 207 |
| | 38 | 43 | 114 | 115 | 163 | 148 | 185 | 206 | 87 | 69 | 73 | 91 | 106 | 102 | 73 | 70 | 92 | 89 | 72 | 61 | 1997 |
| TOTAL | 81 | | 229 | | 311 | | 391 | | 156 | | 164 | | 208 | | 143 | | 181 | | 133 | | 1997 |

Geographic Region

To ensure that validity estimates would not be inflated by age and gender differences in SIPT performance, all SIPT analyses were conducted using standard scores (i.e., each child's scores were represented in standard deviation units, computed using the age- and gender-appropriate norms for each child).

## Construct-Related Validity

Identification of relevant sensory integrative processes and the organization of related behavioral parameters into meaningful theoretical constructs have been accomplished largely through factor analyses of measures including the SIPT, the Southern California Sensory Integration Tests, and related clinical observations. Factor analysis is a statistical technique that identifies groups of test scores that are correlated or covary. For example, we expect that visual form and space tests define a factor and that if a child has a low score on one, it is likely that the child will have low scores on all of them (see Chapter 1).

### FACTOR ANALYSES OF EARLY SENSORY INTEGRATION MEASURES

An early factor analysis of the scores of 100 6- and 7-year-old dysfunctional children on a number of perceptual-motor measures (Ayres, 1965) identified the following symptom complexes: (a) developmental dyspraxia, with major loadings for tactile and motor planning tests; (b) form and space perception deficit, best represented by tests of visual and haptic form and space perception, and kinesthesia; (c) bilateral integration deficit, with highest loadings for right-left discrimination tasks, crossing the body's midline, and bilateral motor coordination; and (d) tactile defensiveness, characterized by tactile defensiveness, distractibility, and poor tactile perception. Similar factors did not emerge from scores on the same measures in a group of 50 age- and sex-matched normal children.

In a subsequent study (Ayres, 1966) of 4- to 8-year-old children, a somatomotor factor linked tactile perception and kinesthesia with motor planning in a mixed group of 92 children (including some dysfunctional children), but not in a group of 164 children with evidence of normal early development. A Q technique factor analysis (Ayres, 1969) of 64 observations for each of 36 learning-disabled children (mean age = 97.7 months, $SD$ = 11.3 months) expanded the identifying markers of the score pattern earlier referred to as bilateral integration deficit. In this analysis, clinically observed postural and ocular responses were statistically associated with the bilateral integration measures.

The tactile, proprioceptive, and visual perception tests tended to share variance in a 1972 factor analysis (Ayres, 1972b) of scores of 148 learning-disabled children (mean age = 92.6 months, $SD$ = 12.0 months) on measures of sensory integration, psycholinguistic ability, academic achievement, intelligence, and postural and ocular responses. Motor planning, hyperactivity, and tactile defensiveness were closely associated. Psycholinguistic and intelligence test scores were significantly correlated.

The close association between praxis and tactile perception was also demonstrated in a later analysis (Ayres, 1977), in which postural and ocular functions again shared variance. Auditory-language abilities loaded on a single separate factor in that analysis.

A study by Ayres, Mailloux, and Wendler (1987) addressed the issue of whether (a) developmental dyspraxia is a unitary function, or (b) there are different types of dyspraxia. Scores on the Southern California Sensory Integration Tests, several auditory-language tests, postural and ocular observations, a block-building test, and early forms of the SIPT Praxis on Verbal Command, Oral Praxis, and Sequencing Praxis tests were analyzed for 182 children known or suspected to be dysfunctional (mean age = 78 months, $SD$ = 17.4 months). Praxis on Verbal Command, Oral Praxis, Sequencing Praxis, block building, and all of the Southern California Sensory Integration Tests except Bilateral Motor Coordination, loaded on a major visuo-somato-praxis factor. Other scores that did not load on this factor included Postrotary Nystagmus, prone extension, supine flexion, and Space Visualization Contralateral Use. The auditory-language tests identified the second factor, on which Praxis on Verbal Command and Sequencing Praxis also had loadings above 0.30. The ability to integrate the functions of the two sides of the body in a series of sequential movements was reflected in a factor with major loadings for Bilateral Motor Coordination, Oral Praxis, and Sequencing Praxis. The authors concluded that the data did not support the existence of either a unitary dyspraxia function or different types of developmental dyspraxia, but rather that the data supported the idea of a general practic function with different practic skills defined by behavioral tasks. The data also supported the idea of a common conceptual component to praxis and visual perception. Throughout all of these pre-SIPT studies, there was a tendency for auditory-language measures to be less closely associated with sensations from the body than were measures of perception and sensory integration.

In summary, the results of the factor-analytic studies with Southern California Sensory Integration Tests and related measures supported the presence of the following constructs: (a) tactile-kinesthesia linked with poor praxis (somatopraxis); (b) form and space perception; (c) postural-ocular scores linked with bilateral integration (defined by Bilateral Motor Coordination, right-left discrimination, and crossing the midline of the body); and (d) tactile defensiveness. Tactile defensiveness is a construct that is not measured by the SIPT. Finally, some of the factor-analytic studies suggested the presence of a more "generalized" construct of poor sensory processing (vestibular-proprioceptive and tactile), praxis, bilateral integration, form of space, and academic achievement.

## FACTOR ANALYSES OF THE SIPT

A number of factor analyses of SIPT scores further clarified the nature of the constructs evaluated by the SIPT. In this discussion, only factor loadings greater than or equal to 0.35 are reported.

**Factor Analysis of the SIPT Normative Sample.** A four-factor solution of a principal components analysis of the SIPT normative sample categorized the tests as those that were primarily visuopractic and those that were primarily somatopractic. The term somatopraxis was derived from findings of a close association between somatosensory (tactile-proprioceptive) processing and motor planning. The use of the term visuopraxis originated in the earlier recognition of a common conceptual link between praxis and visual perception (Ayres et al., 1987). Highest loading tests on the visuopraxis factor were, in decreasing order of magnitude, Constructional Praxis, Space Visualization, Design Copying, Manual Form Perception, Figure-Ground Perception, and Praxis on Verbal Command. Highest loading somatopraxis tests were (in decreasing order of magnitude) Oral Praxis, Bilateral Motor Coordination, Graphesthesia, Postural Praxis, Sequencing Praxis, Standing and Walking Balance, and Finger Identification. The third factor to emerge was a vestibular-somatosensory processing factor. Tests with the highest loadings on the vestibular-somatosensory factor were Postrotary Nystagmus and three somatosensory tests (Kinesthesia, Finger Identification, and Localization of Tactile Stimuli). The fourth factor was a

Kinesthesia-Motor Accuracy doublet. This factor also had a negative loading on Postural Praxis.

**Factor Analysis of Dysfunctional Children.** A principal components analysis of the SIPT scores of 125 children with learning or sensory integrative deficits (mean age = 7.27 years, $SD = 0.97$ years) showed a differentiation of sensory integrative problems into five different categories or patterns. The results of this analysis are shown in Table 8-2.

The first factor to emerge, representing the greatest proportion of the SIPT's variance, was a bilateral integration and sequencing (BIS) factor. The tests representing this factor were Sequencing Praxis, Bilateral Motor Coordination, Graphesthesia, Standing and Walking Balance, Oral Praxis, and Manual Form Perception.

On the second factor, Postrotary Nystagmus had a large positive loading, and Praxis on Verbal Command had the largest negative loading. This relationship suggested that problems in translating verbal directions into body postures is apt to be associated with prolonged postrotary nystagmus. The relationship is consistent with a previous factor analysis (Ayres, 1977) in which the Southern California Postrotary Nystagmus Test had a substantial negative loading on an auditory-language factor. Figure-Ground also had a negative loading on this factor.

Factor 3, somatosensory processing with oral praxis, linked Localization of Tactile Stimuli, Kinesthesia, and Oral Praxis. Factor 4, visuopraxis, was best represented by the form and space perception tests and by the visual construction tests (Design Copying and Constructional Praxis). Factor 5, somatopraxis, was identified by high loading for three praxis tests (Postural Praxis, Constructional Praxis, and Oral Praxis) and one tactile test (Graphesthesia).

**Factor Analysis of a Combined Normal and Dysfunctional Sample.** Scores of a combined sample of 176 normal children and 117 children with learning or sensory integrative deficits (mean age = 7.3 years, $SD = 1.0$ years) were examined in an additional principal components analysis. The first factor to emerge was primarily a somatopraxis/bilateral integration and sequencing factor, with highest loadings for Oral Praxis, Graphesthsia, Bilateral Motor Coordination, Sequencing Praxis, and Standing and Walking Balance, in that order. Praxis on Verbal Command loaded moderately on this factor, as did Postural Praxis.

The second factor was identified as a visuopraxis factor, with highest loadings for Space Visualization, Figure-Ground Perception, Design Copying, Motor Accuracy, and Constructional Praxis. The third factor, vestibular functioning, was defined by a high loading for Postrotary Nystagmus. Finally, the fourth factor, somatosensory processing, was identified with highest loadings for Localization of Tactile Stimuli and Kinesthesia.

In summary, these factor analyses resulted in the identification of a visuopraxis factor (form and space, visual construction, and visuomotor coordination), a somatopraxis factor, a bilateral integration and sequencing factor, and a praxis on verbal command factor associated with prolonged postrotary nystagmus. Additionally vestibular and somatosensory processing factors emerged in several of the analyses, perhaps suggesting an underlying deficit in sensory processing. (Various labels were given to these sensory processing factors.)

## CLUSTER ANALYSIS OF THE SIPT

Cluster analysis is a statistical technique that is conceptually similar to factor analysis. However, cluster analysis is used to identify groups of children who demonstrate similar test score patterns on a battery of tests such as the SIPT (see Chapter 1).

**TABLE 8–2. FACTOR ANALYSIS OF SIPT SCORES OF 125 CHILDREN WITH LEARNING OR SENSORY INTEGRATIVE DEFICITS**

| | FACTOR 1 Bilateral Integration & Sequencing | FACTOR 2 Praxis On Verbal Command | FACTOR 3 Somatosensory Processing & Oral Praxis | FACTOR 4 Visuopraxis | FACTOR 5 Somatopraxis |
|---|---|---|---|---|---|
| Space Visualization [SV] | -.08 | -.11 | -.08 | .64 | .30 |
| Figure-Ground Perception [FG] | .20 | -.36 | .05 | .54 | -.02 |
| Manual Form Perception [MFP] | .38 | -.10 | .12 | .20 | .17 |
| Kinesthesia [KIN] | .24 | .13 | .74 | .02 | -.14 |
| Finger Identification [FI] | .24 | .31 | -.07 | .37 | .30 |
| Graphesthesia [GRA] | .57 | .09 | -.03 | -.04 | .42 |
| Localization of Tactile Stimuli [LTS] | -.27 | -.11 | .83 | .04 | .09 |
| Praxis on Verbal Command [PrVC] | .32 | -.59 | .14 | .06 | .14 |
| Design Copying [DC] | .18 | .00 | .06 | .67 | .06 |
| Constructional Praxis [CPr] | .07 | -.07 | .10 | .38 | .54 |
| Postural Praxis [PPr] | -.07 | -.03 | -.02 | .07 | .89 |
| Oral Praxis [OPr] | .40 | .00 | .37 | -.22 | .51 |
| Sequencing Praxis [SPr] | .78 | .04 | -.02 | .04 | .08 |
| Bilateral Motor Coordination [BMC] | .69 | -.31 | -.04 | .07 | -.10 |
| Standing and Walking Balance [SWB] | .54 | .15 | .16 | .26 | -.07 |
| Motor Accuracy [MAc] | -.03 | .20 | .09 | .78 | -.11 |
| Postrotary Nystagmus [PRN] | .06 | .76 | .04 | .07 | .01 |
| Factor Correlations: 2 | -.08 | | | | |
| 3 | -.26 | .04 | | | |
| 4 | -.37 | .00 | .18 | | |
| 5 | -.34 | .08 | .16 | .31 | |

Using the same sample of 117 dysfunctional and 176 normal children described above, cluster analysis was used to identify distinct groups of children who could be characterized by different score profiles on the SIPT. Both dysfunctional and normal children were included in the sample in order to ensure that the obtained clusters would differentiate between dysfunctional and normal children. The analysis used Ward's method of clustering, which generally produces the most accurate results for the type of data obtained from the SIPT (see, for example, Lorr, 1983).

Cluster solutions were generated to extract from 2 to 10 clusters; a six-cluster solution was determined to be the most appropriate based on both statistical criteria and clinical criteria. Solutions with more than six clusters tended to split the children into very small groups, some of which had only two or three members; solutions with fewer than six clusters combined groups that theoretically and clinically could be delineated.

The six-cluster solution identified the following groups: (a) Low Average Bilateral Integration and Sequencing; (b) Generalized Sensory Integrative Dysfunction; (c) Visuo- and Somatodyspraxia; (d) Low Average Sensory Integration and Praxis; (e) Dyspraxia on Verbal Command; and (f) High Average Sensory Integration and Praxis. The means and standard deviations for each group on all of the 17 major SIPT scores are shown in Table 8–3.

The plotted scores are the cluster group mean scores listed in Table 8–3. Approximately 19 percent of the sample were identified as belonging to the Low Average Bilateral Integration and Sequencing cluster group. This group scored close to the mean on most of the SIPT, but with somewhat lower scores on the five tests that are associated with bilateral integration and sequencing (i.e., Oral Praxis, Graphesthesia, Standing and Walking Balance, Sequencing Praxis, and Bilateral Motor Coordination). Children in this group also had lower scores on Postural Praxis. However, because low scores on Postural Praxis did not emerge in the factor analyses, this score is thought to be less important.

Approximately 12 percent of the sample were identified as belonging to the Generalized Sensory Integrative Dysfunction cluster group. The children in this group tended to score substantially below the mean on all of the SIPT; however, Localization of Tactile Stimuli and Postrotary Nystagmus mean scores were in the average range. Another 12 percent were identified as members of the Visuo- and Somatodyspraxia cluster group. Children in the Visuo- and Somatodyspraxia cluster group also tended to score below the mean on all of the SIPT, but their scores were not nearly as low as the scores of the Generalized Sensory Integrative Dysfunction cluster group.

Approximately 24 percent of the total sample belonged to the Low Average Sensory Integration and Praxis cluster group. This group's SIPT scores tended to fall just below the mean, with the lowest scores (still within average limits) on Postural Praxis, Finger Identification, Sequencing Praxis, Design Copying, and Localization of Tactile Stimuli. The Dyspraxia on Verbal Command cluster group included approximately 10 percent of the total sample. This group's profile of scores was distinguished by the very low scores on Praxis on Verbal Command, and the highest average Postrotary Nystagmus score, in contrast with other scores in the average or low-average range. This group also had low scores on Bilateral Motor Coordination, Sequencing Praxis, Standing and Walking Balance, Design Copying, and Oral Praxis. Finally, 24 percent of the sample belonged to the High Average Sensory Integration and Praxis cluster group. This group tended to score above the mean on all of the SIPT.

TABLE 8–3. SIPT MEANS AND STANDARAD DEVIATIONS FOR THE SIX CLUSTER GROUPS

| Test | GROUP 1 Low Average BIS | | GROUP 2 Generalized SI Dysfunction | | GROUP 3 Visuo-and Somato-dyspraxia | | GROUP 4 Low Average SI & Praxis | | GROUP 5 Dyspraxia on Verbal Command | | GROUP 6 High Average SI & Praxis | |
|---|---|---|---|---|---|---|---|---|---|---|---|---|
| | Mean | SD | Mean | SD | Mean | SD | Mean | SD | Mean | SD | Mean | SD |
| Space Visualization [SV] | -.03 | .67 | -1.36 | .79 | -.90 | .80 | -.32 | 1.03 | -.48 | .87 | .54 | .60 |
| Figure-Ground Perception [FG] | .03 | 1.02 | -1.35 | 1.04 | -.60 | .70 | -.30 | 1.08 | -.81 | .76 | .60 | .89 |
| Manual Form Perception [MFP] | -.13 | .87 | -1.60 | .97 | -.65 | 1.04 | -.09 | 1.17 | -.57 | .72 | .36 | .85 |
| Kinesthesia [KIN] | -.34 | .96 | -1.60 | 1.50 | -1.20 | 1.21 | .14 | .74 | -.78 | 1.20 | .14 | .96 |
| Finger Identification [FI] | .01 | .93 | -1.40 | .97 | -1.01 | 1.12 | -.51 | 1.01 | -.41 | .67 | .43 | .77 |
| Graphesthesia [GRA] | -.81 | .93 | -2.13 | .88 | -1.01 | .91 | -.08 | .93 | -.72 | .80 | .42 | .86 |
| Loc. of Tactile Stimuli [LTS] | -.24 | 1.04 | -.66 | 1.31 | -.41 | .92 | -.43 | 1.14 | -.12 | 1.09 | .61 | .81 |
| Praxis on Verbal Command [PrVC] | .18 | .66 | -2.41 | .84 | -.15 | .68 | -.08 | .93 | -2.38 | .76 | .56 | .49 |
| Design Copying [DC] | -.02 | .74 | -2.11 | .62 | -1.61 | .81 | -.43 | .96 | -1.07 | 1.00 | .74. | .74 |
| Constructional Praxis [CPr] | .16 | .69 | -1.58 | 1.05 | -.88 | .71 | .07 | .62 | -.53 | .58 | .53 | .64 |
| Postural Praxis [PPr] | -.52 | .95 | -2.14 | .93 | -.98 | 1.13 | -.55 | .93 | -.76 | .88 | .53 | .90 |
| Oral Praxis [OPr] | -.94 | .99 | -2.20 | .72 | -.47 | .89 | .13 | .77 | -1.04 | .83 | .24 | .86 |
| Sequencing Praxis [SPr] | -.66 | .90 | -2.06 | .74 | -1.21 | .84 | -.42 | .66 | -1.44 | .97 | .41 | 1.03 |
| Bilateral Motor Coord. [BMC] | -.46 | .79 | -1.46 | .72 | -1.11 | .94 | -.24 | 1.07 | -1.56 | .59 | .47 | .99 |
| Standing/Walking Balance [SWB] | -.77 | .79 | -2.28 | .63 | -1.28 | .94 | .12 | .77 | -1.17 | .85 | .49 | 1.05 |
| Motor Accuracy [MAc] | -.17 | .65 | -1.03 | .48 | -.98 | .39 | -.19 | .73 | -.70 | .45 | .21 | .83 |
| Postrotary Nystagmus [PRN] | -.36 | .88 | -.48 | .84 | -.63 | .78 | .11 | .78 | .47 | .84 | .09 | .71 |

Table 8–4 shows the representation of normal children, children with learning disabilities, and children with sensory integrative deficits in each of the six cluster groups. As expected, most of the normal children had score profiles that matched either the high-average, or two low-average cluster groups. In fact, 88 percent of the normal children fell into one of these three groups (37 percent matched the High Average Sensory Integration and Praxis cluster, 30 percent matched the Low Average Sensory Integration and Praxis cluster, and 21 percent matched the Low Average Bilateral Integration and Sequencing cluster). In contrast, only 3 percent of the children with learning disabilities or sensory integrative dysfunction matched the High Average Sensory Integration and Praxis cluster, and 29 percent matched either the Low Average Bilateral Integration and Sequencing cluster or the Low Average Sensory Integration and Praxis cluster. The remaining 68 percent of the children with learning disabilities or sensory integrative dysfunction matched one of the three dysfunctional cluster groups, and more than 27 percent matched the Generalized Sensory Integration Dysfunction cluster. It should be noted that factor analysis of the dysfunctional sample revealed that the Low Average Bilateral Integration and Sequencing cluster group may be comprised of two groups of children, one group that is normal on the bilateral integration and sequencing factor, and another group that is comprised of children with dysfunction.

## Criterion-Related Validity Evidence

Because the tests in the SIPT are intended for the detection, description, and explanation of current developmental irregularities, rather than for the prediction of criterion scores at a later time, criterion-related evidence is primarily concurrent in nature. In the absence of alternate comparable sensory integration and praxis tests for the same age range against which to compare the SIPT, inferences about the meaning of a given test profile in the current life of a child are best collected through testing children with known, different, and previously determined diagnoses. In this respect, the prior use of the Southern California Sensory Integration Tests and Southern California Postrotary Nystagmus Test with various populations contributes to the evolving ability to derive accurate inferences from SIPT scores. Co-occurrence, of course, *is not to be confused with causation.*

### COMPARISON OF DIAGNOSTIC GROUPS

Means and standard deviations on the SIPT for children in eight different diagnostic groups are shown in Table 8–5. The mean scores of all eight groups combined were below average on all of the SIPT. Scores of some groups show recognizable patterns; in other groups, this is not the case.

**Learning Disability.** For the group of 195 learning-disabled children (mean age = 7.3 years, $SD = 1.0$ years), scores on all tests in the SIPT tended to be below average. The lowest scores were on five of the six praxis tests, and on Graphesthesia and Standing and Walking Balance. By definition, children with learning disabilities have normal IQs. Thus, the high incidence of sensory integrative dysfunction among this group supports the idea that intelligence and sensory integration are relatively distinct constructs.

**Sensory Integrative Dysfunction.** The 36 children with sensory integrative

# TABLE 8–4. REPRESENTATION OF NORMAL, LEARNING-DISABLED, AND SI DEFICIENT CHILDREN IN THE SIX SIPT CLUSTER GROUPS

| | GROUP 1 Low Average BIS | GROUP 2 Generalized SI Dysfunction | GROUP 3 Visuo- and Somatodyspraxia | GROUP 4 Low Average SI & Praxis | GROUP 5 Dyspraxia on Verbal Command | GROUP 6 High Average SI & Praxis | TOTAL |
|---|---|---|---|---|---|---|---|
| Normal Children | 36 | 2 | 13 | 54 | 6 | 65 | 176 |
| Learning-Disabled | 11 | 28 | 13 | 13 | 21 | 3 | 89 |
| SI Dysfunctional | 8 | 4 | 9 | 4 | 2 | 1 | 28 |
| TOTAL | 55 | 34 | 35 | 71 | 29 | 69 | 293 |

TABLE 8-5. SIPT MEANS AND STANDARD DEVIATIONS FOR DIFFERENT DIAGNOSTIC GROUPS

| TEST | Learning-Disabled (n = 195) | | Brain-Injured (n = 10) | | Ment. Retard (n = 28) | | SI Dysf. (n = 36) | | Spina Bifida (n = 21) | | Reading Disorder (n = 60) | | Language Disorder (n = 28) | | Cerebral Palsy (n = 10) | |
|---|---|---|---|---|---|---|---|---|---|---|---|---|---|---|---|---|
| | Mean | SD | Mean | SD | Mean | SD | Mean | SD | Mean | SD | Mean | SD | Mean | SD | Mean | SD |
| Space Visualization [SV] | −.71 | .85 | −1.03 | 1.01 | −1.51 | .97 | −.67 | 1.04 | −.74 | .63 | −.52 | .92 | −.75 | 1.15 | −.85 | .37 |
| Figure-Ground Perception [FG] | −.75 | 1.07 | −1.31 | 1.29 | −1.73 | 1.68 | −.29 | 1.05 | −1.09 | .86 | −.92 | .79 | −.81 | 1.16 | −.68 | .88 |
| Manual Form Perception [MFP] | −1.02 | 1.23 | −1.90 | 1.30 | −2.79 | .32 | −.46 | .99 | −1.91 | 1.25 | −.99 | 1.10 | −1.17 | 1.14 | −.65 | .21 |
| Kinesthesia [KIN] | −1.09 | 1.36 | −1.69 | 1.59 | −2.73 | .55 | −.60 | 1.08 | −1.12 | 1.30 | −1.30 | 1.02 | −1.01 | 1.48 | −.60 | 1.54 |
| Finger Identification [FI] | −1.02 | 1.03 | −.80 | 1.01 | −1.90 | .89 | −.73 | 1.05 | −.53 | 1.06 | −1.02 | 1.02 | −1.04 | 1.00 | −1.60 | 1.28 |
| Graphesthesia [GRA] | −1.37 | 1.14 | −1.57 | 1.15 | −2.42 | .69 | −1.09 | 1.06 | −1.94 | .69 | −.63 | 1.18 | −1.17 | 1.01 | −1.28 | 1.47 |
| Loc. of Tactile Stimuli [LTS] | −.65 | 1.20 | −1.18 | 1.09 | −1.63 | 1.77 | −.61 | 1.20 | −1.38 | 1.12 | −.33 | 1.07 | −.86 | 1.04 | −1.80 | .94 |
| Praxis on Verbal Command [PrVC] | −1.40 | 1.36 | −1.58 | 1.50 | −3.00 | .00 | −.49 | 1.25 | −.99 | 1.24 | −1.01 | 1.32 | −1.74 | 1.38 | −.63 | 1.52 |
| Design Copying [DC] | −1.60 | 1.12 | −1.43 | 1.35 | −3.00 | .00 | −.86 | 1.05 | −2.05 | 1.13 | −1.24 | 1.27 | −1.33 | 1.11 | −2.33 | .99 |
| Constructional Praxis [CPr] | −.91 | .95 | −.83 | 1.02 | −2.17 | .53 | −.46 | .95 | −1.18 | 1.09 | −.60 | .88 | −.78 | .93 | −1.00 | .95 |
| Postural Praxis [PPr] | −1.44 | 1.13 | −2.28 | 1.00 | −2.74 | .61 | −1.05 | 1.33 | −1.59 | .83 | −1.42 | 1.01 | −.92 | 1.08 | −1.73 | 1.07 |
| Oral Praxis [OPr] | −1.37 | 1.17 | −2.34 | .88 | −2.67 | .66 | −.77 | 1.23 | −2.05 | .79 | −.70 | 1.10 | −1.30 | .99 | −1.58 | 2.41 |
| Sequencing Praxis [SPr] | −1.48 | .98 | −1.56 | 1.11 | −2.36 | .74 | −1.17 | .87 | −1.13 | 1.00 | −.78 | .83 | −1.36 | .84 | −.93 | .76 |
| Bilateral Motor Coord. [BMC] | −1.15 | .99 | −1.68 | .91 | −1.85 | .49 | −.71 | 1.16 | −1.18 | .81 | −.58 | .92 | −1.47 | .54 | −1.23 | .86 |
| Standing/Walking Balance [SWB] | −1.58 | 1.11 | −2.17 | 1.17 | −2.87 | .31 | −1.46 | .98 | −2.98 | .11 | −.61 | 1.01 | −1.31 | 1.00 | −2.73 | .32 |
| Motor Accuracy [MAc] | −1.04 | 1.02 | −1.97 | .97 | −2.44 | .83 | −.89 | 1.00 | −1.23 | 1.16 | −.47 | .86 | −.67 | 1.00 | −1.98 | .83 |
| Postrotary Nystagmus [PRN] | −.12 | 1.22 | 1.09 | 1.46 | −1.04 | 1.44 | .84 | 1.00 | n/a | n/a | −.21 | .80 | −.05 | .77 | .19 | .31 |

217

dysfunction (mean age = 6.9 years, $SD$ = 1.1 years) tended to score in the low-average range on most of the tests, but were considerably lower than average on Graphesthesia, Postural Praxis, Sequencing Praxis, and Standing and Walking Balance. This pattern may reflect a selective factor in the referral and acceptance of children for treatment of sensory integrative dysfunction. As in the learning-disabled group, fairly large standard deviations on some of the tests indicated considerable heterogeneity within this group. Different patterns of scores may have been obscured by the computation of mean scores across a fairly heterogeneous group of children.

**Reading Disorder.** The mean SIPT scores of 60 children with reading disorders (mean age = 7.1 years, SD = 0.9 years) fell largely in the low-average range, but scores were considerably lower than average on Postural Praxis, Kinesthesia, and Design Copying. The mean scores for this group generally fell somewhere between those of children with learning disabilities and children with sensory integrative dysfunction. The group with reading disorders differed more from these two groups on Standing and Walking Balance than on any of the other tests, suggesting that the children in this group had better vestibular-proprioceptive sensory integration.

**Language Disorder.** The SIPT means and standard deviations of 28 children with language disorders (mean age = 6.6 years, $SD$ = 1.6 years) indicated some impairment in the areas tested. More than half the scores were considerably below average, and the score pattern was a fairly good approximation of the profile for the Dyspraxia on Verbal Command cluster group. This suggests that children matching this cluster group profile may have left hemisphere rather than sensory integrative deficits.

*The remaining four groups have identified central nervous system abnormalities or damage that are associated with obvious sensory, neuromotor, or cognitive deficits.* If we can administer the SIPT to groups of children with known sensory, neuromotor, or cognitive impairments, and can show that expected test scores are low, we can use this evidence to support the hypothesis that the SIPT are tests of neurobehavioral functioning. *However, this does not mean that the low scores on these tests obtained by these children necessarily reflect sensory integrative dysfunction*

**Mental Retardation.** Scores in the SIPT for a sample of 28 children with mental retardation (mean age = 7.1 years, $SD$ = 1.3), were consistently low. This may suggest that many of these tests have a cognitive component. However, it also is likely that the same neural conditions that lead to mental retardation also influence SIPT scores. Their highest mean SIPT score (excluding Postrotary Nystagmus) was slightly below the seventh percentile on Space Visualization (i.e., their mean score was approximately −1.5). In this group of children with mental retardation, the mean scores on all six praxis tests were below the third percentile (i.e., all scores were lower than −2.0). Their low tactile and vestibular-proprioceptive scores may reflect brain abnormalities rather than poor sensory integrative functioning, per se.

**Spina bifida.** The scores of 21 children with a diagnosis of spina bifida (mean age = 7.5 years, $SD$ = 0.9 years) were below average on all of the SIPT. Excluding scores on Standing and Walking Balance (for neuromotor rather than sensory integration-related reasons), the lowest scores suggested the presence of visuo- and somatodyspraxia. Visual perception tasks with little practic demand (Space Visualization and Figure-Ground Perception) were easier for these children than were visual space perception tasks that require practic ability (Design Copying and Constructural Praxis). Bilateral integration and sequencing ability was poor (Oral Praxis, Bilateral Motor Coordination, Sequencing Praxis, and Graphesthesia).*

**Traumatic Brain Injury.** Mean scores of six boys and four girls who were victims of traumatic brain injury (mean age = 7.6 years, $SD$ = 0.8 years) were generally low to very low. The standard deviation of the SIPT scores in this group tended to be fairly high, suggesting rather large differences among these children. Nevertheless, some general patterns were evident. The Postrotary Nystagmus score, which was unusually prolonged, was consistent with the belief that brain injury may decrease the inhibition on the vestibulo-ocular reflex. In addition, the pattern of SIPT scores indicated that the sensory processing and neuromotor status of these children at the time of testing was poor. Their generally poor performance should be interpreted with caution, because the sample size was quite small, and because performance on these tests may be impaired by primary sensory and neuromotor deficits.

**Cerebral Palsy.** For the sample of 10 children with cerebral palsy (mean age = 6.1 years, SD = 1.4 years), the majority of scores were quite low. The scores on all tests with a motor component are assumed to be depressed by the neuromotor incoordination typical of cerebral palsy. This group as a whole had trouble on tests of visuopraxis and somatopraxis, but in this instance, the depressed scores may have been due to higher-level damage. Poor tactile perception also is associated with brain damage. The possibility that some scores were lowered by the neuromotor deficits was supported by relative strengths in form and space perception tasks that do not involve motor execution, and in following the verbal instructions of Praxis on Verbal Command.

## COMPARISON OF THE SIPT WITH OTHER TESTS

Another approach to the evaluation of test validity is to correlate test scores on alternate measures, of which some are presumed to assess similar abilities (convergent validity) and others are presumed to assess different abilities (divergent validity). The pattern of correlations is then examined to determine whether or not the obtained results are consistent with these theoretical expectations.

Both the SIPT and the Kaufman Assessment Battery for Children (K–ABC) (Kaufman & Kaufman, 19833) were administered to a combined sample of normal children, children with learning disabilities, and children with sensory integrative disorders. The K–ABC is a standardized intelligence test that is also used to screen for level of achievement. Correlations of the subscales on the SIPT and the K–ABC are shown in Table 8–6. As expected, the SIPT measures of sequential processing (especially Sequencing Praxis and Bilateral Motor Coordination) have higher correlations with the K–ABC Sequential Processing scale than with the Simultaneous Processing scale and, in fact, have the highest correlations of any of the SIPT tests

---

*Editor's Note:* The authors appear to suggest that children with spina bifida have sensory integration dysfunction. We believe that this may reflect an inappropriate interpretation of the SIPT scores. For children with spina bifida, low scores do not necessarily reflect dyspraxia or bilateral integration and sequencing deficits, per se. Rather, this supports literature that children with spina bifida have visuomotor as well as gross motor (including bilateral) deficits. Finally, the basis for computation of a mean Standing and Walking test score is unclear. The Standing and Walking Test was not administered to the children with spina bifida (A. Price, personal communication, November 14, 1988).

**TABLE 8–6. PEARSON PRODUCT-MOMENT CORRELATIONS BETWEEN SIPT SCORES AND STANDARDIZED K-ABC SCORES**

| SIPT Test | | | | | K-ABC Scale | | | |
| --- | --- | --- | --- | --- | --- | --- | --- | --- |
| | Arithmetic | Riddles | Decoding | Understanding | Sequential Processing | Simultaneous Processing | Mental Proc. Composite | Achievement |
| | | | | Results for a Group of Normal (n = 47) Children | | | | |
| Space Visualization [SV] | .24* | .41* | .21 | −.20 | .17 | .20 | .23 | −.02 |
| Figure-Ground Perception [FG] | .12 | .46* | .26* | .19 | .28* | .15 | .25* | .05 |
| Manual Form Perception [MFP] | .04 | −.01 | −.07 | −.23 | .30* | .15 | .26* | −.13 |
| Kinesthesia [KIN] | .20 | .28* | .36* | .27* | .22 | .03 | .19 | .27* |
| Finger Identification [FI] | .09 | .07 | −.09 | −.35* | −.16 | .19 | .01 | −.06 |
| Graphesthesia [GRA] | .01 | −.09 | −.02 | .00 | −.06 | −.14 | −.15 | .16 |
| Loc. of Tactile Stimuli [LTS] | .11 | .03 | .10 | .04 | .03 | .08 | .15 | .11 |
| Praxis on Verbal Command [PrVC] | .14 | .22 | .10 | −.03 | .21 | .18 | .28* | .24* |
| Design Copying [DC] | .21 | .29* | .43* | .24* | .20 | .15 | .25* | .17 |
| Constructional Praxis [CPr] | .11 | .14 | .15 | −.06 | .22 | .29* | .36* | −.10 |
| Postural Praxis [PPr] | .16 | .15 | .14 | .12 | .28* | .02 | .19 | .14 |
| Oral Praxis [OPr] | .00 | .33* | −.04 | .14 | .06 | .13 | .19 | −.05 |
| Sequencing Praxis [SPr] | .23 | .16 | .45* | .10 | .46* | .38* | .46* | .17 |
| Bilateral Motor Coord. [BMC] | .34* | .20 | .45* | .53* | .31* | .20 | .32* | .06 |
| Standing/Walking Balance [SWB] | .21 | .16 | .18 | .23 | .15 | −.01 | .07 | .38* |
| Motor Accuracy [MAc] | −.16 | .23 | .21 | .28* | .05 | −.03 | .12 | .02 |
| Postrotary Nystagmus [PRN] | −.08 | −.21 | −.02 | .41* | .04 | −.26* | −.19 | .16 |

## Results for a Group of Learning-Disabled (n = 35) Children

| | | | | | | | |
|---|---|---|---|---|---|---|---|
| Space Visualization [SV] | .13 | .15 | -.06 | .27 | .28* | .33* | .02 |
| Figure-Ground Perception [FG] | .41* | .33* | .12 | .30* | .45* | .48* | .47* |
| Manual Form Perception [MFP] | .30* | -.10 | -.23 | .15 | .57* | .51* | .05 |
| Kinesthesia [KIN] | .45* | .13 | .02 | .36* | .41* | .47* | .22 |
| Finger Identification [FI] | -.30* | -.12 | .03 | -.17 | -.12 | -.21 | -.32* |
| Graphesthesia [GRA] | .21 | .18 | .00 | .32* | .27 | .36* | .11 |
| Loc. of Tactile Stimuli [LTS] | .07 | .02 | .27 | .09 | .09 | .03 | .06 |
| Praxis on Verbal Command [PrVC] | .41* | .11 | .26 | .44* | .31* | .47* | .41* |
| Design Copying [DC] | .51* | .27 | .22 | .17 | .49* | .45* | .37* |
| Constructional Praxis [CPr] | .59* | .11 | .03 | .26 | .44* | .44* | .24 |
| Postural Praxis [PPr] | .41* | .08 | .00 | .25 | .46* | .47* | .13 |
| Oral Praxis [OPr] | .40* | .23 | .18 | .45* | .55* | .63* | .29* |
| Sequencing Praxis [SPr] | .49* | .47* | .48* | .47* | .15 | .37* | .40* |
| Bilateral Motor Coord. [BMC] | .24 | .38* | .32* | .29* | .14 | .24 | .32* |
| Standing/Walking Balance [SWB] | .50* | -.03 | .09 | .36* | .34* | .44* | .21 |
| Motor Accuracy [MAc] | .28* | .22 | .35* | -.01 | .20 | .14 | .24 |
| Postrotary Nystagmus [PRN] | .04 | -.15 | -.16 | -.12 | .19 | .08 | -.13 |

## Results for a Combined Group of Normal (n = 47), Learning-Disabled (n = 35), and SI Disordered (n = 9) Children

| | | | | | | | |
|---|---|---|---|---|---|---|---|
| Space Visualization [SV] | .47* | .41* | .43* | .12 | .43* | .50* | .19* |
| Figure-Ground Perception [FG] | .54* | .61* | .50* | .30* | .55* | .53* | .26* |
| Manual Form Perception [MFP] | .56* | .49* | .37* | .15 | .54* | .59* | .15 |
| Kinesthesia [KIN] | .67* | .54* | .54* | .36* | .59* | .58* | .36* |
| Finger Identification [FI] | .33* | .27* | .28* | .02 | .22* | .24* | .12 |
| Graphesthesia [GRA] | .55* | .36* | .50* | .28* | .51* | .43* | .31* |
| Loc. of Tactile Stimuli [LTS] | .39* | .27* | .32* | .10 | .30* | .27* | .21* |
| Praxis on Verbal Command [PrVC] | .68* | .68* | .53* | .41* | .63* | .65* | .24* |
| Design Copying [DC] | .73* | .60* | .64* | .46* | .57* | .66* | .34* |
| Constructional Praxis [CPr] | .70* | .56* | .53* | .30* | .57* | .68* | .24* |
| Postural Praxis [PPr] | .57* | .46* | .44* | .30* | .55* | .52* | .28* |
| Oral Praxis [OPr] | .60* | .57* | .51* | .39* | .59* | .61* | .24* |
| Sequencing Praxis [SPr] | .66* | .46* | .65* | .45* | .67* | .63* | .33* |
| Bilateral Motor Coord. [BMC] | .56* | .45* | .59* | .54* | .56* | .51* | .26* |
| Standing/Walking Balance [SWB] | .68* | .59* | .48* | .42* | .58* | .54* | .44* |
| Motor Accuracy [MAc] | .62* | .59* | .61* | .49* | .52* | .51* | .29* |
| Postrotary Nystagmus [PRN] | .04 | .05 | .08 | .16 | .12 | .08 | .14 |

*p<.05

221

with the Sequential Processing scale in the normal control group. Furthermore, the SIPT tests that should, in theory, require little or no sequential processing (i.e., Finger Identification, Localization of Tactile Stimuli, and Postrotary Nystagmus) generally show the lowest correlations with the K–ABC Sequential Processing scale.

In general, the more basic tactile tests in the SIPT show the lowest correlations with the K–ABC scales, while the complex praxis tests generally have the highest correlations. The processes that are common to both the K–ABC and the SIPT praxis tests are probably of a *complex cognitive nature*. As shown in Table 8–6, the overall pattern of correlations was similar for the normal and dysfunctional children, although the magnitude of the correlations differed somewhat across the two subsamples.

Because many of the tests in the SIPT are revisions of tests that were included in the earlier Southern California Sensory Integration Tests (Ayres, 1972), correlations between these tests in the Southern California Sensory Integration Tests and other relevant measures may provide some additional evidence for the validity of the SIPT. For example, parts of Luria-Nebraska Neuropsychological Battery, Children's Revision (Golden, Hemmeke, & Purisch, 1980) assess parameters that are similar to those assessed by the Southern California Sensory Integration Tests. Both tests were designed to evaluate neurological dysfunction. Kinnealey (1989) administered the tactile-kinesthetic sections of both tests to 30 8-year-old normal children and 30 8-year-old children with learning disabilities, and obtained a correlation of 0.73 ($p < 0.001$) between the total scores. The total tactile score for the Southern California Sensory Integration Tests was a sum of the $z$ scores for each of the somatosensory (tactile and kinesthesia) tests; the $t$ score for the tactile section of the Luria was used as the total score for that test. In a comparable study of the motor tests of the Luria and the Southern California Sensory Integration Tests, Su and Yerxa (1984) obtained a correlation of 0.83 ($p < 0.001$) between total scores on the two tests in a sample of 30 8-year-old dysfunctional children who had been referred to three private occupational therapy clinics for evaluation or treatment of sensory integrative dysfunction.

Although the Bruininks-Oseretsky Test of Motor Proficiency (Bruininks, 1978) is a test of motor skill rather than sensory integration, it does contain a number of tests requiring practic ability. Ziviani, Poulsen, and O'Brien (1982) administered both the Southern California Sensory Integration Tests and the Bruininks-Oseretsky to 32 boys and 27 girls with learning disabilities (aged 4 years, 10 months to 12 years, 2 months), and obtained significant correlations between the Bruininks-Oseretsky Fine Motor Scale and 13 of the Southern California Sensory Integration Tests. Fewer of the Southern California Sensory Integration Tests correlated significantly with the Bruininks-Oseretsky Gross Motor Scale. However, the overall pattern of correlations suggested that the two tests share a common practic-postural domain.

Scores on the Bender-Gestalt Test (Bender, 1938) predicted a Southern California Sensory Integration Tests space perception composite score ($r = 0.65$, $p < 0.01$) in a group of children (mean age = 84.8 months, $SD = 12.8$ months) with suspected sensory integrative dysfunction (Kimball, 1977). The Bender-Gestalt did not correlate significantly with tests of postural and bilateral integration.

## EVIDENCE SUPPORTING INDIVIDUAL TEST VALIDITY

Although SIPT score profiles are usually interpreted as a whole, or as an overall pattern that can be related the SIPT cluster groups, inferences sometimes must be drawn from the relationships among a smaller number of scores. To explore the meaning of these relationships, a number of correlational and factor analyses were generated to explore various relationships among the tests in the SIPT. Appendix 8-A summarizes some of the most important of these statistical relationships. Correlations are based on the combined sample.

# RELIABILITY

*Interrater reliability* indicates the extent to which a child's test scores agree when his or her performance is evaluated, recorded, and scored by different examiners. Most tests have some margin for human error. For example, examiners may differ in the accuracy and precision with which they measure the time it takes a child to perform a task, or the leniency with which they evaluate the accuracy of the child's performance. A high interrater reliability coefficient is an indication that the child's score will be very similar when his or her performance is evaluated by different examiners. *Test-retest reliability* indicates the extent to which test scores for an individual are consistent across different testings over time. Insofar as the constructs assessed by the SIPT are assumed to be fairly stable over time, a good measure of these constructs should have fairly high test-retest reliability. The reliability statistics for the SIPT are summarized in Table 8-7.

To evaluate interrater reliability, the SIPT was administered to 63 children from the age of 5 years, 0 months to 8 years, 11 months (50 boys, 13 girls, mean age = 7.26 years, SD = 1.04 years). This sample included 19 children with diagnosed reading disorders, 41 children with other learning disabilities, and 3 children with spina bifida. Eight examiners participated in the interrater reliability study, and each child's performance on the SIPT was evaluated, rated, and scored by two different examiners. All of the reliability coefficients were very high, ranging from 0.94 to 0.99. These reliability coefficients, summarized in Table 8-7, indicate that different examiners should be able to obtain similar results from the tests. It should be noted, however, that all of the examiners in the interrater reliability study had completed a comprehensive SIPT administration course. Interrater reliabilities probably would be considerably lower among untrained examiners.

The test-retest reliability of the SIPT was evaluated in a sample of 41 dysfunctional children (24 boys, 17 girls, mean age = 6.5 years, SD = 1.3 years) and 10 normal children (four boys, six girls, mean age = 6.8 years, SD = 1.4 years). Each child was tested twice with the SIPT, with an interval of 1 to 2 weeks between testings. To ensure that the reliability coefficients would not be inflated by age differences in test performance, all coefficients were computed using standard scores (derived from the age- and gender-appropriate norms for each child). The test-retest reliability coefficients are shown in Table 8-7.

As a group, the praxis tests had the highest test-retest reliabilities, but reliabilities for most of the other tests were acceptably high. However, 4 of the 17 tests did show rather low test-retest reliability. These included Postrotary Nystagmus, two of the somatosensory tests (Kinesthesia and Localization of Tactile Stimuli), and one visual test (Figure-Ground Perception). The SIPT test-retest reliabilities for Kinesthesia and Localization of Tactile Stimuli are quite similar to those reported for the earlier Southern California Sensory Integration Tests version of these tests (Ayres, 1980). The reliability of the SIPT Figure-Ground Perception test is slightly higher than the reported reliability of the Southern California Sensory Integration Tests version of Figure-Ground Perception.

**TABLE 8–7. SIPT RELIABILITY STATISTICS**

| | Interrater Reliability | |
| --- | :---: | :---: |
| | *r* | **(n)** |
| SPACE VISUALIZATION [SV] Time-Adjusted Accuracy | .99 | (63) |
| FIGURE-GROUND PERCEPTION [FG] Accuracy | .99 | (58) |
| MANUAL FORM PERCEPTION [MFP] Total Accuracy | .99 | (47) |
| KINESTHESIA [KIN] Total Accuracy | .99 | (60) |
| FINGER IDENTIFICATION [FI] Total Accuracy | .95 | (62) |
| GRAPHESTHESIA [GRA] Total Accuracy | .96 | (54) |
| LOCALIZATION OF TACTILE STIMULI [LTS] Total Accuracy | .99 | (59) |
| PRAXIS ON VERBAL COMMAND [PrVC] Total Accuracy | .98 | (62) |
| DESIGN COPYING [DC] Total Accuracy | .97 | (58) |
| CONSTRUCTIONAL PRAXIS [CPr] Total Accuracy | .98 | (63) |
| POSTURAL PRAXIS [PPr] Total Accuracy | .96 | (62) |
| ORAL PRAXIS [OPr] Total Accuracy | .94 | (63) |
| SEQUENCING PRAXIS [SPr] Total Accuracy | .99 | (51) |
| BILATERAL MOTOR COORDINATION [BMC] Total Accuracy | .96 | (48) |
| STANDING AND WALKING BALANCE [SWB] Total Score | .99 | (60) |
| MOTOR ACCURACY [MAc] Weighted Total Accuracy | .99 | (62) |
| POSTROTARY NYSTAGMUS [PRN] Average Nystagmus | .98 | (56) |

# Test-Retest Reliability

| | Combined Sample | | | | | | Learning-Disabled Sample | | | | | |
| | Test | | Retest | | | | Test | | Retest | | | |
| | Mean | SD | Mean | SD | r | (n) | Mean | SD | Mean | SD | r | (n) |
|---|---|---|---|---|---|---|---|---|---|---|---|---|
| SPACE VISUALIZATION [SV] Time-Adjusted Accuracy | -.42 | 0.93 | -.25 | 1.17 | .69 | (49) | -.58 | .87 | -.48 | 1.11 | .62 | (39) |
| FIGURE-GROUND PERCEPTION [FG] Total Accuracy | -.67 | 1.24 | -.28 | 1.02 | +.56 | (47) | -.90 | 1.23 | -.41 | 1.02 | +.54 | (38) |
| MANUAL FORM PERCEPTION [MFP] Total Accuracy | -.99 | 1.10 | -.34 | 1.24 | +.70 | (31) | -1.07 | 1.14 | -.43 | 1.25 | +.69 | (26) |
| KINESTHESIA [KIN] Total Accuracy | -.94 | 1.31 | -.55 | 1.19 | +.50 | (46) | -1.29 | 1.19 | -.76 | 1.15 | +.33 | (37) |
| FINGER IDENTIFICATION [FI] Total Accuracy | -.52 | 1.33 | -.62 | 1.28 | .74 | (46) | -.67 | 1.33 | -.76 | 1.27 | .75 | (38) |
| GRAPHESTHESIA [GRA] Total Accuracy | -.28 | 1.37 | -.21 | 1.37 | .74 | (42) | -.60 | 1.37 | -.55 | 1.31 | .72 | (32) |
| LOCALIZATION OF TACTILE STIMULI [LTS] Total Accuracy | -.42 | 1.08 | -.29 | 1.24 | .53 | (47) | -.65 | 1.02 | -.54 | 1.16 | .54 | (37) |
| PRAXIS ON VERBAL COMMAND [PrVC] Total Accuracy | -.87 | 1.34 | -.61 | 1.43 | +.86 | (48) | -1.17 | 1.31 | -.91 | 1.44 | +.88 | (38) |
| DESIGN COPYING [DC] Total Accuracy | -.47 | 1.45 | -.08 | 1.60 | +.93 | (36) | -.68 | 1.50 | -.36 | 1.64 | +.94 | (27) |
| CONSTRUCTIONAL PRAXIS [CPr] Total Accuracy | -.39 | 1.12 | -.42 | 1.10 | .70 | (51) | -.54 | 1.17 | -.56 | 1.09 | .67 | (41) |
| POSTURAL PRAXIS [PPr] Total Accuracy | -.52 | 1.30 | -.12 | 1.46 | +.86 | (49) | -.65 | 1.37 | -.30 | 1.50 | +.88 | (39) |
| ORAL PRAXIS [OPr] Total Accuracy | -.47 | 1.53 | -.25 | 1.43 | +.90 | (49) | -.76 | 1.50 | -.52 | 1.41 | +.89 | (39) |
| SEQUENCING PRAXIS [SPr] Total Accuracy | -.77 | 1.16 | -.55 | 1.22 | +.84 | (47) | -1.03 | 1.10 | -.74 | 1.23 | +.84 | (38) |
| BILATERAL MOTOR COORDINATION [BMC] Total Accuracy | -.74 | 1.07 | -.52 | 1.14 | +.82 | (45) | -1.08 | .82 | -.76 | 1.08 | +.77 | (36) |
| STANDING AND WALKING BALANCE [SWB] Total Score | -1.50 | 1.42 | -1.68 | 1.33 | .86 | (48) | -1.88 | 1.32 | -2.06 | 1.19 | .80 | (38) |
| MOTOR ACCURACY [MAc] Weighted Total Accuracy | -.44 | 1.20 | -.43 | 1.20 | .84 | (45) | -.59 | 1.27 | -.53 | 1.29 | .84 | (35) |
| POSTROTARY NYSTAGMUS [PRN] Average Nystagmus | .03 | .77 | .11 | .67 | .48 | (39) | -.03 | .87 | .12 | .72 | .47 | (29) |

+Indicates significant practice effects on retest ($p < .05$).

It should be noted that the test-retest reliability coefficient of 0.49 for Postrotary Nystagmus is considerably lower than the test-retest coefficients previously obtained in normal children for the identical Southern California Postrotary Nystagmus Test. Although it is conceivable that the test-retest reliability of Postrotary Nystagmus is negatively affected when it is administered after other tests in the SIPT, the coefficient of 0.49 is probably an underestimate of the actual reliability of this test. For example, Ayres (1975) reported a 2-week test-retest reliability coefficient of 0.83 in a sample of 42 children presumed to be normal. Kimball (1981) obtained a test-retest reliability coefficient of 0.80 in a sample of 63 normal children (ages 5 through 9 years), with a test-retest interval of approximately $2\frac{1}{2}$ years. Punwar (1982) reported a 0.82 test-retest reliability coefficient in a sample of 56 normal children, aged 3 through 10 years, tested 2 weeks apart. And Dutton (1985) reviewed the published Southern California Postrotary Nystagmus Test reliability data and found that the test-retest reliability coefficients ranged from 0.79 to 0.81 for normal 4- to 11-year-old children.

# INTERPRETATION OF SIPT RESULTS

The SIPT was designed to *assist* in the clinical understanding of children with *mild to moderate irregularities* in learning and behavior. SIPT results should never be used as the sole source of information when making diagnostic judgments. In particular, the clinician should have: (a) a clear and comprehensive description of the presenting problem; (b) a relevant history of the child; (c) a general knowledge of the child's intellectual capacity, language development, and academic achievement; (d) any pertinent psychological and medical diagnoses; and (e) clinical observations, including those of ocular and postural responses, defensive reactions to tactile and other sensory stimuli, and degree of gravitational security. The SIPT scores should be interpreted in light of all of these additional sources of information.

## Interpretation of Full and Partial Profiles

The *WPS Test Report for the SIPT* provides comprehensive descriptive information about the child's performance on each of the 17 SIPT. In addition, the *WPS ChromaGraph for the SIPT* compares the child's overall pattern of SIPT scores with the patterns that characterize the six different diagnostic clusters described below.

### DEFICIT IN BILATERAL INTEGRATION AND SEQUENCING

It is assumed that the score constellation of this SIPT cluster group presents the purest and clearest picture of the bilateral integration and sequencing deficit. Although the mean scores for this SIPT cluster group were all within average range, this group shows the prototypic pattern of deficit in the bilateral integration and sequencing function. This group tends to score in the low-average range on Oral Praxis, Standing and Walking Balance, Sequencing Praxis, Bilateral Motor Coordination, Graphesthesia, and Postural Praxis. In contrast, this group tends to score in the average to high-average range on Figure-Ground Perception, Finger Identification, Praxis on Verbal Command, Design Copying, and Constructional Praxis. Contrast between scores on the bilateral integration and sequencing tests, *when they fall below the normal range*, and the rest of the tests is an important criterion in diagnosis.

When symptoms characterizing a bilateral integration and sequencing deficit appear along with other sensory integrative or practic deficits, scores on the tests that are associated with bilateral integration and sequencing functions may be described as part of the total picture, or they may be described separately if a bilateral integration and sequencing deficit is clearly present. In general, the diagnosis of bilateral integration and sequencing deficit should be made only when there are no other conditions that would account for the child's performance (e.g., low tactile scores associated with somatodyspraxia). Moreover, when low bilateral integration and sequencing scores are associated with low Praxis on Verbal Command scores and prolonged nystagmus, the low bilateral integration and sequencing scores are not interpreted as a bilateral integration and sequencing deficit.

## VISUO- AND SOMATODYSPRAXIA

Members of this group generally score lowest on Design Copying, Standing and Walking Balance, Sequencing Praxis, Kinesthesia, Bilateral Motor Coordination, Postural Praxis, Motor Accuracy, Graphesthesia, and Finger Identification, in that order. They generally score highest on Praxis on Verbal Command. This group has the lowest Postrotary Nystagmus score of the six groups. Whereas both visuo- and somatopraxis scores were low for children in this cluster, children likened to this cluster on the WPS ChromaGraph may demonstrate low scores in only visuopraxis or in only somatopraxis. Further, as was discussed earlier, the visuopraxis scores should be delineated instead as form and space perception, visuomotor coordination, or visual construction deficits.

## DYSPRAXIA ON VERBAL COMMAND

This type of dysfunction is the most discrete and least variable in its manifestation among children. The major identifying feature of the dyspraxia on verbal command profile is the contrast between a very low Praxis on Verbal Command score and a relatively high Postrotary Nystagmus score. This group also has low scores on Design Copying, Oral Praxis, Sequencing Praxis, Bilateral Motor Coordination, and Standing and Walking Balance. Equally important in characterizing the dyspraxia on verbal command profile are average to low-average scores on the rest of the tests, which include the somatosensory, the visual form and space, and the visuopraxis tests. As discussed elsewhere in this chapter, dyspraxia on verbal command disorder is believed to be associated with higher level, rather than sensory integrative dysfunction.

## GENERALIZED SENSORY INTEGRATIVE DYSFUNCTION

This group tends to score far below average on all of the SIPT. It is characterized by consistently low level of performance, rather than by any kind of discrete pattern of performance. Careful analysis of scores of children in this group suggests that they demonstrate, and are better identified as having, severe deficits in visuo- and somatopraxis or bilateral integration and sequencing.

## LOW-AVERAGE SENSORY INTEGRATION AND PRAXIS

This group also is characterized by its general level of performance, rather than by any distinguishing *pattern* of scores. Children in this group tend to fall in the low-average range on most of the tests in the SIPT.

## HIGH-AVERAGE SENSORY INTEGRATION AND PRAXIS

Like those of the previous two groups, members of this group are distinguished by their general level of performance, and not by any distinguishing pattern of scores. Children in this group tend to fall in the average to high-average range on most of the tests in the SIPT.

## PARTIAL PATTERNS

Sometimes only part of the SIPT cluster group profile fits the child's profile. At other times, there is only a partial, but recognizably meaningful, score pattern. And, occasionally, there is no SIPT cluster group profile, but only the child's profile plotted on the ChromaGraph. These cases require a different interpretative approach.

Study of a large number of factor analyses (unpublished data) revealed natural linkages among tests. These partial patterns also appeared on some of the children's profiles. In one analysis, low Postrotary Nystagmus shared variance with low Design Copying, Constructional Praxis, Space Visualization, Finger Identification, Motor Accuracy, Manual Form Perception, and Figure-Ground Perception. The pattern suggests that inefficient central nervous system processing of vestibular input sometimes may be associated with poor form and space perception.

Another analysis showed a strong relationship among Space Visualization, Figure-Ground Perception, Design Copying, Motor Accuracy, and Constructional Praxis. Two or more of these tests could identify a visual form and space perception deficit, with or without dyspraxia. The term "visual construction deficit" could be used when Design Copying and Constructional Praxis scores are low. The term "visuomotor coordination deficit" could be used when Motor Accuracy and Design Copying scores are low. "Poor visual form and space perception" could be used when Space Visualization and Figure-Ground score are low (see also, Table 1–1).

Postural Praxis and Oral Praxis appeared as essentially a doublet in several analyses, indicating a likely linkage. In a number of analyses, the somatosensory tests correlated with each other and independent of praxis, suggesting a sensory integrative deficit without dyspraxia. In other analyses, Postrotary Nystagmus correlated with the somatosensory tests, suggesting a vestibular-somatosensory processing deficit.

Readers interested in additional information concerning the interpretation of individual tests are referred to the SIPT manual (Ayres, 1989b). However, it is important to remember that interpretation is always based on clusters of test scores that, when considered together, can be interpreted in a meaningful manner. Some of the SIPT have limited reliability when considered in isolation. Therefore, when several scores assessing the same construct are low, diagnosis can be made with more confidence.

Finally, diagnostic judgments should never be made without confirming evidence obtained from the child's current performance at home and in school, relevant history, other available test scores, and clinical observations of ocular and postural responses, sensory defensiveness, and gravitational security. The art of interpretation of the SIPT is discussed in Chapter 9.

## REFERENCES

Ayres, A. J. (1965). Patterns of perceptual-motor dysfunction in children: A factor analytic study. *Perceptual and Motor Skills, 20,* 335–368.

Ayres, A. J. (1966). Interrelation among perceptual-motor functions in children. *American Journal of Occupational Therapy, 20,* 68–71.

Ayres, A. J. (1969). Relation between Gesell developmental Quotients and latter perceptual-motor performance. *American Journal of Occupational Therapy, 23,* 11–17.

Ayres, A. J. (1972a). *Southern California Sensory Integration Tests* manual. Los Angeles: Western Psychological Services.

Ayres, A. J. (1972b). Types of sensory integrative dysfunction among disabled learners. *American Journal of Occupational Therapy, 26*, 13–18.

Ayres, A. J. (1975). *Southern California Postrotary Nystagmus Test* manual. Los Angeles: Western Psychological Services.

Ayres, A. J. (1977). Cluster analyses of measures of sensory integration. *American Journal of Occupational Therapy, 31*, 362–366.

Ayres, A. J. (1978). Learning disabilities and the vestibular system. *Journal of Learning Disabilities, 11*, 18–29.

Ayres, A. J. (1980). *Southern California Sensory Integration Tests* manual: Revised 1980. Los Angeles: Western Psychological Services.

Ayres, A. J. (1989a). Forward. In L. J. Miller (Ed.), Developing norm-referenced standardized tests [Special issue]. *Physical and Occupational Therapy in Pediatrics, 9*(1).

Ayres, A. J. (1989b). *Sensory Integration and Praxis Tests.* Los Angeles: Western Psychological Services.

Ayres, A. J., Mailloux, Z., & Wendler, C. L. (1987). Developmental dyspraxia: Is it a unitary function? *Occupational Therapy Journal of Research, 7*, 93–110.

Bender, L. (1938). *A visuo-motor gestalt test and its clinical use* (Research Monograph No. 3). New York: American Orthopsychiatric Association.

Bruininks, R. H. (1978). *Bruininks-Oseretsky Test of Motor Proficiency.* Circle Pines, MN: American Guidance Services.

Dutton, R. E. (1985). Reliability and clinical significance of the Southern California Postrotary Nystagmus Test. *Physical & Occupational Therapy in Pediatrics, 5*, 57–67.

Gesell, A., & Amatruda, C. S. (1974). *Developmental Diagnosis.* New York: Paul B. Hoeber.

Golden, C. J., Hemmeke, T. A., & Purisch, A. D. (1980). *The Luria-Nebraska Neuropsychological Battery.* Los Angeles: Western Psychological Services.

Kaufman, A. S., & Kaufman, N. L. (1983). *Kaufman Assessment Battery for Children.* Circle Pines, MN: American Guidance Service.

Kimball, J. G. (1977). The Southern California Sensory Integration Tests (Ayres) and the Bender Gestalt: A creative study. *American Journal of Occupational Therapy, 31*, 294–299.

Kimball, J. G. (1981). Normative comparison of the Southern California Postrotary Nystagmus Test: Los Angeles vs. Syracuse data. *American Journal of Occupational Therapy, 35*, 21–25.

Kinnealey, M. (1989). Tactile functions in learning-disabled and normal children: Reliability and validity considerations. *Occupational Therapy Journal of Research, 9*, 3–15.

Lorr, M. (1983). *Cluster analysis for social scientists.* San Francisco: Jossey-Bass.

McAtee, S. M. (1987). *A correlational study of the Design Copying atypical approach parameters and the Southern California Sensory Integration Tests: A pilot study.* Unpublished master's thesis, University of Southern California, Los Angeles.

Punwar, A. (1982). Expanded normative data: Southern California Postrotary Nystagmus Test. *American Journal of Occupational Therapy, 36*, 183–187.

Silberzahn, M. (1975). Sensory integrative function in a child guidance population. *American Journal of Occupational Therapy, 29*, 28–34.

Su, R. V., & Yerxa, E. J. (1984). Comparison of the motor tests of SCSIT and the L–NNBC. *Occupational Therapy Journal of Research, 4*, 96–107.

Ziviani, J., Poulsen, A., & O'Brien, A. (1982). Correlation of the Bruininks-Oseretsky Test of Motor Proficiency with the Southern California Sensory Integration Tests. *American Journal of Occupational Therapy, 36*, 519–523.

# APPENDIX 8-A

# Validity of Individual SIPT Scores

## TACTILE AND VESTIBULAR-PROPRIOCEPTIVE SENSORY PROCESSING TESTS

Kinesthesia correlated most consistently with Sequencing Praxis, Standing and Walking Balance, Constructional Praxis, Design Copying, Motor Accuracy, and Oral Praxis, suggesting a possible proprioceptive link with each of these tasks. In factor analyses, Kinesthesia loaded highest on (and helped to identify) somatosensory processing factors.

Finger Identification correlated most strongly with Graphesthesia and with visuo- and somatopraxis tests, and had the lowest correlations with Praxis on Verbal Command. In factor analyses, Finger Identification loaded most strongly on (a) somatopraxis and somatosensory processing factors, (b) visuopraxis factors, and (c) factors reflecting positive correlations between Postrotary Nystagmus and somato-sensory processing.

Graphesthesia correlated most strongly with tests that identified the bilateral integration and sequencing function, but it also correlated substantially with Postural Praxis and with the visual construction tests. In factor analyses, Graphesthesia loaded consistently and strongly on bilateral integration and sequencing factors. It also loaded substantially on somatopraxis factors. These loadings possibly point to the sensitivity of Graphesthesia to deficits in complex tactile processing and in translating complex stimuli into planned bilateral action sequences.

Localization of Tactile Stimuli correlated most strongly with Kinesthesia, Bilateral Motor Coordination, and Oral Praxis. In factor analyses, Localization of Tactile Stimuli loaded strongly on somatosensory processing factors. A considerable link between Localization of Tactile Stimuli and Oral Praxis was also demonstrated in one of the three factor analyses. The data reaffirmed the close relationship between tactile processing and certain practic abilities.

Correlations between Postrotary Nystagmus and the other tests in the SIPT were fairly weak. In a sample of 125 children with sensory integrative deficits, Postrotary Nystagmus had a significant negative correlation with Praxis on Verbal Command; in a combined sample of 117 children with learning disabilities or sensory integrative deficits and 176 matched children from the normative sample, Postrotary Nystagmus had significant, but low, positive correlations with Finger Identification, Motor Accuracy, and Graphesthesia.

Standing and Walking Balance correlated significantly with many of the other tests in the SIPT, suggesting that some process needed for body balance also may contribute to performance on the other tests in the SIPT. The strongest associations were with the bilateral integration and sequencing function, proprioception, and visual construction. The most likely basis for these relationships was the degree of integration of sensation from the vestibular and proprioceptive systems. Analyses suggested that Standing and Walking Balance was more apt to be low when duration of postrotary nystagmus is prolonged than when duration of postrotary nystagmus is depressed, but that relationship was not invariable. In fact, Standing and Walking Balance performance, as well as the other tests of bilateral integration and sequencing were apt to be depressed in each of the domains of sensory integrative dysfunction identified, suggesting a vulnerability of body balance to dysfunction. However, when a bilateral integration and sequencing deficit is associated with high (prolonged) Postrotary Nystagmus, the problem is thought to be due to higher-level dysfunction.

## FORM AND SPACE PERCEPTION AND VISUOMOTOR COORDINATION TESTS

The adjusted Space Visualization score correlated best with Design Copying, Constructional Praxis, and Motor Accuracy. Space Visualization loaded well on visuopraxis factors, suggesting a strong visual space perception component.

The Figure-Ground Perception accuracy score consistently loaded on visuopraxis factors, and the data indicated that Figure-Ground is primarily visual in its assessment and that there is little or no praxis involved in the task. Of the 17 tests in the SIPT, Figure-Ground Perception is the least related to somatosensory processing. Figure-Ground performance was sometimes associated with the same conditions that contributed to high (prolonged) Postrotary Nystagmus scores.

Manual Form Perception loaded primarily on visuopraxis factors, indicating a haptic form perception component with a strong visualization component. The test also showed some linkage to somatosensory processing and to bilateral integration and sequencing factors.

Motor Accuracy (preferred and non-preferred hand scores) correlated most strongly with Design Copying, Sequencing Praxis, Space Visualization, Oral Praxis, Bilateral Motor Coordination, Constructural Praxis, and Standing and Walking Balance. This suggests that visuomotor coordination may be linked with form and space perception, bilateral integration and praxis, and visual construction. In the normative sample of 1,750 children, both preferred and non-preferred hand scores correlated significantly with almost all of the other scores and subscores on the SIPT, indicating that the test taps a *fundamental sensorimotor process* related to most of the SIPT. This may indicate that poor visuomotor coordination is an end product of sensory integrative dysfunction. In factor analyses, Motor Accuracy loaded most strongly and consistently on visuopraxis factors.

## PRAXIS TESTS

The Praxis on Verbal Command accuracy score was the major identifying test of both a Praxis on Verbal Command factor and the dyspraxia on verbal command cluster group. In both instances, low Praxis on Verbal Command scores were apt to be associated with abnormally increased Postrotary Nystagmus. Notable positive Praxis on Verbal Command correlations were with Design Copying, Constructional Praxis, and Postural Praxis. In addition, there were substantial correlations with

Bilateral Motor Coordination, Sequencing Praxis, Standing and Walking Balance, and Oral Praxis. These latter correlations do not necessarily stem from the same condition that is central to the bilateral integration and sequencing function. That is, when Postrotary Nystagmus scores are high and Praxis on Verbal Command scores are low, low scores on the tests of bilateral integration and sequencing are presumed to be due to higher level dysfunction.

Of all the tests in the SIPT, Design Copying appears to have one of the highest saturations on a common visual construction element. It particularly taps visual construction of two-dimensional space, and was correlated most highly with Constructional Praxis, Space Visualization, Motor Accuracy, and Sequencing Praxis. In the factor analyses, Design Copying accuracy held one of the highest loadings on the factor it helped to identify as visuopraxis, and on the function it helped to identify as visuo- and somatopraxis. All the Design Copying atypical approach parameters consistently loaded on praxis factors.

Constructional Praxis correlated positively and significantly with all other tests in the SIPT except Postrotary Nystagmus. Highest correlations were with Design Copying, Postural Praxis, and Sequencing Praxis. Constructional Praxis loaded most strongly on the visuopraxis and somatopraxis factors. Overall, the data suggest that three-dimensional construction involves more than visual space perception and that Constructional Praxis assesses a basic visuo- and somatopraxis skill.

Postural Praxis correlated positively with most of the other SIPT, indicating high saturation of a common praxis element in this test. Correlations with Oral Praxis, Sequencing Praxis, Graphesthesia, Design Copying, and Constructional Praxis were particularly strong. Postural Praxis loaded substantially on somatopraxis factors.

Oral Praxis correlations and factor loadings demonstrated three major links with Oral Praxis performance: (a) somatosensory; (b) bilateral integration and sequencing; and (c) motor planning ability. Oral Praxis loaded strongly on somatopraxis factors and on bilateral integration and sequencing factors.

Sequencing Praxis was most highly correlated with the tests that define the bilateral integration and sequencing function, with the visuopraxis tests, and with the somatopraxis tests. The correlations suggest that Sequencing Praxis evaluates a central practic ability that subserves most aspects of praxis under evaluation by the SIPT. Sequencing praxis consistently carried high loadings on the bilateral integration and sequencing factor in numerous factor analyses.

## BILATERAL INTEGRATION AND SEQUENCING TESTS

Bilateral Motor Coordination correlated most strongly and positively with the other tests that identify the bilateral integration and sequencing function, especially with Sequencing Praxis, Oral Praxis, and Graphesthesia. Bilateral Motor Coordination also correlated with the visuomotor coordination tests (Motor Accuracy and Design Copying). Finally, Bilateral Motor Coordination had a positive association with Praxis in Verbal Command.

The Space Visualization Contralateral Use score discriminated effectively between 49 dysfunctional and 49 matched normal children ($p < 0.05$). In a group of 1,750 normal children, Space Visualization Contralateral Use scores correlated significantly with the majority of the other SIPT scores. The highest correlations were with the arm and feet items of Bilateral Motor Coordination. The positive association between Space Visualization Contralateral Use and Bilateral Motor Coordination also emerged in factor analyses, emphasizing the bilateral integration aspect of Space Visualization Contralateral Use. The data also linked low Space Visualization Contralateral Use scores to right-left and reversal drawing approaches in Design Copying, and to poor somatosensory processing. These correlations support the interpretation of Space Visualization Contralateral Use as a reflection of the functional integration of the two sides of the body.

Dysfunctional children tend to have lower Preferred Hand Use scores, indicating that they exhibit less strong hand preference than do normal children. In both the dysfunctional and normal samples, boys exhibited weaker hand preference than girls. Correlations between Preferred Hand Use and Space Visualization Contralateral Use ranged from 0.47 to 0.52 ($p < 0.001$).

Additional data support the idea that limitations in development of unilateral hand preference may be associated with poor functional integration of the two sides of the body, with right-left reversals, with diminished preferred-hand visuomotor coordination, and with depressed duration of postrotary nystagmus. These associations were not necessarily strong, and could easily be overshadowed by other linkages in the dysfunctional child.

The high correlation of the Bilateral Motor Coordination arm items with the Space Visualization Contralateral Use score emphasized and supported the bilateral integration interpretation of this test. In factor analyses, Bilateral Motor Coordination loaded strongly on the somatopraxis factors and helped identify the bilateral integration and sequencing factors. In some factor analyses, Bilateral Motor Control and Postural Praxis loaded strongly on the same factor, suggesting that Bilateral Motor Coordination performance may depend in part on a more general somatopractic ability.

# CHAPTER 9

# The Interpretation Process

**Anne G. Fisher, ScD, OTR**
**Anita C. Bundy, ScD, OTR**

*Interpret — 1: to explain or tell the meaning of: present in understandable terms 2: to conceive in the light of individual belief, judgement, or circumstance.*

*G. & C. Merriam, 1981*

## PURPOSE AND SCOPE

In previous chapters, we have presented the theory of sensory integration and its related evaluation technology: the Sensory Integration and Praxis Tests (SIPT) (Ayres, 1989; Chapter 8) and related clinical observations of sensorimotor behavior (Chapters 4 through 7). In this chapter, we will demonstrate how this information is applied to the process that we use to interpret the results of an evaluation. We will do this by presenting a case report of Steven, a boy who was recently referred to us for evaluation. We will recount the process that we went through to determine (a) that Steven had sensory integrative dysfunction, (b) the specific nature of his sensory integrative dysfunction, and (c) how his sensory integrative dysfunction appeared to interfere with his ability to perform daily life tasks. Finally, we will demonstrate how the results of an evaluation can be presented to parents or teachers.

Assessment involves gathering the relevant information about the individual being tested. *Interpretation involves making meaning of the assessment results.* In the case of sensory integrative dysfunction, we use our knowledge of theory, the results of the SIPT, clinical observations of relevant sensorimotor behavior, and relevant information obtained from the client, his or her family, and the teacher. When they are available, additional test scores are considered as well. In all instances, the information obtained is made meaningful by interpreting it in relation to the reason for referral and the goals of the client, the family, and the teacher. That is, in interpreting the results of an evaluation of sensory integrative functioning, we want to explain the presenting problems by using sensory integration theory, when appropriate. In subsequent treatment planning, we want to set goals with the family and the client, and create activities, based on the theory of sensory integration, to meet those goals.

Interpretation of the results of an evaluation of sensory integrative dysfunction is an art, based on a thorough understanding of the strengths and limitations of sensory integration theory and its related evaluation technology. In large part, because interpretation is based on meaningful clusters of scores that, when considered together, suggest dysfunction within a given domain, an important part of the interpretation process is analyzing the results to determine if any such clusters are present. In this process, related information that is relevant to the client, but not to the identification of sensory integrative dysfunction, is identified and temporarily set aside. Only after domains of dysfunction are identified should meaningful clusters of scores be used to provide a basis for explaining the presenting behavior of the client. Finally, when meaningful clusters cannot be identified, or when there is more about the presenting problems that we *can't* explain than that we can explain, we must acknowledge that perhaps sensory integration is not the theoretical framework that provides the best model for understanding the client and his or her problems.

# THE REFERRAL AND DEVELOPMENTAL HISTORY

Steven was $6\frac{1}{2}$ years old at the time of his initial referral to occupational therapy for evaluation of suspected sensory integrative dysfunction. His referral was initiated by his mother, who knew quite a bit about occupational therapy because her sister is an occupational therapist.

Steven's mother, Mrs. P, telephoned us to discuss Steven and to inquire about the possibility of an evaluation. "I don't know what any of this means," she said, "but I want to tell you how Steven is different from my other three children." Mrs. P then related the following story of Steven's development from the time of his birth. As she progressed, we asked her a few questions to help her focus her story on the relevant aspects of Steven's early childhood and the effect of his problems on his life and his family. We also listened carefully for evidence that an evaluation of sensory integrative functioning was indeed warranted.

Steven was a full-term infant and his birth was uncomplicated. From the time of his first feeding, however, Mrs. P felt that there was something different about him. Steven was a cranky, irritable baby who seemed to dislike cuddling and handling. He had some difficulty nursing because of a weak suck and because he tired quickly. His sleep cycles were erratic and he did not sleep for more than 4 hours at a time until he was almost 2 years of age. Even at 6 years of age, he seldom slept more than 6 hours.

Steven's "crankiness" and difficulty sleeping were complicated by chronic middle-ear infections that began in infancy and persisted throughout his early childhood; tubes inserted in his ears reduced the frequency of the ear infections. Steven's mother had hoped that his other problems also were due to his ear infections. However, she soon realized that Steven persisted in being "somehow different" from her other children.

As an infant, Steven attained most motor milestones "at the latter end of normal." He sat independently at 8 months and walked at 15 months. He never crawled on hands and knees. Before he learned to walk, Mrs. P felt that Steven was frustrated by his inability to get around his environment; he cried a great deal of the time. Mrs. P remembered feeling relieved when Steven learned to walk because his disposition seemed to improve markedly. However, she recalled that her relief was short-lived. The ambulatory Steven was in constant motion. He was "into everything"; he fell frequently, bumped into things, and knocked everything over.

Despite Steven's often difficult behavior and frequent outbursts of temper, Mrs.

P described him as a loving and loveable child. She felt that he was quite bright. His language skills had developed ahead of schedule and she indicated that he had a highly developed sense of humor.

As he grew older, it became more and more apparent to his family how different Steven really was. Steven was the second of four children. Although all four children were active, Mrs. P stated that Steven's activity, unlike that of his siblings, often seemed without purpose. She described Steven as running from place to place and thing to thing without ever stopping to engage in an activity for more than a few seconds. Mrs. P related that Steven's behavior became markedly worse when there were a lot of people around or when a situation was very noisy. As a result, the family had stopped taking him to shopping malls and avoided many restaurants. They also had noticed that when he ate certain foods he became even more active, so they controlled his diet carefully.

By the time Steven was 5 years of age, and as the time drew closer when he would begin school, Mrs. P became more and more concerned about Steven's poor motor skills. Although he seemed to use his right hand slightly more often than his left, Mrs. P observed that Steven tended to use whichever hand was closest to the object at the moment. He continued to look awkward when he walked and ran. He still bumped into things and fell a lot. He was unable to catch a ball even as well as his 3-year-old brother, and his throwing looked awkward and was similarly inaccurate. He didn't seem to know how to pump himself on a swing (although he loved to be pushed and would swing for hours on end). He had difficulty propelling a small bicycle (with training wheels) in a straight line.

Although Steven expressed some interest in coloring, doing artwork, and doing puzzles, Mrs. P did not feel that he was very good at those "preschool" activities, which his 4-year-old sister did much better than Steven. Mrs. P described that while engaged in those activities, Steven often laid his upper body on the table; sometimes he fell off the chair. Whenever he got his hands even slightly dirty, he had to wash them immediately. Further questioning clarified that Steven often responded adversely to light touch stimuli. Mrs. P felt that his dislike of such things as glue or fingerpaint on his fingers was related to this sensitivity to touch.

Mrs. P expressed her concerns about Steven's development and his level of activity to the pediatrician when Steven went for his kindergarten physical examination. The physician recommended trying Steven on a small dosage of Ritalin; the family agreed. The medication seemed to help Steven to attend better and Mrs. P believed it was beneficial to her son. However, while he was able to attend slightly better, his activity level remained very high; he continued to be overly sensitive to touch and noise, and his coordination was not improved.

Steven entered kindergarten at age 5 $\frac{1}{2}$. His teacher really enjoyed Steven's sense of humor and genuinely liked him. Since she seemed to understand Steven's needs, and easily accommodated to them, Steven's kindergarten year was a success. Mrs. P was delighted that Steven seemed to be doing well, but at the same time, she was worried that he seemed to be getting further and further behind his peers in terms of his motor coordination and his school readiness skills; his activity level had not diminished. She further worried that, although he had his brother and sisters to play with at home, he did not have any friends of his own, either at school or in the neighborhood. Mrs. P was concerned that Steven would not be able to succeed as well in first grade as he had in kindergarten because he would have to be in school for the whole day and the demands on him would be greater. She also was concerned that a new teacher might not be as understanding as his kindergarten teacher, and might not be willing to make the adaptations to the classroom routine that had enabled Steven to succeed in kindergarten. The school personnel were more optimistic and tried to assure Mrs. P that Steven was bright and that he would do fine in school.

Mrs. P's concerns were warranted, however. Steven's first days in first grade were a "disaster." He came home expressing that he hated school. He developed stomach aches and found many excuses to be able to remain at home. His work was poor and his behavior was worse. His teacher began to send home notes indicating that Steven was having difficulty finishing his work on time, his handwriting was illegible, and he erased his papers until there were holes in them. On other occasions, he would get frustrated and tear up his papers. Steven's teacher wondered about having him tested for eligibility for special education services. It was at that point that Mrs. P discussed Steven with her sister, who recommended that she have him evaluated for sensory integrative dysfunction, and Mrs. P contacted us.

When asked what she felt were the difficulties that hindered Steven the most, Mrs. P replied that she was particularly worried that he would grow up having a very poor self-image. She felt his distractibility, his clumsiness, and his lack of friends caused him the greatest difficulty in school and at home and contributed to his feelings that he couldn't do anything right.

## THE EVALUATION

We listened carefully to Mrs. P's concerns about Steven. We scheduled an appointment for a formal evaluation for Steven because several aspects of Mrs. P's description of Steven suggested that an evaluation of sensory integrative functioning was warranted. In particular was her description of a child who, in her opinion, had gross and fine motor coordination problems. Another important aspect of her story that prompted us to evaluate Steven was the obvious impact of his activity level on his school and family behavior. We wondered if there might be a sensory integrative basis for his increased activity level and his distractibility.

### Classroom Observation

At our request, Mrs. P also made arrangements for us to observe Steven at school and to spend a little time with his teacher. Since one of Mrs. P's major concerns was Steven's behavior in school, we felt that the opportunity to observe him within a natural context would enhance our ability to meaningfully interpret our test results, and possibly to provide the teacher as well as his mother with recommendations that would help both them and Steven.

We observed Steven during reading group, while he did an arithmetic activity, during lunch, and at recess. We paid careful attention to the effects of the various environments on Steven's performance.

The first grade classroom was a busy place. Steven was one of 33 students in a class with one teacher and a teacher's aide. Because Steven was having difficulty attending to his work, his seat was in the front corner of the room, beside the teacher's desk. As a result, there was a steady stream of children passing his desk all day long to get help or instruction from the teacher. Steven was observed on several occasions to follow directions that were given to another child standing beside his desk rather than to continue with his own assignment. Also, because his seat was on a "major traffic aisle," a few children bumped into his desk on their way back to their own seats. When this happened, Steven was provoked and sometimes hit at the child, which resulted in Steven's being disciplined.

Steven's arithmetic assignment required that he cut out squares of paper on which numbers were drawn, and then paste them in spaces for the answers to the problems on a second sheet of paper. Steven's skills with the scissors, although slow and labored, were adequate for the task. However, after he had pasted the first square onto the answer sheet, he became so preoccupied with removing the paste that remained on his fingers that he did not complete the assignment. Instead, he spent his time picking paste off his fingers and watching what the other kids were doing.

His performance in reading group was markedly better. Steven, his teacher, and four of his classmates all gathered in one corner of the room, their backs to the class. Steven was able to contribute to the group appropriately. However, he fell out of his chair twice and was reprimanded for his sitting posture on several occasions.

At lunch, Steven seemed completely overwhelmed by the noise and the number of children in the cafeteria. He had extreme difficulty opening his milk container, and finally used so much force on it that he spilled milk on the table and again was reprimanded for not paying attention. Although he sat with other kids in his class, he did not interact with them at all. Instead, Steven spent most of his time looking around at the other kids, and when lunch was over, he had eaten only half of his sandwich and one bite of fruit.

Steven and his classmates then went outside for recess before beginning the afternoon's activities. On the playground, Steven raced around, seemingly without purpose. He again did not interact with any of his classmates; he did not attempt to join the more organized games that many were playing, nor did any of his classmates ask him to join a team.

After lunch, when we had the opportunity to discuss Steven with his teacher, she indicated that the morning's activities we had observed were typical examples of Steven's behavior. She expressed extreme frustration with Steven because she felt he could do much better if he tried harder. Her greatest concerns pertained to his behavior, especially his distractibility and activity level, and his not finishing his work on time.

## Sensory Integration and Praxis Tests

The following week, we evaluated Steven using the SIPT and the related clinical observations that have been described in Chapters 4 to 8. Steven's scores on the SIPT are shown in Table 9–1.

## Clinical Observations

Steven found it difficult to sit for prolonged periods of time during the SIPT. He particularly disliked the tactile tests and rubbed his arms and hands immediately following the application of the stimuli. He also made a number of excuses as to why we should quit testing during that portion of the evaluation.

Steven was given the Touch Inventory for Elementary School Aged Children (TIE) (Royeen & Fortune, 1990; see also Chapter 5). He received a raw score of 69 (of 78 possible); when this score was compared with those of the normative sample, we

## TABLE 9-1. STEVEN'S SENSORY INTEGRATION AND PRAXIS TEST RESULTS

| Test | SD Score |
|------|----------|
| Space Visualization (SV) | −1.47 |
| SV Contralateral Use | −1.05 |
| SV Preferred Hand Use | −.62 |
| Figure-Ground Perception | .67 |
| Manual Form Perception | −1.25 |
| Kinesthesia | −.24 |
| Finger Identification | −.81 |
| Graphesthesia | −2.13 |
| Localization of Tactile Stimuli | 1.34 |
| Praxis on Verbal Command | .92 |
| Design Copying | −1.69 |
| Constructional Praxis | −2.32 |
| Postural Praxis | −1.52 |
| Oral Praxis | −2.72 |
| Sequencing Praxis | −3.00* |
| Bilateral Motor Coordination | −2.21 |
| Standing and Walking Balance | −2.04 |
| Motor Accuracy | −1.42 |
| Postrotary Nystagmus | −1.43 |

*Scores lower than −3.0 are reported by Western Psychological Services as −3.0.

noted that 100 percent of the normative sample responded in ways that suggested that they were *less* tactually defensive than Steven.

Steven also had difficulty with many of the clinical observations associated with vestibular-proprioceptive functioning (see Chapter 4). Although he was able to assume portions of the prone extension posture, his head was not fully erect and he complained that his neck hurt. He also flexed his legs sharply at the knees after only a few seconds. He was able to maintain this approximation of the prone extension posture for only about 8 seconds. Steven was slightly better at performing supine flexion than at performing prone extension. He was able to assume the posture without assistance; however, his head lagged slightly as he did so. He maintained supine flexion for 12 seconds.

Not surprisingly, Steven also demonstrated hyptonia of extensor muscles. Observation of his standing posture revealed marked lordosis and a tendency to lock his knees. Proximal stability, observed in quadruped, also was found to be poor. Steven's scapulae winged bilaterally, and he tended to lock his elbows and externally rotate his arms at the shoulders to mechanically improve his stability. His trunk sagged slightly. Finally, he had apparent difficulty modulating force when opening his milk container.

Steven's ability to maintain his equilibrium was slightly better than his ability to maintain tonic postures. When seated on a large ball that the therapist tipped slowly, Steven moved his trunk and limbs in appropriate compensatory ways to prevent his falling off the ball. He particularly liked this activity and asked to repeat it several times. When asked to stand on either a flat board or a tilt board and to reach for an object placed at shoulder height but slightly out of reach, he was able to lift his uphill, contralateral foot from the board, but he flexed his uphill leg more than 30° at the knee (see Figure 4-11). When he was tilted laterally while standing on a small tilt board, he persisted in not flexing his uphill leg (see Figure 4-8).

Steven demonstrated no signs of gravitational insecurity. In fact, he enjoyed riding on moving equipment and being tipped upside down or placed in precarious positions. He also demonstrated no evidence of an aversive response to vestibular stimulation.

We observed Steven for signs of difficulty with bilateral projected action sequences (Chapter 4) by asking him to catch a tennis ball that was thrown or bounced to him from a number of different directions and by asking him to perform various hopping and jumping tasks. Steven never caught the ball unless it was thrown directly into his outstretched hands. When asked to jump across the room (on two feet), Steven was unable to make both feet land at precisely the same time. When we created a path for Steven to jump in by placing 12 inch hoops on the floor, Steven's jumping noticeably deteriorated. He was unable to perform this task in a smooth fashion and stopped before executing each new jump. His performance on jumping jacks, symmetrical stride jump, and reciprocal stride jump was below −1.0 SD during both the learning and performance phases, based on the means and standard deviations reported by Magalhaes, Koomar, and Cermak (1989). Finally, he appeared to have difficulty crossing the midline with either hand, but the left seemed somewhat worse than the right.

Upon completion of our evaluation, we asked Steven about school and what he did when he was at home. In spite of Steven's verbal abilities, it was hard for him to articulate his likes and dislikes or to talk of his concerns about his perceived difficulties in school or his lack of friends. He did tell us that he really didn't like school, but that he guessed that his favorite subject was reading. He was unable to specify for us any play activity he particularly enjoyed. He also indicated that he was often the last person chosen when teams were picked at school. He did agree that he liked riding on playground equipment, and that he didn't like going to the mall with his mother. When asked who were his best friends, he said that his younger brother and sister were his best friends.

## Other Information

When they are available, the results of evaluations by other professionals can be helpful in interpreting the results of an occupational therapy evaluation of sensory integrative functioning. In Steven's case, the only evaluation result that was available to us were his scores on the Weschler Intelligence Scale for Children–Revised (WISC–R) administered by the school psychologist as part of the process of determining if Steven was to be eligible for special education services. His verbal IQ was reported to be 130 and his performance IQ was reported to be 114.

## INTERPRETING THE RESULTS

At this point, we had quite a lot of information about Steven. Our task was to begin to organize this information in a manner that would help us to interpret his test results. We did this in two stages. In the first stage, we made a list of the relevant information conveyed by his mother and his teacher, as well as obtained through our observation of his behavior at school and during testing (Table 9–2).

One of our goals in preparing the list shown in Table 9–2 was to clearly separate (a) the more global information that pertains to Steven's *presenting problems* and *sensorimotor history* (Table 9–2, section I), (b) the *relevant background information*

**TABLE 9–2. SUMMARY OF THE RELEVANT INFORMATION OBTAINED BY PARENT AND TEACHER REPORT AND THROUGH OBSERVATION OF STEVEN'S SCHOOL AND SENSORIMOTOR BEHAVIOR**

I. STEVEN'S PRESENTING PROBLELMS
  A. *Parental and teacher concerns*
  Feeling that he can't do anything right and is growing up with a poor self-image
  Distractibility:
    Behavior became worse in crowded or noisy situations
    Follows directions given to other children standing close to his desk
    Easily disrupted/distracted by other children
  Activity level:
    Once ambulatory; in constant motion
    Runs from place to place without stopping to engage in activity
    Behavior becomes worse in crowded or noisy situations
    Races around playground seemingly without purpose
    Difficulty sitting still for prolonged periods
  Clumsiness (see C., Sensorimotor development)
  Lack of friends
  Not finishing his school work on time
  B. *Related behavior*
  Hates school; developed stomach aches and other excuses to remain at home
  Gets frustrated and tears up his papers
  Does not play or interact with friends or classmates
  Sometimes hits at other children who bump into him
  C. *Sensorimotor development*
  Difficulty nursing — weak suck, tired quickly
  Sat independently at 8 months, walked at 15 months; never crawled
  Fell frequently, bumped into things, knocked things over
  Seemed to prefer right hand, but tended to use hand closest to objects
  Awkward when he walked and ran
  Unable to catch; throwing awkward, inaccurate
  Didn't know how to pump himself on a swing
  Loved to be pushed on swing, would swing for hours on end
  Difficulty propelling a bicycle (with training wheels)
  Problems with coloring, artwork, and puzzles
  Laid his upper body on the table when coloring, etc.
  Fell off chair
  Illegible handwriting
  Erased his papers until there were holes in them
II. RELATED BACKGROUND INFORMATION
  A. *Developmental history*
  Full-term, uncomplicated birth
  Cranky, irritable baby who disliked cuddling and handling
  Erratic sleep cycles, did not sleep for more than 4 hours until age 2
  Seldom sleeps more than 6 hours
  History of chronic middle-ear infections
  B. *Strengths*
  Loving and loveable child
  Mother feels that he is bright
  Language skills developed ahead of schedule
  Sense of humor
  C. *Strategies that already have been tried*
  Tubes inserted into his ears
  Control of diet did not resolve his problems
  Ritalin helped attention but not activity level
  Desk placement at front of room near his teacher
  Disciplined for his behavior
  Performance better in small group, back to the class
III. RELATED TEST RESULTS
  Verbal IQ 130; performance IQ 114 (WISC–R)
IV. EVALUATION OF SENSORY INTEGRATIVE FUNCTIONING
  A. *Behaviors observed during the school observation*
  Scissor skills slow and labored, but adequate for task
  Fell out of chair
  Difficulty opening milk container

*(continued)*

**TABLE 9–2. SUMMARY OF THE RELEVANT INFORMATION OBTAINED BY PARENT AND TEACHER REPORT AND THROUGH OBSERVATION OF STEVEN'S SCHOOL AND SENSORIMOTOR BEHAVIOR** (*continued*)

B. *Clinical observation of postural-ocular movements*
  Poor prone extension posture
  Head lag when assuming supine flexion
  Hypotonia of extensor muscles
  Lordotic standing posture, tendency to lock his knees
  Poor proximal stability in quadruped
  Equilibrium better than static, controlled postures
  Deficient tilt board response
  Used too much force to open milk container
C. *Clinical observation of bilateral integration and sequencing abilities*
  Difficulty with bilateral and projected action sequences (catching a ball, jumping with two feet together, jumping jacks, etc.)
  Difficulty crossing the midline
D. *Clinical observation of somatopractic abilities*
  Unable to maintain supine flexion
E. *Indicators of poor sensory modulation*
  Responded aversely to light touch stimuli
  Dislike of glue or fingerpaint on his fingers
  Sensitive to noise
  Rubbed arms and hands following application of tactile stimuli
  Made excuses to quit testing during tactile tests
  Touch Inventory for Elementary School-Aged Children (TIE) score of 69
  No gravitational insecurity
  No evidence of an aversive response to vestibular stimulation

that might be important for us to consider when interpreting or making recommendations regarding the results of Steven's evaluation of sensory integrative functioning (Table 9–2, sections II and III), and (c) the *specific information* about Steven's sensory integrative functioning obtained from our evaluation (Table 9–2, section IV). More specifically, Steven's presenting problems and sensorimotor history were the major reason for his referral. Our goal was to determine if sensory integrative dysfunction was contributing to these behavioral problems. Therefore, we separated related information from his *specific* sensory integration evaluation results to ensure that we didn't use the history and referral information to justify the presence of dysfunction. That is, we were seeking to determine if our interpretation of his test results might help us to better understand Steven's presenting problems.

While this may seem obvious, to do otherwise would have been equivalent to using circular reasoning. That is, we would be saying both that Steven exhibited certain traits that indicated that he had sensory integrative dysfunction, and that his sensory integration dysfunction caused these symptoms or traits (e.g., his activity level and his distractibility indicated that he had tactile defensiveness; his tactile defensiveness caused his high activity level and his distractibility). Instead, we wanted to be able to explain significant numbers of his presenting problems using our knowledge of sensory integration theory (e.g., Steven's aversive responses to touch and to noise suggested that he had a problem modulating tactile and auditory information; since we knew that sensory modulation disorders have been associated with a tendency to be distractible or overly active, we hypothesized that Steven's problems with modulation of sensory inputs were contributing to his behavior problems).

The second stage in organizing the information we had obtained about Steven was to examine Table 9-2, section IV, and his SIPT results (Table 9-1) to look for meaningful patterns of behavior that were suggestive of dysfunction within specific domains of sensory integrative functioning. As we proceeded, we were aware that some of Steven's test results would not fit into a meaningful cluster of behavior, and we remained cognizant that such isolated observations would not help us to clarify Steven's problems.

To facilitate the process of looking for meaningful clusters of test scores indicative of dysfunction, we developed and used the SIPT Interpretation Worksheet, marking a plus (+) if there was evidence of a problem and a minus (−) if the test score indicated normal performance (see Table 9-3). We left the space blank if we did not assess that specific behavior. Evidence of possible dysfunction was defined as a SIPT score below −1.0 SD (see also Chapter 8), or a clinical observation of sensorimotor behavior considered deficient for a 6½-year-old child.

Now that Steven's test scores were organized on the SIPT Interpretation Worksheet, we were ready to begin the actual interpretation process. When we examined the pattern of pluses and minuses within each box (Table 9-3), we noted that the pluses predominated in every instance. As we began to apply our understanding of the theory of sensory integration, we began the art of interpretation. To guide us in this process, we developed and used the Model for Interpretation of the SIPT and related clinical observations shown in Figure 9-1. Although *not considered disorders of sensory integration*, the SIPT can contribute to the identification of right or left hemisphere dysfunction (see Chapter 7). Therefore, the end products of higher level dysfunction also are included on Figure 9-1. As we soon were to see, a predominance of pluses, when interpreted appropriately, did not mean that Steven had dysfunction in every domain.

Since we were evaluating Steven for sensory integrative dysfunction, we began by examining his data for evidence of a sensory processing deficit. We remained aware that evidence suggesting an underlying deficit in processing, and interpreting either vestibular-proprioceptive or tactile sensory information, had to be present if we were to conclude that Steven's problems were the result of a sensory integrative (rather than higher level) deficit.

It was readily apparent that Steven had several scores that were suggestive of central vestibular-proprioceptive processing deficits. More specifically, Steven's pattern of performance suggested to us that he had a *postural-ocular movement disorder*. As is always the case when identifying whether or not there are vestibular-proprioceptive disorders, our interpretation relied heavily on our clinical observation of sensorimotor behaviors. We were not surprised about his normal score on the Kinesthesia test because we recalled that Kinesthesia is a measure of passive joint movement and not proprioception (see Chapter 4).

When we examined Steven's tactile test scores, the results were less clear. Two of Steven's four tactile discrimination test scores (Graphesthesia and Manual Form Perception) were below −1.0 SD. But we were aware that Graphesthesia also is a major indicator of bilateral integration and sequencing (projected action sequencing), and that Manual Form Perception also is a test of form and space perception. Since both of Steven's more "pure" or discrete tactile discrimination test scores (Localization of Tactile Stimuli and Finger Identification) were within normal limits, we decided to examine the domains of (a) bilateral integration and sequencing, and (b) form and space perception, before deciding whether or not Steven's low tactile test scores reflected inadequate tactile discrimination. We felt that his Graphesthesia

**TABLE 9–3. SIPT INTERPRETATION WORKSHEET**

| Postural-Ocular Movement Disorder | +/− | Tactile Discrimination | +/− |
|---|---|---|---|
| Standing and Walking Balance | + | Localization of Tactile Stimuli | − |
| Postrotary Nystagmus | + | Finger Identification | − |
| Kinesthesia | − | Manual Form Perception | + |
| Prone extension | + | Graphesthesia | + |
| Proximal joint stability | + | | |
| Extensor muscle tone | + | | |
| Equilibrium | + | | |
| Neck flexion in supine | + | | |
| Postural adjustments | | | |
| Poor modulation of force | + | | |
| Diminished awareness of body position or movement | | | |

| Sensory Modulation Disorders | +/− | Bilateral Integration and Sequencing (BIS) | +/− |
|---|---|---|---|
| Gravitational insecurity | − | Bilateral Motor Coordination | + |
| Aversive response to movement | − | Sequencing Praxis | + |
| Touch Inventory (TIE) | + | Oral Praxis | + |
| Tactile defensiveness | + | Graphesthesia | + |
| Other sensory modulation deficits | + | Standing and Walking Balance | + |
| (e.g., aversive response to sound, smell) | | (Postural Praxis) | + |
| Avoidance of sensory experiences | | (Praxis on Verbal Command) | − |
| | | SV Contralateral Use | + |
| | | SV Preferred Hand Use | − |
| | | Mixed/delayed hand preference | + |
| | | Crossing midline of body | + |
| | | Right-left confusion | |
| | | Projected action sequences | + |
| | | Bilateral motor skills | + |

| Somatodyspraxia | +/− | Dyspraxia on Verbal Command | +/− |
|---|---|---|---|
| Meaningful BIS cluster | + | Praxis on Verbal Command | − |
| Postural Praxis | + | Postrotary Nystagmus (prolonged) | − |
| Meaningful tactile cluster | − | (Bilateral Motor Coordination) | + |
| (Meaningful postural-ocular cluster) | + | (Sequencing Praxis) | + |
| Supine flexion | + | (Standing and Walking Balance) | + |
| Sequential finger touching | | (Oral Praxis) | + |
| In-hand manipulation | | | |
| Diadokokinesia | | | |

## VISUAL PERCEPTION AND VISUOMOTOR

| Form and Space Perception | +/− | Visual Construction | +/− | Visuomotor Coordination | +/− |
|---|---|---|---|---|---|
| Space Visualization | + | Design Copying | + | Motor Accuracy | + |
| Figure-Ground Perception | − | Constructional Praxis | + | Design Copying | + |
| Constructional Praxis | + | Other constructional ability measures | | Other visuomotor test scores | |
| Design Copying | + | | | | |
| Manual Form Perception | + | | | | |
| Other visual perceptual test scores | | | | | |

Note: Tests scores that are listed in parentheses may be low when dysfunction is present, but *low scores are not considered to be major indicators of dysfunction.*

+ = score that is a positive sign suggesting that dysfunction is present.

− = score that is a negative sign refuting the presence of dysfunction.

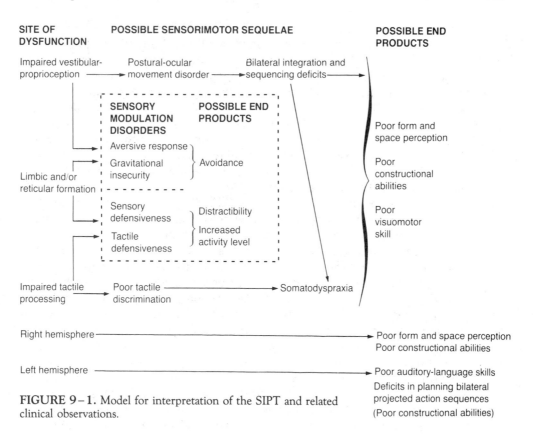

SITE OF
DYSFUNCTION

POSSIBLE SENSORIMOTOR SEQUELAE

POSSIBLE END
PRODUCTS

Impaired vestibular-
proprioception

Postural-ocular
movement disorder

Bilateral integration and
sequencing deficits

SENSORY
MODULATION
DISORDERS

POSSIBLE END
PRODUCTS

Aversive response ⎤
Gravitational      ⎬ Avoidance
insecurity         ⎦

Limbic and/or
reticular formation

Sensory
defensiveness ⎤ Distractibility
              ⎬
Tactile       ⎦ Increased
defensiveness    activity level

Poor form and
space perception

Poor
constructional
abilities

Poor
visuomotor
skill

Impaired tactile
processing

Poor tactile
discrimination

Somatodyspraxia

Right hemisphere ——————————————————→ Poor form and space perception
                                      Poor constructional abilities

Left hemisphere ———————————————————→ Poor auditory-language skills
                                      Deficits in planning bilateral
                                      projected action sequences
                                      (Poor constructional abilities)

FIGURE 9-1. Model for interpretation of the SIPT and related
clinical observations.

score was more likely to be related to his low bilateral integration and sequencing test scores (rather than form and space perception test scores) because, although Graphesthesia has a tactile form and space component, the SIPT data did not suggest that this test was a strong indicator of form and space perception (see Chapter 8). However, we felt that his low Manual Form Perception score was more likely associated with his low form and space perception test scores. As a result, we concluded that Steven did not have a meaningful cluster of test scores suggestive of a deficit in tactile discrimination.

Steven did not have a problem with *modulation* of vestibular-proprioceptive sensory information; he demonstrated no evidence of gravitational insecurity or aversive responses to movement. However, both parental report and our observation of Steven confirmed that Steven had tactile defensiveness and that he was sensitive and overly responsive to noise. Therefore, we concluded that Steven had a *tactile and auditory sensory modulation disorder.*

Having concluded that there was, indeed, evidence to support the conclusion that Steven did have sensory integrative deficits, we were ready to begin to examine the relationship between these sensory processing deficits and any deficits that he might have in other domains assessed by the SIPT (see Fig. 9-1). Examination of the scores indicative of a deficit in bilateral integration and sequencing (see Chapter 4) revealed strong evidence of a problem in this area. In fact, the only scores in this section that were within normal limits were Praxis on Verbal Command and Space Visualization Preferred Hand Use; Praxis on Verbal Command may be low in children with bilateral integration and sequencing deficits, but a low score is not commonly associated with deficits in this domain.

As we moved on to examine the evidence supporting and refuting the presence of a deficit in somatopraxis, we were reminded that the major distinguishing characteristics of somatopraxis are (a) the presence of deficits in both bilateral projected action sequences and more input-dependent, responsive motor actions (see Table 4–1), and (b) a related deficit in tactile or tactile-proprioceptive (somato-) processing (see Chapter 6). Postural Praxis is the best indicator of an input-dependent practic deficit; however, this test score may be low in children with just the projectional, bilateral integration and sequencing component (see Chapter 4). Furthermore, because we had concluded that Steven did not have a deficit in tactile discrimination, we had to reject the possibility that he had a somatopractic disorder.

When we examined the domain of dyspraxia on verbal command, the decision to conclude that Steven did not have a deficit in this area was much easier to make. This type of dysfunction is characterized by abnormally high (prolonged) durations of Postrotary Nystagmus and low Praxis on Verbal Command scores. Steven had depressed nystagmus durations and normal Praxis on Verbal Command scores. The only scores in this domain that were low were those also associated with deficits in planning and producing bilateral projected action sequences. Such deficits can be associated with impaired processing of vestibular-proprioceptive inputs at subcortical levels (i.e., sensory integrative based deficits in bilateral integration and sequencing), or with cortical dysfunction involving motor planning areas (i.e., *non*-sensory integrative based deficits in motor planning). In fact, Steven had a *relative* strength in translating verbal commands into motor actions.

So far, we had concluded that Steven had deficits in interpreting normally the sensory information derived from active movement of his body in space (vestibular-proprioception) and that these deficits were associated with difficulty in planning and producing bilateral and projected action sequences (see Fig. 9–1). The final phase of our interpretation of his test scores was to determine if he had any of the commonly associated end products of sensory integrative dysfunction: deficits in form and space perception, deficits in visuomotor coordination, and deficits in visual construction. Although we noted that Figure-Ground Perception was a relative strength, we concluded that Steven's other test scores suggested that he had problems in all three areas. When test scores in all three areas are low, it is common for the test scores to be likened (statistically) to the cluster group that contained children with a pattern of dysfunction Ayres called visuodyspraxia (see Chapter 8). However, as we have discussed elsewhere (see Chapters 1, 7, and 8), the use of the terms visuodyspraxia or visuopraxis should be avoided, and, instead, the deficit areas described in behavioral terms. Thus, we concluded that Steven's sensory integrative problems were associated with deficits in form and space perception, visuomotor coordination, and visual construction.

## REPORTING THE RESULTS

Reporting the results of Steven's evaluation of sensory integrative functioning involved communicating the results in a manner that would be meaningful to his parents and his teacher, and that would help them to "reframe" his behavioral problems (where appropriate) in terms of his sensory integrative deficits. In this process, we were careful to refer to the results of our *occupational therapy evaluation* of sensory integrative functioning. The reader also may have noticed that we have avoided the use of the term hyperactivity. Although Steven had been diagnosed as hyperactive by his pediatrician, *hyperactivity is a medical diagnosis*, and the height-ened activity level seen in children with sensory integration dysfunction is not necessarily equivalent to the medical condition of hyperactivity or attention deficit disorder.

We prepared a written report and we met with Mrs. P to talk with her about the results of Steven's evaluation. The content of both the written and verbal reports was similar; however, the written report also included a brief summary of his relevant history and his presenting problems. We also described the methods we used to assess Steven, explaining that we used both standardized tests and clinical observa-tion to evaluate (a) Steven's ability to meaningfully interpret sensory information about touch and about movement of his body in space, (b) his ability to use this information to plan and produce motor actions, and (c) Steven's visuomotor, form and space perception, and visual construction skills. In both reports, we were careful to present our results in terms that would be meaningful to Mrs. P or to Steven's teacher. Because it was the more detailed of the two reports, we present the sum-mary of our oral presentation of the results here.

Both Mrs. P and Steven's teacher had expressed major concerns about Steven's distractibility and the level of his activity. Therefore, we began our report of Steven's evaluation with a discussion of the relationship between sensory integrative dys-function and distractibility and activity level. We explained that an individual who has sensory integrative dysfunction has difficulty with the meaningful interpretation of sensory information coming in from the environment. Often those individuals seem to be unable to "screen out" irrelevant information; thus, they behave as though they are attempting to pay attention to, and to act on, all the information coming in from the environment at any given time. To elucidate the difference between Steven's experience and ours, we used the example that all of us were wearing clothing and that our clothing was providing a source of continual sensory stimulation. However, unlike Steven, we were able to screen out that stimulation and not pay attention to it unless someone began to talk about clothing or something about a piece of clothing went awry (e.g., the clothing became twisted or got wet).

We also discussed with Mrs. P that, although there was noise in the hallway where other clients passed to and fro, we were not consciously aware of that noise (until one of us brought it up in conversation); rather, we were able to concentrate on the conversation we were having. We explained that the results of Steven's testing suggested that he had difficulty modulating or screening out irrelevant sensory information and attending only to that information that was most important at the moment (e.g., his mother's or his teacher's instructions, his schoolwork, the particu-lar game he had elected to play). Thus, he appeared to be highly distractible and to run from thing to thing. Since his distractibility apparently was caused by his inability to screen out irrelevant stimuli, it became markedly worse when the amount of stimulation was greater. Thus, it was understandable that his behavior deterio-rated in busy places such as shopping malls or crowded restaurants; similar difficul-ties occurred when Steven's classmates congregated around the teacher's desk, all waiting for different instructions.

We also explained to Mrs. P that it was likely that Steven's difficulties with touch stemmed from a similar source. When Steven became "overwhelmed" by too much stimulation (which was much of the time), he began to translate light touch nega-tively. The more people touched him, either accidentally or to try to control his behavior, the more stimulation he received and the less able he became to cope with that stimulation. Thus, his distractibility and increased activity, caused by his inability to screen out irrelevant stimulation, became a part of a vicious cycle as his parents or teacher provided additional stimulation (touch) to try to control it. We also suggested that Steven's "lashing out" at other children when they accidentally bumped him was related to his inability to interpret the affective aspects of touch meaningfully.

Mrs. P also was concerned that Steven was growing up feeling that he couldn't do anything right. She believed that his negative self-concept was caused, in part, by the number of reprimands he received for his behavior during a typical day. Although his parents tried hard to emphasize Steven's accomplishments, it was still necessary, for his own safety, to attempt to control his behavior. Thus, a lot of "don't do that's" were directed toward Steven each day. This situation was even worse at school, where Steven's teacher's strategy for controlling his behavior was to reprimand him.

Mrs. P also believed that Steven felt bad about himself because he knew that his motor skills were not even as good as those of his younger brother and sisters. He was aware that he had no friends and that he was never included in games because no one wanted him on their team. Mrs. P was at a loss to deal with this problem because she knew that Steven's appraisal of his motor skills was fairly accurate. However, she hoped we could provide her with some information to help her understand what caused his motor incoordination. Further, she hoped that we would suggest some type of treatment to improve Steven's skills.

We agreed with Mrs. P's perceptions of Steven's poor self-concept as being related to both the need to reprimand him for his behavior and to his motor incoordination. With regard to his motor incoordination, we explained that Steven seemed particularly unable to interpret the sensations that came from his body as he moved through space. Without launching into a major description of vestibular-proprioception or of factor analysis, we explained that many children who had this type of dysfunction seemed to demonstrate coordination problems similar to Steven's. That is, we believed that Steven's difficulties with catching and throwing a ball, with jumping, with knowing how much force to use when playing with a toy or when erasing on his paper, with deciding which hand to use to write, and with his posture were all related to Steven's difficulties interpreting the sensory information that should be telling him about the position and movement of his body in space.

Because Mrs. P seemed particularly interested in therapy to alleviate some of Steven's difficulties, we discussed different ways that an occupational therapist could provide services to Steven and the benefits she might expect from each type of service. We told her that, if we were to provide direct service for Steven using the principles of sensory integration theory, we would involve him in a number of activities in which we provided him with opportunities for *controlled* sensory intake; these activities would require that Steven be actively involved, attempting new skills and mastering those that were emerging. We told her that we would carefully construct the activities so that they would address both the needs she had expressed and those that we had identified through testing.

We also cautioned Mrs. P that, while we believed Steven's skills would improve markedly, all of us (the therapists, the family, and the teacher) would have to work very hard with Steven to improve his self-image. That is, an improvement in Steven's skills would not automatically result in an improvement in his self-concept. Mrs. P agreed; she expressed her willingness to try to think of creative ways to facilitate Steven's participation with the children in the neighborhood. We discussed the need to talk frequently with her to discuss his progress in therapy and at home, as well as any new problems that might arise.

We also recommended to Mrs. P that the occupational therapist at Steven's school serve as a consultant to Steven's teacher. Because of the nature of Steven's difficulties and the realistic constraints on the therapist at school, we believed that Steven's direct service could be best provided in a private clinic. However, the services of the consultant at school also would be invaluable to Steven's success there. That is, in much the same way that we had interpreted Steven's difficulties to Mrs. P, the consultant could explain Steven's problems in school to his teacher by providing her with some knowledge of Steven's underlying sensory integrative dysfunction. Once Steven's behavior had been "reframed" for the teacher, the consultant could provide her with whatever ongoing assistance was necessary to enable Steven to succeed in school *despite* the limitations imposed by his sensory integrative dysfunction.

We explained to Mrs. P that the consultant might help the teacher to reorganize the classroom space so that Steven was less distracted by the other children. Further, the therapist might help the teacher to adapt assignments so that Steven could express what he was learning in the easiest way possible. For example, perhaps Steven's arithmetic assignments could be completed by having him write the answer, rather than by gluing it to the page. We told Mrs. P that we would share the information we had gained in our evaluation with the school occupational therapist.

We had given Mrs. P a great deal to think about. She expressed that she was relieved that finally someone had provided her with an explanation that seemed to fit *so many* of Steven's problems. We encouraged her to take the information home and discuss it with her husband and, perhaps, with her sister who was an occupational therapist. Although we had made numerous recommendations, including the provision of treatment provided through both direct service and consultation, we made sure she understood that the decisions were hers to make. We told her that the next step in the process, if she decided to pursue part or all of our recommendations, would be to request the services of an occupational therapist at school and to meet together to set goals for Steven's treatment. We also encouraged her to call us if any further questions arose.

## SUMMARY

In this chapter, we have presented the process of interpreting or making meaningful the results of an occupational therapy evaluation of sensory integration functioning. An important component of this process was to reframe the presenting problems of the child in terms that were easily understood by the family, and also in keeping with the unique perspective of occupational therapy and sensory integration theory. In subsequent chapters, we will discuss in more detail the process of setting goals with the family and the teacher, and then providing treatment using direct service (Chapters 10 and 11) and consultation (Chapter 12).

When we talked with Mrs. P again the next week, she told us that she had decided to follow our recommendations and that she had already begun the process of requesting occupational therapy services for Steven at school. She was eager to make an appointment for herself and her husband to begin to develop goals with us for Steven's treatment. The results of that process are the focus of Chapter 11.

# REFERENCES

Ayres, A.J. (1989). *Sensory Integration and Praxis Tests.* Los Angeles: Western Psychological Services

C. & G. Merriam. (1981). *Webster's new collegiate dictionary.* Springfield, MA.

Magalhaes, L. C., Koomar, J., & Cermak, S. A. (1989). Bilateral motor coordination in 5- to 9-year-old children: A pilot study. *American Journal of Occupational Therapy, 43,* 437–443.

Royeen, C. B., & Fortune, J. C. (1990). TIE: Touch Inventory for School Aged Children. *American Journal of Occupational Therapy, 44,* 155–160.

# CHAPTER 10

# The Art and Science of Creating Direct Intervention from Theory

Jane A. Koomar, MS, OTR
Anita C. Bundy, ScD, OTR

*Integration means the creation of an inner unity, a center of strength and freedom so that a being ceases to be a mere object acted upon by outside forces, and becomes, instead, a subject, acting from its own inner space.*

*Schumaker, 1977, p. 13*

When a client enters a treatment room, we must be prepared to respond in a variety of ways simultaneously. We immediately engage in a "dialogue" with the client, during which we listen, observe, and communicate. We learn about the client's readiness to begin the treatment session and the state of his or her central nervous system. We establish a "playful" interaction in which we engender the trust of the client by providing cues that assure him or her that we will not require more than he or she can give. We collaborate with the client to create activities that tap the client's inner drive to explore and master and that promote the client's self-direction and growth. We skillfully adjust the activities so that they provide the "just right challenge," and we facilitate the flow of one activity into another as the session progresses. This is the *"art" of therapy*, which relies heavily on our clinical experience and training, our observation and communication skills, and our intuition.

We also create a sequence of activities that (a) logically reflect sensory integration theory, (b) address the client's underlying dysfunction, and (c) facilitate the attainment of his or her goals. This is the *"science" of therapy*. It is derived from our understanding of sensory integration theory and our knowledge of how that theory applies to *this particular client*.

In order to provide *effective direct intervention*, based on the principles of sen-

---

The authors wish to acknowledge the contributions of Gretchen Dahl Reeves to the case materials in this chapter.

sory integration theory, there must be a "marriage" of the art and the science of therapy, set in the context of meaningful objectives. As in all good marriages, the relationship between art and science is fluid. One may predominate for a time, but both make equal contributions to the effectiveness of a session and to the long-term outcome of intervention. The meaningful objectives give direction to our intervention.

## PURPOSE AND SCOPE

In this chapter, we provide guidelines for creating direct intervention based on the art and science associated with sensory integration theory. We begin this chapter with a discussion of the art of therapy. Then we discuss the creation of activities to address specific problems related to sensory integrative dysfunction. Finally, we address practical considerations in making recommendations for intervention and for beginning intervention programs. These basic topics provide the foundation for intervention programs based on sensory integration theory. In this chapter, we focus on the creation of activities for one-on-one direct intervention. In subsequent chapters, we will illustrate the process of intervention with one child and we will generalize the intervention principles of the *consultation* and the *integrated (combined) approaches*.

## THE ART OF THERAPY

We are guided in the creation of direct intervention by the postulate that we can enhance the functioning of the client's nervous system (and thereby lay foundations for improved motor or academic learning) by providing the client with opportunities to take in enhanced sensory information in the context of active participation in activities that are meaningful to the client and that elicit adaptive behaviors (see Chapter 1). This treatment postulate appears to be fairly simple. Its implementation, however, is complex. The orchestration of each treatment session is an art. The art is reflected in (a) decisions about where to begin intervention; (b) the skillful adjustment of activities so that they provide the just-right challenge; (c) the creation of activities that tap the client's inner drive and promote the client's self-direction and growth; (d) the transition, or flow, of one activity into another; (e) the therapist's relationship with the client; and (f) decisions about when to discontinue intervention. We also believe that helping the client to understand the impact of sensory integrative dysfunction on his or her daily life reflects the art of therapy.

Because it is so difficult to learn, the art of therapy requires considerable discussion. We will discuss each of the many ways in which this art is manifested in intervention. However, we believe that *the best way to master the art of therapy is in the context of a mentoring relationship with an experienced therapist.*

### Deciding Where to Begin Intervention

Once we have concluded that a client's presenting difficulties can be explained in some meaningful way by sensory integration theory, and have set specific objectives, together with the client and his or her caregivers (see Chapter 12), we are confronted with decisions about the area or areas to "target" as we begin our intervention. In intervention, we seek to (a) lay a firm foundation on which increasingly complex adaptive behaviors can be built, and (b) influence the client's belief that he or she has the skills needed to perform activities that he or she either values or must accomplish (see Chapter 2).

For clients with sensory integrative dysfunction, the term "foundation" refers both to the processing of vestibular-proprioceptive and tactile information, and to sequelae such as postural competence, bilateral integration and sequencing abilities, and praxis (see Fig. 9-1). We believe these are foundations on which occupational performance can be built. Frequently, clients have difficulty in many areas. For some clients, intervention must begin with a focus on assisting the client to respond more appropriately to sensory input.

Melanie is a 5-year-old child who exhibited several classroom behaviors that were particularly problematic. Melanie's teacher reported that Melanie constantly moved around the classroom, rarely maintaining a seated position for more than a few moments at a time. When she did sit at her desk, she was "all slumped over with her nose practically touching her paper." Several times she had fallen out of her chair as she worked on a paper.

The teacher also said that Melanie constantly manipulated any object she found in the classroom (such as items on the teacher's desk). Both the teacher and Melanie's classmates found these behaviors annoying.

Another socially inappropriate behavior that Melanie developed was climbing up onto the shelf above the coat rack in her classroom and jumping off. The teacher was very puzzled by this behavior because Melanie did not appear to do it to seek attention. In fact, she seemed somewhat oblivious to the reactions of her teacher and peers when she engaged in this unusual behavior. When asked directly why she did this, Melanie replied, "it feels good to jump."

Melanie had great difficulty getting herself dressed, she was a sloppy eater, and her ability to control a crayon was very poor. She was not able to pump a swing or to skip, despite frequent opportunities to learn these skills. The occupational therapy assessment, which included the Sensory Integration and Praxis Tests (SIPT) (Ayres, 1989) and clinical observations of neuromotor performance, revealed that Melanie had poor tactile and vestibular-proprioceptive processing, low muscle tone, delayed equilibrium reactions, deficits in bilateral integration and sequencing, and poor praxis.

In order to meet the more specific educational objectives that the members of Melanie's educational team had set for her, Melanie's occupational therapist was guided by the following general goals for intervention.

1. Improve Melanie's ability to process incoming tactile and vestibular-proprioceptive information and help her to decrease her socially inappropriate behavior (jumping from unsafe surfaces, manipulating others' possessions, etc.).
2. Improve Melanie's postural stability and equilibrium reactions and help her to sit appropriately during classroom activities.
3. Improve Melanie's bilateral and practic abilities and help her to develop greater ease and effectiveness in using tools needed to do her schoolwork (e.g., scissors, crayons), performing age-appropriate and valued motor skills (e.g., pump the swing and skip), and performing self-care tasks.

When Melanie began treatment, we focused on the first general area. Because our assessment revealed that Melanie did not have a very well-developed body scheme, we focused on providing her with controlled opportunities to take in enhanced sensory information. We believed that the development of a sound body scheme would form a foundation for the other skills and abilities we hoped she would acquire.

In particular, we provided her with many opportunities to participate in activities that incorporated linear movement and provided resistance to her movements. Melanie especially liked activities that involved swinging prone in the frog swing (Fig. 10–1). We also provided her with many opportunities to take in tactile input, such as hiding her body in the bubble ball bath (Fig. 10–2) and finding large objects buried in a box filled with dried beans and rice.

We focused on improving Melanie's ability to process incoming sensations in order to help her to be able to act more appropriately in her classroom and to develop a better body scheme. However, by having Melanie perform many activities in a prone position, we also began to work on improving her extensor muscle tone and postural stability.

As we did with Melanie, we almost always address several different areas simultaneously in treatment, with our primary focus on one or two areas at a time. As treatment progressed with Melanie, and she showed signs of improved processing of sensation by demonstrating more complex adaptive behaviors, we began to change

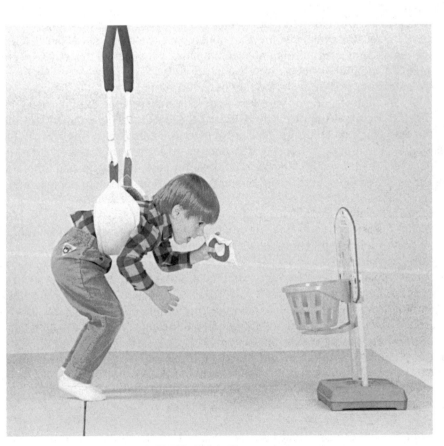

FIGURE 10–1. Frog swing.

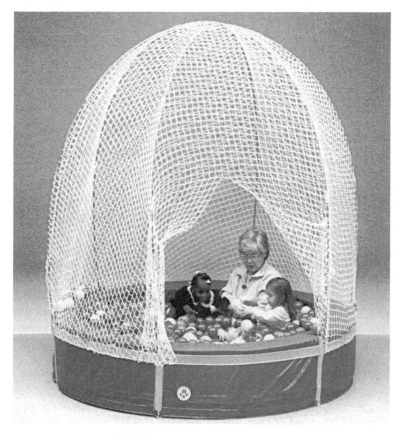

FIGURE 10–2. Bubble ball bath.

the focus of her intervention toward improving her postural and practic abilities. Although from the beginning Melanie had great difficulty with praxis, it would have been of little use to focus our efforts on facilitating Melanie's abilities to sequence projected actions (an aspect of praxis) before she had demonstrated that she was developing the important prerequisite of a more well-developed body scheme. We already had observed that Melanie's attempts to learn to skip had not resulted in her mastering skipping; her sensory foundation seemed to be inadequate to enable her to benefit from practice of this difficult skill.

At the same time, we would not want to focus *exclusively* on helping Melanie to develop an improved body scheme without paying any attention to the other skills and abilities that we would expect her to develop *simultaneously*. Development is a complex process. Although we believe that the development of a body scheme is related to an individual's ability to perform practic acts, body scheme is not fully developed before practic acts emerge. As body scheme is refined, praxis also becomes more highly developed; conversely, as the individual becomes more skilled, he or she develops a more complete body scheme. The two are intertwined; they codevelop in the spiral process described in Chapter 1. We must create intervention that reflects our belief in this principle.

## The Just Right Challenge

We often are advised that if we consistently are able to create the just right challenge, our clients will be *motivated* to engage in therapy and will demonstrate *noticeable improvements* in their adaptive behavior during each treatment session. When we speak of the just right challenge, we refer to activities that prompt our clients to stretch just a little beyond their current abilities, but that are not so difficult as to generate frustration or poor quality of response.

However, as commonsensical as these statements may seem, they portray a deceptively simple picture of one of the most difficult aspects of intervention. They give rise to questions that even expert therapists find difficult to answer *explicitly*. For example, what does the just right challenge look like?

In response to this question, one experienced therapist said, "The child gets a kind of wide-eyed look and an open smile. He often remarks, 'I *did* it!' He wants to show his mother the activity."

Any therapist who has experienced the effects of creating the just right challenge will recognize that verbal descriptors are far too simplistic to capture the real feelings that we get when witnessing a challenge unfold into a success. What is missing is the very real *sense* that we get when the client begins to work *with*, not against, the equipment. It is difficult to use words to describe the pervasive involvement with, and commitment to, mastering the challenges that pervade the treatment area. Instead, we may speak of the client's desire to repeat an activity, and his or her expressions of mastery, because these things are easier to describe.

Even if we could easily describe the experience of the just right challenge, our words would not help us to create it. Hence, the advice we gave at the beginning of this section — implementing effective intervention is best learned in the context of a mentoring relationship with an experienced therapist.

The inexperienced therapist does not need a mentor to learn to recognize the just right-challenge. He or she needs a mentor to (a) reflect on those experiences when the just right challenge did *not* happen, (b) provide guidance so that his or her skills can be refined in such a way that the probability of creating the just right challenge is increased, and (c) provide a model for successfully and consistently creating that challenge.

## Motivation: Tapping the Client's Inner Drive

Generally, a client demonstrates his or her motivation to do an activity by becoming totally involved in it. However, apparent lack of motivation for an activity may take several forms. Certainly, some clients (particularly children) verbalize that they don't want to do an activity because "it's boring" or "it's baby stuff." Some children try to divert our attention by attempting to engage us in a conversation or another activity. Others may withdraw from the activity and seek a protected space, such as inside a stack of inner tubes or a barrel. Still others become increasingly anxious or overly active and disorganized in their behavior. When a client expresses, either verbally or non-verbally, that he or she does not want to perform an activity, we must seek to discern the reason for this apparent lack of motivation, since the cause suggests the remedy.

In our experience, a client's "lack of motivation" in treatment usually means that (a) the activity we have created is too difficult, (b) the client has the necessary skill, but *perceives* that the activity is too difficult, or (c) the client is overstimulated.

Clearly, if the activity is too difficult, we must modify the demands of the activity until they more closely match the client's skills. However, if the activity is not too difficult, but the client believes that it is, we must decide whether to (a) modify the activity so that the client believes he or she can accomplish it, or (b) try to entice or cajole the client into attempting the activity in order to "teach" the client that he or she truly does possess the needed skill. The decision to modify or to cajole and entice is dependent on (a) which of these two approaches best fits our style of interacting with this particular client, and (b) how adamantly the client seems to be refusing.

If we decide to cajole or entice the client into trying the task, we must take care not to enter into a "power struggle" with the client. We must remember that the primary purpose in this approach is to help the client discover skills that he or she possesses, not to force the client into doing something he or she clearly does not feel able to do. If the client cannot be convinced easily to try the task, we "dump" the plan and move on to another activity.

If the reason that the child is "unmotivated" to perform the activity is that he or she is overstimulated (as is often the case with children who seek protected spaces or who become overly active and disorganized), we must respect the child's need for quiet time. It usually is best for us to express our understanding of the child's need for "space" and to allow the child to remain in the protected area as long as he or she feels the need. Some children, if asked, will express their desire to terminate the session and go home. Again, we need to express to the child that this may be an adaptive and desirable behavior when he or she feels overwhelmed; if the session is terminated, we should not do it in a punitive fashion.

Another significant challenge to our "artistic" ability is in striking a balance between allowing the client freedom to explore, initiate, and choose activities and imposing structure. Although the client who has a strong inner drive may be motivated, and able, to select many appropriate activities independently, in most cases we need to "impose" enough structure to assist the client to develop increasingly complex adaptive behaviors. We may need to intervene with physical or verbal prompts or with slight alterations to an activity.

## Discontinuing and Modifying Activities

Another important, but difficult, aspect of the art of therapy is knowing when to discontinue, or modify, an activity. We discussed this briefly in an earlier section; here we expand and clarify that discussion. We believe that it is desirable to remain with a given activity as long as the client demonstrates continued motivation to participate and improvements in adaptive behavior. Certainly, we should not discontinue an activity because *we* are bored or because we are fearful that a particular treatment session lacks variety. In deciding when to discontinue or modify an activity, the client must be our guide. As long as the client remains totally involved in a carefully selected activity, it is likely that he or she is benefiting from that activity.

Sometimes an activity *clearly* is either too easy or too hard for a client. Although the "cues" that a client gives when an activity is too easy may be quite different from those that he or she gives when an activity is too hard, the solution often is the same — modification.

Modification, when it can be done readily, usually is preferable to dumping the activity, because it is less disruptive to the flow of the session. Further, if an activity is too hard, but not out of the realm of possibility for a client (as often is the case), we sometimes can make the activity temporarily a little easier, keeping in mind the goal of gradually grading it back to the original task. In this way, the client is able to see clear signs of progress during the session.

Of course, sometimes it is necessary to dump an activity that is either too easy or too hard. This occurs most often when the task lacks flexibility; that is, it does not inherently allow for modification either by varying the position of the client or the desired outcome. For example, while a Sit 'N' Spin (Fig. 10–3) sometimes may be useful in intervention, it is not readily adaptable because the client can do only a limited number of different things on it and only in the sitting position.

If it is necessary to discontinue an activity, we should take the responsibility for the "mistake" so that the client does not have additional reason to believe that his or her skills have, once again, caused an activity to fail. It is easy enough for us to say, "This really is too hard. That was *my* mistake. Let's do something different."

We may find that there are times when a client simply needs to repeat an activity many times in order to develop some new skill or to master the activity. Don, an 11-year-old boy who was dyspraxic, had particular difficulty sequencing the steps of an activity. While prone in a net swing, he attempted to propel himself forward with his hands to hit a suspended punching bag. He had great difficulty sequencing his pushing off the mat to reach the target. When we tried to making subtle modifications to the activity, however, they seemed only to disrupt his efforts rather than to make the task easier. When we "left him alone," he was able to "get it all together" and succeed at the activity. Apparently, for Don, the critical factor for success was the opportunity to repeat the motions several times; it took about 5 minutes of practice before he was able to consistently propel himself forward and hit the punching bag.

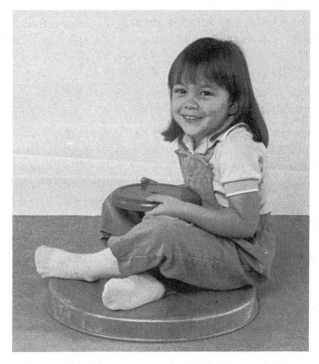

FIGURE 10–3. Sit 'N' Spin.

Once he established the sequence and could make contact with the punching bag, he remained eagerly engaged in the activity for an additional 15 minutes. If we had given up on the activity too soon and not given him the time he needed to master the sequence, we would not have allowed him to meet a challenge of which he was capable.

It often is possible to ask older children and adults whether or not *they* would like to continue an activity (although that sometimes disrupts their concentration and the flow of the activity). The real problem for us in trying to decide whether or not to modify an activity is with younger clients. If the activity is too hard for a young child, and if we do not react quickly enough to alter the demands of the task, the child may become frustrated or discouraged. It may then be difficult to re-engage the child during that treatment session and, possibly, during subsequent treatment sessions as well.

Activities that are *too easy* do not challenge the client to stretch his or her skills and, therefore, are not particularly useful for treating the client's sensory integrative dysfunction. Further, most clients, recognizing that the activity does not present a challenge, become bored with it quickly. Often the client, especially if asked, may suggest modifications to make it a bit more difficult. We must remember, however, that while very easy activities are not beneficial for improving sensory integration, those activities still may have *therapeutic* value. Sometimes a client benefits emotionally from performing an activity that he or she has mastered and especially enjoys, particularly if that activity is valued by the child's peers or family.

When a treatment session is most effective, the therapist and the client flow from one activity to another like skilled dancers responding to changing pieces of music. At certain times, *we* take the lead and modify an activity or initiate a new one. At other times, we follow the client's lead and surreptitiously incorporate challenges, as needed.

Jerry, a 10-year-old boy who had significant motor planning problems, frequently requested activities he had previously mastered. He most often would select activities that allowed him to use his relatively strong postural extensor muscles rather than activities that challenged his weak flexors.

During one treatment session, he asked to play a game where he rode prone on a scooter board down a ramp (Fig. 10–4) in order to "steal jewels from the queen's castle while she slept." We wanted to involve Jerry in an activity that encouraged movement into *flexion.* Our task with Jerry, as with many of our clients who seem fearful of failure, is to "capture" their motivation and to invest it in a slightly more challenging activity.

Thus, after a few minutes of Jerry's riding down the ramp, we announced that the queen had decided she must find a better way to protect her jewels because he was simply too good at stealing them from the wall of her castle. She had decided to put them in a moat filled with alligators that could only be reached by flying overhead on a "helicopter" (the T-swing) (Fig. 10–5). Moving Jerry's story into a new activity allowed us to maintain his interest and enthusiasm while providing a greater challenge to flexion.

Moving fluidly from one activity to another results in a treatment session that looks and feels playful. To the untrained observer, this may appear to be less structured than are other kinds of intervention programs. Parents and teachers sometimes misinterpret the playful nature of the treatment session and question the "validity" of the intervention. (Can anything that much fun *really* be doing any good?) It is therefore important to express clearly the purpose of the treatment

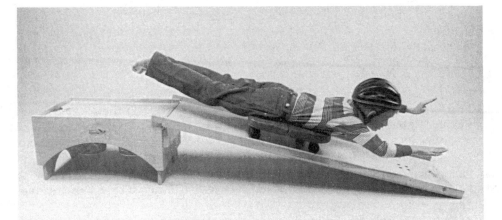

FIGURE 10-4. Scooter board and ramp.

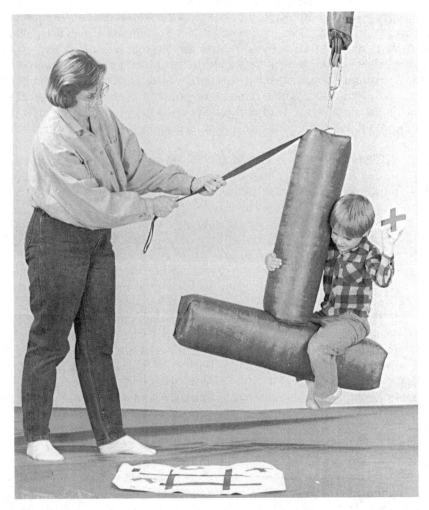

FIGURE 10-5. T-swing.

activities and the benefits of playful, fluid sessions to the important others in a client's life.

## Therapeutic Interactions

We are important therapeutic "tools." Each of us possesses different styles for interacting with clients. Our styles of interacting affect our clients, and we may need to alter our inherent styles to best suit the needs of each client.

### ESTABLISHING A SAFE ENVIRONMENT

In intervention based on the principles of sensory integration theory, the client is asked to engage in sensorimotor activities that may expose his or her vulnerabilities. This can be very threatening or even frightening for some clients. In order for those clients to engage fully in the therapeutic process, we must engender their trust. That is, we must provide the client with the sense that we understand his or her abilities and needs and that we will assure that he or she is safe, both physically and emotionally.

At a very basic level, all clients need to believe that the equipment they use in treatment is safe and that they are safe on it. We need to remain near enough to the client during activities to promote and maintain safety, yet far enough away to allow the client to be self-directed and challenged.

At first, some clients may be fearful of or resistant to becoming involved in challenging activities. It may be necessary to allow young children time to observe someone else performing an activity before we ask them to do it. Inviting interaction with the activity through pretend play often is a successful strategy. One therapist began a session with a particularly timid child by putting a stuffed animal in the swing and saying, "My bunny *loves* to swing. Do *you* want to push her"? A little later, she asked the child, "Would *you* like a turn on the swing now"?

With many children, we have found that becoming directly involved in the activity with the child is a successful strategy. There are many ways to become a part of an activity that we have created with a client. For example, we might swing together, or sit in a cozy spot while exploring tactile materials.

### INCORPORATING COMPETITION

Clients sometimes request that we engage in competitive games with them. However, we have found that some clients are particularly sensitive to failure and unable to successfully "handle" the stress of true competition. An example of an activity that we have used with children who seem particularly sensitive to failure involves throwing "food" (beanbags) to the "baby fish in the pond" (inner tube). When the food goes outside the pond, the big fish in the ocean gladly eat it! Throwing at a target is a common component of competitive games, but in this case it's not who wins, but whether or not the fish eat that becomes the outcome. In activities such as this, there is no competition and very little risk of failure.

Another example of an activity involving minimal competition also involves throwing beanbags or balls into a container. In this activity, each time the client hits the target with the beanbag, he or she gets a point; however, when the client misses the target, *we* get the point. We design and adapt these activities carefully to ensure that the client succeeds most of the time.

Sometimes the activities that we create with a client *require* that we engage in friendly competition. For example, each of us may try to knock over a row of blocks that the other is "defending." Children can sense it when we are not trying hard enough or are letting them win. Thus, we should minimize our deliberate failures (e.g., "bad shots"). Instead, we can "handicap" ourselves by increasing the distance to our targets or by setting up more targets for ourselves. Another strategy we have found useful for minimizing the discrepancy between our level of skill and that of our clients is to change places with them midway through a game (Schaefer & Reid, 1986). In this way, they begin to play from the position of relative advantage that they gained when they took over our lead. Children usually accept these strategies, especially if we remind them that we have a lot more chance than they do to practice the game.

## ASSUMING "ADVERSARIAL ROLES"

Sometimes children request that we play an imaginary "adversarial role" as part of an activity. Although we may assume the adversarial role created by the child (e.g., the monster or the "bad guy"), we believe that it usually is better to play an assistive role. Instead of being the bad guy, we join the "good" team and, with the client, go after the bad guy. We try to relegate the adversarial role to a punching bag or other inanimate object. We do this particularly when our clients are vulnerable or become overly threatened or frightened when we assume a negative role.

## PROVIDING VERBAL PRAISE, FEEDBACK, AND INSTRUCTIONS

Another aspect of therapeutic interaction is our use of language. Ayres (1972) felt that it was not always necessary to provide *verbal* praise. She felt that the expression on a therapist's face often was sufficient, and that the client's own knowledge of success was the most important "reinforcer." However, verbal praise can be very important to some clients. We often serve as a "barometer" of the subtle improvements in our clients of which they might otherwise be unaware.

For this, and other reasons, we feel that it is very important to give accurate *verbal feedback* to our clients. Clients use our verbal feedback in a number of positive ways. Many use it as a basis for modifying inaccurate perceptions of their movements and body position in space. For example, one client we treated felt as though she were falling each time her postural muscles contracted in response to movement. Our verbal feedback helped her to understand that those muscle contractions were actually equilibrium reactions that *prevented* her from falling.

Some clients seem unable to use the body's feedback to perceive the movements they have accomplished. They may rely on our verbal feedback, especially during the early stages of intervention, to learn how they have moved. For example, Kerry, a 12-year-old girl who completed a forward flip on a trapeze bar for the first time, was cheered by her therapist. Kerry appeared pleased, but then asked, "What did I do?" When the therapist verbalized what Kerry had done, and gave her physical cues, she was able to repeat her performance successfully.

We often give *verbal instructions* in the form of encouragement with clients who approach an activity somewhat impulsively. If a client rushes into an activity, fails, and then immediately stops trying, we might say, "I think you can do it better. I'm going to help you. This is the place to learn."

Finally, sometimes we need to use verbal instruction to modify a client's behavior, such as to help a child discontinue an undersirable action. We have found that positive instructions often are more successful than negative commands. For example, "put your foot here" often works better than "stop kicking" (Ayres, 1985). Luria (1961) indicated that children younger than 5 years of age routinely have difficulty discontinuing an action in response to a verbal command. It is likely that children who have a delayed language are much older than 5 years before they can respond reliably to a verbal command to stop an action.

## Strategies for Helping Clients Understand Sensory Integrative Dysfunction

It is important that we enable our clients to understand the impact of their sensory integrative dysfunctions and the purpose of their interventions, and that we help them to develop strategies to adapt to, and compensate for, these dysfunctions. By the time they reach 6 or 7 years of age (and often earlier), most of our clients are aware that they are somehow different than other children. They usually notice that they are unable to perform activities and skills that come easily to other children or that they get into trouble more often. Although they already are trying as hard as they can, many of our clients have received repeated feedback from adults that they could do better if they tried harder. In response, many clients develop "explanations" for their failures. They have never heard of sensory integration theory. As far as they know, other people process sensory information from their bodies and from the environment in the same way they do. Thus, they come to believe that the reason they cannot do certain things well is because they are "bad," "lazy," or "dumb."

We have found that many clients experience immense relief when we use sensory integration theory to provide explanations for their difficulties — in language they can readily understand. One client's mother reported that it was as though someone had taken a huge weight off her 7-year-old son's shoulders. "He's like a different kid," she said. "I guess I never realized how much he worried about not being able to do things as well as the other kids."

We begin explaining their sensory integrative dysfunction to our clients when we report the results of their evaluations. We also begin to elicit from them their own perceptions of the things they do well and the things they are not so good at doing. Most importantly, we also elicit from them their explanations of why they think they are good or bad at particular things. We ask our clients if they have ever talked to their parents or teachers about these matters and, if so, how their parents or teachers have explained them. We try to "reframe" the explanations using sensory integration theory. We are very careful to use words that the clients will understand.

Our explanations do not end with the evaluation. We continue to discuss their sensory integrative dysfunction, as opportunities present themselves, throughout the intervention process. In so doing, we hope to help them not only to understand the impact of their sensory integrative dysfunction better, but also to develop strategies to compensate for their dysfunction. We first "check out" the strategies we suggest to a child with the child's parents or teachers, to be certain that they understand the rationale behind the strategies and that they agree with them. As much as possible, we develop those strategies *with* the client and with his or her parents or teachers.

One strategy that we have used successfully with children who become overly active and highly distractible during treatment is to say, "When you feel like this, it is a good time to go into a quiet place." We then create a safe, enclosed space for the client, such as underneath a large cushion or inside a carpeted barrel. Thus, we teach the client that an appropriate way to deal with too much sensory stimulation is to go to a place where that stimulation is minimized. When the child has calmed down sufficiently, we often use the opportunity to talk to him or her about the difficulty of concentrating when too much is going on in a place. We explain that, in an enclosed space, it is easier to be calm and to concentrate because not so many things are happening all at the same time.

When we suspect that a child engages in twisting locks of hair or chewing on shirt collars, outside of treatment, in order to provide him- or herself with sensory input, we might suggest that the client chew bubble gum or engage in other activities that provide proprioceptive input, such as jumping on a mini-trampoline. Some clients find that pulling on both ends of a piece of rubber tubing (that they can carry in their pockets) helps to "relieve built-up tension."

We feel that it is very important that clients with sensory integrative dysfunction become able to explain their difficulties to others so that they can shape their own environments and minimize the impact of their difficulties. Billy, a 4-year-old who was quite tactually defensive, demonstrated unusual understanding of his difficulties and the purpose of his treatment. Billy found it useful to "brush" himself when he became agitated at home. One day, Billy asked his father why he didn't wear his wedding ring. When his father responded that he didn't like the feeling of things on his hands, Billy promptly produced his brush and told his father that if he brushed his hands he might be able to wear his ring. Not only was he able to assist himself, he was able to share the information he had learned about himself in an attempt to assist his father.

## Discontinuing Intervention

When a client has reached his or her objectives in treatment and many of the day-to-day interferences of sensory integrative dysfunction have been minimized or eliminated, the client's intervention is discontinued. When we decide it is time to stop intervention, we are most interested in a client's ability to function adequately and easily in his or her routine daily roles and tasks. Whether or not sensory integrative dysfunction interferes with a client's functional abilities is the critical factor in deciding to begin or discontinue intervention.

Ideally, clients receive treatment as long as they continue to benefit in a meaningful way. However, despite careful evaluation of the degree to which a client's sensory integrative dysfunction interferes with his or her life, often it is difficult to predict the total duration of intervention that will be required to minimize or eliminate that interference. The minimum duration of intervention usually is 6 months; in our experience, most commonly, clients receive intervention for 1 to 2 years. A few clients may continue to benefit from intervention for 3 or more years.

We recommend that clients be reevaluated every 3 to 6 months to determine what progress has been made toward meeting the objectives for treatment and to specify clearly any new objectives that may have emerged. More formal assessments of progress, using standardized instruments, also may be warranted periodically.

During the course of intervention, periods of "plateauing" may occur for several weeks, followed by periods of significant progress. This may reflect a period of time during which the client is consolidating, or integrating, the gains he or she has made. Although currently there are no studies that have examined the effectiveness of treating clients for an initial period of time, then discontinuing treatment during periods of plateauing, this provides an interesting hypothesis to examine through research. We have had some success with this strategy.

As we consider whether or not a client's intervention can be discontinued, we remember that a client may master certain skills in the clinic before these same or similar skills are mastered in other settings. This may indicate that, while the skill is emerging, the client is not yet able to use it automatically or without assistance. It also may indicate that the client does not yet believe, or know, that he or she has developed this new skill or that a particular new skill developed in the clinic is the same skill required in other situations.

When we do decide to discontinue intervention, we prepare the client and his or her caregivers for the possibility that evidence of the sensory integrative dysfunction may recur when the client is under stress, such as when learning a new complex skill or during activities that provide strong sensory input. Scott, an 8-year-old boy who had received extensive treatment for severe gravitational insecurity, had shown tremendous gains, particularly in his play. He had learned to climb the jungle gym, descend the slide, ride a two-wheeled bike, roughhouse with his parents, and tumble with other children — effortlessly and without fear. However, when his parents took him sledding for the first time, they found that he was fearful of a moderately steep hill that his younger siblings did not find fear-inducing. In this case, Scott's day-to-day functioning was adequate for most play and social activities. However, in an unfamiliar situation where he felt that he had little control, some of the gravitational insecurity still could be seen.

Because of our ongoing consultation with them, Scott's parents understood his reaction. We had discussed with both Scott and his parents the reasons that he was afraid of certain activities; we helped them to develop strategies, ahead of time, to minimize that stress. Because Scott really wanted to go sledding, he and his father went to a smaller hill to "get warmed up." Later, they returned to the bigger hill and one of his parents rode with Scott on a two-person sled until he developed a sense of control over the movement.

Scott did not need further intervention from us. When a particular activity resulted in his becoming overly fearful, Scott and his family evaluated whether or not the activity was important for him and for them. If it was important, they worked together to grade the activity so that Scott could master it.

## Summary

The art of therapy is a multifaceted phenomenon. Much of the success of our direct intervention depends on our "artistic" ability. We have discussed many aspects of the art of therapy, including (a) deciding where to begin treatment, (b) creating the just right challenge, (c) tapping the client's motivation, (d) discontinuing and modifying activities, (e) forming a therapeutic relationship, (f) helping client's to understand their sensory integrative dysfunction, and (g) discontinuing our intervention. In the following section, we will discuss the creation of activities based on sensory integration theory. Although this section speaks primarily to the science of intervention, effective intervention involves much more than designing a sequence of activities; it is the art that holds it all together.

## IMPLEMENTING INTERVENTION

In this section, we will depict and discuss activities that we have found to be successful for addressing specific areas of difficulty. Clearly, we cannot describe *every* activity that a therapist might develop in any given area. Rather, our goal is to provide the reader with *ideas* for activities and with a *systematic method for evaluating activities* in order to determine what they might be used to accomplish.

Rarely will any activity meet only one objective. The difficult task for us is to determine which, of all the possible inherent uses that an activity might have, is the one that is *most appropriate* for this particular client *at this particular point* in his or her intervention. Since we frequently alter activities during a treatment session, we must have a clear idea of what we hope to achieve through a particular activity in order to be able to alter it appropriately. As much as possible, we will attempt to point out some of the multiple uses for the activities we discuss.

We begin by discussing activities that can be used to provide the client with opportunities to take in enhanced sensory information. Then we discuss the treatment of a number of manifestations of sensory integrative dysfunction. These include (a) sensory modulation disorders, (b) sensory discrimination disorders, (c) postural-ocular movement disorders, and (d) practic disorders.

Before we present those activities, however, we want to discuss a related and important point. That is, that direct intervention is only one of the ways in which we can deliver occupational therapy based on the principles of sensory integration theory. Consultation with "significant others" (typically parents, teachers, and other professionals) in the client's life also is a very powerful approach to intervention. In consultation, we offer sensory integration theory as a "frame" through which the consultees are helped to view the client's behaviors in a new way. Based on their new understanding of the client's behavior, consultees work together with us to develop new, more effective strategies for interacting with the client. This approach to intervention is discussed in more detail in Chapter 11.

## Designing Activities that Offer Opportunities for Enhanced Sensory Intake

Our abilities to create effective intervention based on the principles of sensory integration theory depend heavily on our working knowledge of the vestibular-proprioceptive and tactile systems. Thus, we begin our discussion of creating activities to meet specific goals with a brief review of critical aspects of the opportunities for enhanced vestibular-proprioceptive and tactile intake that influence our selection of activities. (Vestibular-proprioceptive and tactile processing deficits are reviewed in greater detail in Chapters 4 and 5, respectively.) Then, we apply this information to the creation of activities for the treatment of selected disorders of sensory modulation and sensory discrimination.

All of our comments should be prefaced by a word of caution. No matter what type of opportunities for enhanced sensory intake we incorporate in the activities we create, we must be vigilant observers of our clients' behaviors in response to that intake. We must have clear goals in mind and select forms of sensory intake (using theory as our guide) that will help our clients to attain those goals. Much is known about what we can expect from various types of sensory intake; therefore, we can approach the creation of treatment activities in a logical fashion, based on accepted principles of sensory integration theory. However, much also is *unknown* about the use of intervention that incorporates opportunities for enhanced sensory intake. Further, we know that clients' responses to sensory input are individually determined. Thus, the "accepted principles" can serve only as guidelines. They can never replace the knowledge we gain by watching our clients carefully and by talking with them regularly.

## ENHANCED VESTIBULAR-PROPRIOCEPTIVE INTAKE

When creating activities to provide a client with controlled opportunities to take in enhanced vestibular-proprioceptive information, we remember that the vestibular system *is* a proprioceptor. That is, it provides us with valuable information about the positions and movements of our heads in space. Therefore, anytime we create activities involving movement, we are creating opportunities for our clients to take in vestibular-proprioceptive information.

However, when we create activities designed to provide clients with controlled opportunities to take in vestibular-proprioceptive information, we must also remember that there are many different kinds of vestibular-proprioceptive receptors. Each receptor is particularly sensitive to a different kind of information. Although we cannot isolate these receptors, there are times in treatment when we want to *emphasize* the provision of stimulation to one or more of them in particular.

There are three aspects to vestibular-proprioceptive intake, which we commonly incorporate into activities for the treatment of sensory integrative dysfunction, that are particularly important to consider. These are: (a) type of movement (i.e., linear vs. angular), (b) speed of movement (i.e., slow vs. fast), and (c) the presence of resistance to active movement.

Slow and linear movements (and also steady-state information), related to head position and the force of gravity, are detected by the otolith organs of the vestibular system. Fast and angular movements are detected by the semicircular canals. Resistance to movement is detected by receptors in the muscles. However, another critical source of proprioception is corollary discharge (see Chapter 4). Thus, the opportunity to take in enhanced sensory information should always involve *active* movement by the client.

Because different receptors are particularly sensitive to different kinds of sensory information, activities can be designed to emphasize stimulation to specific receptors. This enables us to choose activities that will facilitate the specific behavioral response desired. For example, swinging *very slowly* back and forth while prone in the net will stimulate primarily the otolith organs and facilitate tonic postural responses, while spinning rapidly in the net will stimulate primarily the semicircular canals and facilitate phasic postural responses (see Fig. 4–2).

Most treatment activities provide multiple sources of sensory information. For example, pulling on an elastic cord to enable oneself to swing rapidly back and forth in the net, provides stimulation to the semicircular canals, the otolith organs, *and* the muscle receptors. While many activities stimulate more than one type of vestibular-proprioceptive receptor, it is clear that a client propelling him- or herself back and forth in the net by means of an elastic cord is having a very different kind of sensory experience than the client who is spinning in the net. We also expect that their behavioral responses to the two activities will be very different.

## PROVIDING OPPORTUNITIES FOR ENHANCED TACTILE INTAKE

As with vestibular-proprioceptive stimulation, there are certain characteristics of tactile stimulation that we should consider when creating activities to provide clients with controlled opportunities to take in enhanced tactile information. Of particular importance is whether the tactile input offered is light touch, deep touch-pressure, or discriminative touch. For many clients, light touch seems to be translated as noxious and may be overarousing, whereas firm pressure generally is thought to be calming and to have an organizing effect for the client (see Chapter 5). Discriminative touch is associated with haptic perception and somatopraxis (see Chapter 6). Again, however, clients' responses are very individualized.

## Addressing Sensory Modulation Disorders

When an individual overresponds, underresponds, or fluctuates in response to sensory input in a manner disproportional to that input, we say that the individual has a sensory modulation disorder. Disorders of sensory modulation occur in both the vestibular-proprioceptive and tactile systems. In this section, we will discuss the treatment of four common types of sensory modulation disorders: (a) tactile defensiveness, (b) gravitational insecurity, (c) aversive responses to movement, and (d) poor sensory registration.

### TREATING TACTILE DEFENSIVENESS

Tactile defensiveness, as the name suggests, is a disorder of processing tactile input, particularly light or unexpected touch. Individuals who are tactually defensive often describe the desire for a "fight or flight" response to forms of touch that non-tactually defensive individuals would readily tolerate, or even find pleasurable. In our experience, individuals who are tactually defensive also commonly are defensive to auditory or other forms of sensory information. Thus, as we discussed in Chapter 5, the more general term, sensory defensiveness, is commonly used to describe the collection of symptoms seen in these individuals

In this section, we will concentrate on intervention for tactile defensiveness as this is the form of sensory defensiveness that has been described most clearly in the literature (Ayres, 1972, 1979; Fisher & Dunn, 1983). However, we also will provide some suggestions for addressing the broader problem of sensory defensiveness.

**Treatment Activities (and Materials).** We believe that activities that provide controlled opportunities for the client to simultaneously take in enhanced vestibular-proprioceptive and tactile information may provide the best foundation for reducing the client's tactile defensiveness. These opportunities are provided, at least in part, by covering swings and other equipment in the treatment area with various textured materials (e.g., carpeting, corduroy, sheepskin). When the individual lies on, sits on, or firmly hugs the equipment, during an activity, he or she receives deep touch-pressure. Carefully designed activities that inherently provide both tactile and vestibular-proprioceptive sensory information are recommended, based on the belief that tactile (and sensory) defensiveness may be the result of overarousal in the central nervous system, and that modulation of the client's level of arousal may be accomplished by a combination of calming influences.

Throughout treatment, we observe the client's behaviors in response to various types of sensory information in order to find the best combination of sensory experiences for reducing tactile and sensory defensiveness. In addition to the various types of tactile and vestibular-proprioceptive experiences that can be built into an activity, we can experiment with the modulation of our speaking voices, the level of lighting, and adjustments to any other sensory information that seem to influence the client.

Whereas, in general, clients who are tactually defensive seem to respond best to slow linear movements, deep touch-pressure, and subdued voices and lighting, some clients may find other kinds of intake to be more calming. In the treatment of tactile (and sensory) defensiveness, as in the treatment of all types of sensory integrative dysfunction, the responses of the client are our best guide.

Sometimes, we elect to concentrate on activities that provide opportunities to take in *primarily* enhanced tactile information with a client who is tactually defensive. We may make this decision for a number of reasons, including that the client seems to crave kinds of tactile information not readily incorporated into more complex activities, or that the client's tactile (or sensory) defensiveness does not seem to have been reduced (or seems to be increased) by certain activities that apparently provide too much stimulation.

We have found a variety of treatment materials helpful when developing activities that provide opportunities for the client to take in enhanced tactile information, with the goal of decreasing tactile defensiveness. These include wide paint brushes for brushing the skin, textured mitts for scrubbing the skin (Fig. 10–6), powder, shaving cream and lotion for rubbing onto the skin, large containers of plastic bubble balls in which clients can move around, boxes filled with dried beans or rice in which objects can be hidden, large pillows and mats that clients can bury themselves underneath, large therapy balls that the therapist can roll firmly over the client's back and legs (Fig. 10–7), and vibrators that clients can use on their arms and legs.

**General Guidelines for Providing Tactile Experiences.** As with all forms of sensory intake, some general guidelines can assist us when designing activities that include opportunities for clients to take in enhanced tactile information. However, as with all guidelines, there are exceptions; we also will discuss some of these.

First, we usually find that tactile activities are most beneficial when the client,

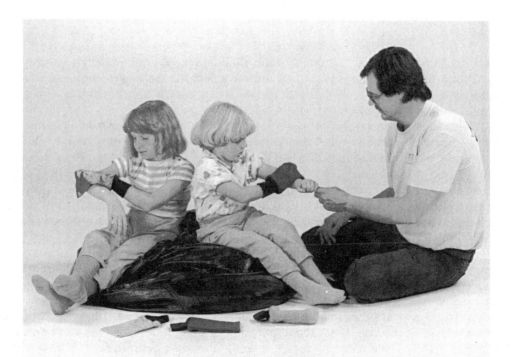

FIGURE 10–6. Textured mitts.

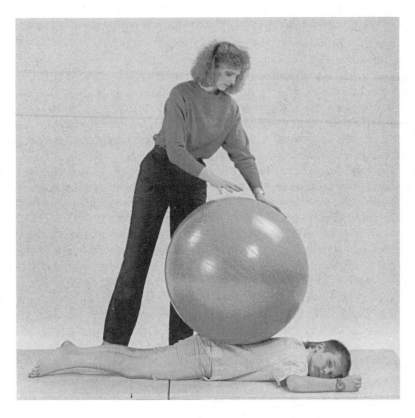

FIGURE 10–7. Large therapy ball.

rather than the therapist, administers the stimulation. When the client administers the stimulation, he or she is in control and can select the areas of the body on which to apply it, the type of intake desired, the relative pressure with which it is administered, and the length of time it will be applied.

Second, while deep touch-pressure usually is the type of enhanced tactile intake most commonly recommended for decreasing tactile defensiveness, some clients may prefer light, rapid stimulation; we interpret this as indicating that their thresholds for tactile intake are exceedingly low (Ayres, 1972). Ayres hypothesized that some clients actually may perceive light touch as deep touch-pressure. Because some individuals seem to crave light touch, it is important to experiment with different types of tactile experiences to determine what is more readily effective for the treatment of each client.

Third, we have noticed that clients usually find deep touch-pressure (and other forms of enhanced tactile intake) to be most acceptable when applied to their arms and legs rather than to their faces or other body areas. Although defensive reactions may occur in response to light touch to any area of the body, it usually is not necessary to provide enhanced tactile stimulation to all parts of the body during treatment. We have found that the application of deep touch-pressure to the arms and legs usually is sufficient to decrease tactile defensiveness. Ayres (1972) postulated that deep touch-pressure has a central inhibitory effect. Therefore, although the treatment is applied to specific body areas, it may have a more general effect.

Fourth, clients also seem to find tactile stimulation to be more tolerable if it is applied in the direction of hair growth. Moving against the hairs often seems to be more arousing than calming.

Fifth, our clients sometimes find that a quiet, enclosed area (e.g., an empty appliance box lined with pillows) is the most beneficial place for the administration of enhanced tactile stimulation, such as with a paint brush, textured mitt, or vibrator. We believe enclosed spaces often are preferred by our clients because other forms of sensory information, particularly threats of unexpected touch, are minimized.

Finally, the desired outcome of activities in which enhanced tactile stimulation is provided is that a client's tactile (and sensory) defensiveness is reduced. This should enable the client to concentrate better and to behave in a more organized, and less tactually defensive, fashion. If such is not the outcome of these activities, clearly they should be discontinued. Negative effects of enhanced sensory intake may not appear immediately following an activity; in fact, those effects may be delayed for several hours (Fisher & Bundy, 1989). *We must communicate regularly with our clients and their caregivers to be certain that our treatment actually is having the desired effect.*

**Special Notes on Vibration.** We have found vibration from a battery-operated or electric body massager to be a particular favorite for some clients who have tactile defensiveness. All of the guidelines specified above for the use of enhanced tactile intake also apply to this discussion of vibration. However, because it is requested so often, it warrants a little further discussion.

Vibration is considered to be a form of both touch-pressure and artificial proprioception. It is a very potent stimulus and should be used *cautiously.*

Sometimes clients want to put the vibrator in their mouths or on their ears. Since these areas of the body are so sensitive, we interpret this as a desire for unusually powerful stimulation. Most clients who seek this form of stimulation will administer it to themselves for a short time and then put the vibrator down in favor of some other activity; we interpret this as a signal that the client has had enough and *never* encourage him or her to continue with this activity. However, some clients seem to be (a) unaware of when they have taken in enough information, or (b) unable to provide us with reliable cues that they have had enough. We believe that *unless clients reliably demonstrate that they are aware of the amount and type of sensory intake they can safely tolerate, using the vibrator on the face should be avoided.*

**Special Notes on Treatment Directed at the Mouth and Face.** When a client's mouth or entire face is particularly hypersensitive to touch, we have found that deep touch-pressure, administered carefully to these areas, can be beneficial. There are a number of ways to provide stimulation to the mouth of a client who has extreme sensitivity there. For infants and young children, we may provide deep pressure to the roof of the mouth or gums with our fingers or other soft rounded object, such as the Nuk tooth brush. Older children and adults can be taught to provide deep touch-pressure to the insides of their own mouths. We have found that clients seem to enjoy a variety of types of whistles for this purpose (Fig. 10–8). As clients hold the whistles in their mouths, they provide themselves with deep touch-pressure. Some clients like to bite on knotted rubber tubing as a means of providing deep touch-pressure to their mouths. Another favorite activity is to blow into a rubber strip that is stretched across the mouth, thus creating "raspberries." This activity provides vibration to the lips and face.

**Imposing Tactile Stimulation.** In general, we recommend that enhanced tactile stimulation be administered by the client. However, sometimes it may be beneficial

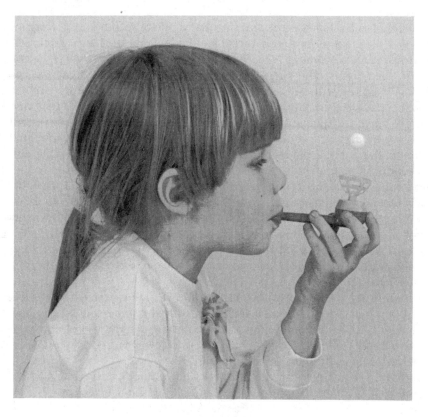

FIGURE 10–8. Whistle.

or necessary for us to administer the stimulation in an attempt to "break through" the client's defensiveness. This decision usually is made when working with particular clients who seem to benefit from frequently scheduled administrations of tactile stimulation. We emphasize that, although *imposed* deep touch-pressure has been reported anecdotally to be beneficial (see, for example, the case of Lydia in Chapter 5), it should be prescribed and used cautiously. No research has yet been undertaken to examine the effectiveness of this procedure with tactually defensive individuals.

Wilbarger (1988) has described a systematic technique for providing deep touch-pressure to clients. She has recommended using a surgical scrub brush to rub quickly on the client's arms and legs (Fig. 10–9), followed by applying joint compression to the ankles, knees, hips, wrists, elbows, shoulders, toes, and fingers. Wilbarger does not allow the client to withdraw from the tactile stimulation, but she instructs clients who are verbal to tell her how hard or soft she should scrub. The entire procedure takes approximately 2 minutes.

Wilbarger (1988) has claimed that this procedure is effective for decreasing tactile defensiveness when it is used six or more times per day for a period of several days (up to 2 weeks). After this period of intensive input, she recommends that clients do "maintenance treatment."

Although highly successful with some clients we know, this technique may elicit aggressiveness, severe withdrawal, crying, or other adverse responses in other

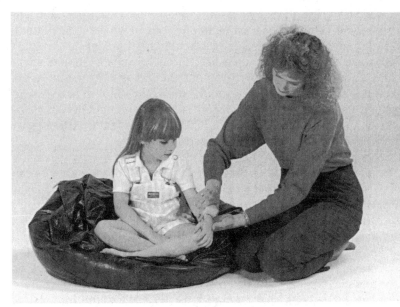

FIGURE 10–9. Surgical scrub brush.

clients. As with all procedures, imposed scrubbing should be discontinued if the effects are negative.

## TREATING GRAVITATIONAL INSECURITY

Gravitational insecurity is described as a "primal fear" response to changes in head position or disturbances to the base of support (May, 1988). In our experience, gravitational insecurity is one of the most devastating types of sensory integrative dysfunction. Gravity is a pervasive phenomenon. When a client is terrified of moving against gravity, as happens whenever he or she changes position, the client can become easily "paralyzed" by the demands of daily life.

Gravitational insecurity is thought to result from a disorder of modulating input to the otolithic organs of the vestibular system (Fisher & Bundy, 1989). In Chapter 4, we speculated that gravitational insecurity may be associated with poor development of a body scheme and an inability to resolve sensory conflict. Thus, our treatment of gravitational insecurity centers on activities that provide opportunities for our clients to take in controlled linear vestibular and proprioceptive information. The client's active participation in treatment activities is important for the development of body scheme; when the activity also provides resistance to the client's movements (as happens, for example, when propelling a swing), the resulting proprioceptive intake is heightened.

**General Guidelines.** It is especially important that we *control* the amount of vestibular-proprioceptive information taken in by our clients. Clients who are afraid of moving, of having their heads out of the upright position, often perceive very small movements to be much larger than they actually are. Further, although *we* may think that a swing is moving in a straight line, clients who are gravitationally insecure may perceive even an almost imperceptible arc as "going around in circles." We need to be aware that our client's perceptions are *real*, and to alter treatment activities so that they do not elicit the fear response we are trying to eliminate.

Clients who are gravitationally insecure need a lot of support and encouragement from therapists. They must trust us implicitly and we must earn that trust. We have found two strategies that have been particularly helpful for developing the trust of clients who are gravitationally insecure. First, the client should always be in control of the amount and type of movement that occurs during an activity. This means that, at least initially, activities should allow the client to keep his or her feet near the ground so as to be able to stop the activity immediately if he or she so desires. Usually, that is most easily accomplished if the client is sitting on a swing or lying prone over a frog swing or a suspended inner tube.

After clients have worked through some of their fear of being other than upright, we usually begin to create activities that they can do while prone. Clients can control the amount of movement provided when they are prone in a swing if they are given handles or elastic ropes by which to propel themselves (Fig. 10–10) or if they are very close to the mat. Some clients feel most "secure" when using the therapist's outstretched hands to swing themselves.

Second, in our experience, clients who are gravitationally insecure seem especially to fear movements into backward space. We believe that they are especially fearful when they move backward because they cannot see where they are going. Of course, all swings move backward *half* the time. We have found that stacking cardboard blocks (or other lightweight objects that are easily knocked over) behind the swing, at a distance that the client approves, often helps the client to overcome some of the initial fear of moving backward. Perhaps having prior knowledge of an end

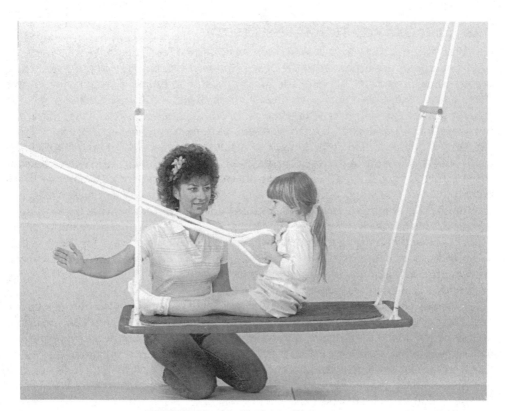

FIGURE 10–10. Platform glider swing.

point for the backward movement helps to resolve some of the sensory conflict that the client seems to experience. The distance can be increased gradually as he or she becomes less fearful. This gives both the client and the therapist a measure of improvement and often enables intervention to progress at a more rapid rate.

**Suggested Activities.** We have used successfully a number of activities in the treatment of gravitational insecurity with both children and adults. For example, young children, while sitting or lying, may benefit from swinging and bouncing in a frog swing. This swing allows the child to stop the movement quickly and easily by placing his or her feet on the mat below. Other activities that may be beneficial include swinging back and forth, either prone or seated on a platform glider swing, or prone in a dual swing; walking up and down an incline (such as a ramp); riding prone on a scooter board in a linear direction; and bouncing up and down on a mini-trampoline or bounce pad (Fig. 10–11).

When riding on a platform or bolster swing, it is preferable to have the swing

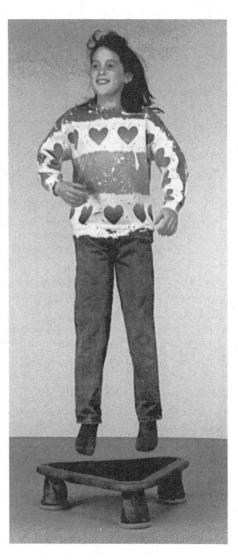

FIGURE 10–11. Bounce pad.

suspended from two suspension points to allow for smooth linear movement and to minimize rotational movements, which often are fear-inducing. When seated, it also is important that the client be able to put his or her feet on the floor easily in order to control the movement of the swing.

In our experience, most gravitationally insecure clients initially prefer pieces of equipment that provide maximum stability and support. However, we occasionally have seen clients who prefer riding equipment like the dual swing, which provides little support to the trunk and limbs, but gives pressure to the shoulder and hip joints when the client is prone. This activity seems to be most enjoyable when the straps of the swing are made from rubber inner tubes.

Beth, a 7-year-old first grader, initially responded to many kinds of movement by making her body rigid and complaining that she was afraid. She avoided swings, slides, and climbers on playgrounds and refused to participate in physical education. After watching Beth, we felt that her responses were caused by gravitational insecurity. As we created activities to use in Beth's treatment, we incorporated linear vestibular input and activities that provided resistance to her movements. We gradually introduced these activities, creating increasingly greater challenges for Beth.

Initially, Beth was willing only to ride in a seated position on the platform glider swing, or to bounce and swing back and forth in the frog swing. The glider swing offered a firm base of support, and the frog swing allowed her to place her feet on the floor easily and quickly in order to control the movement. The course of her treatment was very gradual; it was crucial that Beth feel safe. She also needed to develop a trusting relationship with us before she could begin to be challenged by activities requiring more movement.

As Beth became more willing to try new challenges, her therapist rode with her on a plastic mat down a ramp. Over the course of several sessions, Beth became more confident with this activity, until she finally was able to slide down alone. Eventually, we were able to introduce riding down the ramp on a scooter board. Beth performed this activity cautiously at first; gradually, she began to ride down the ramp freely. She began to express her enjoyment of the scooter.

Beth progressed to being able to ride on equipment that moved less predictably. She liked lying prone on the bolster swing while being swung side to side. Later, she began to release her hold on the bolster swing and land on a "crash pad" underneath (Fig. 10-12). As her gravitational insecurity diminished, she began to seek more movement experiences outside of the clinic, on playground equipment and in gym class. She began to enjoy gross motor play with other children. In addition, her parents reported that they had a better sense of her "true personality" now that she felt more secure with movement. They reported that Beth seemed to be more outgoing and increasingly self-confident.

## TREATING AVERSIVE RESPONSES TO VESTIBULAR INPUT

Another vestibular-proprioceptive modulation problem is intolerance (aversive responses) to vestibular input. Aversive responses to movement are hypothesized to be due to lack of modulation of input to the semicircular canals (Fisher & Bundy, 1989). In Chapter 4, we speculated that aversive responses may be related to an impairment of the ability to use vestibular-proprioceptive information to resolve sensory conflicts. Aversive responses are manifested as vertigo (sensation of self-movement), nausea, or vomiting in response to movements that normal individuals readily tolerate. Aversive responses also may be accompanied by sweating and pallor, and avoidance of movement activities (particularly those involving angular

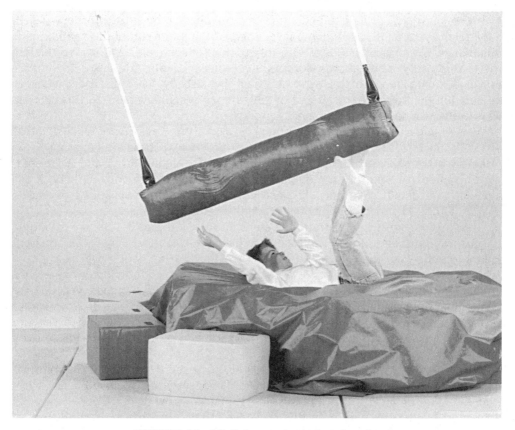

FIGURE 10-12. Bolster swing and crash pad.

movement). An increase in arousal and restlessness following movement also *may suggest* the presence of aversive responses to movement.

We have found that activities that provide enhanced *linear* vestibular information and resistance to the client's active movements are helpful when treating aversive responses. Thus, the activities described above for the treatment of gravitational insecurity also can be used for the treatment of aversive reactions to vestibular stimuli.

The goal of intervention is to help the client to be able to tolerate common movement experiences, such as riding in a car or on a swing, without feeling sick or dizzy. We have found that individuals who show persistent signs of aversive responses to movement, which prevent them from participating in daily life activities and impede their progress in treatment, sometimes respond positively to a non-sensory integrative treatment technique known as vestibular habituation training. Vestibular habituation training is a prescribed and carefully monitored program of desensitization to movement (Fisher & Bundy, 1989).

## Treating Diminished Sensory Registration

Sensory registration is a term that has not been described clearly in sensory integration theory. In Chapter 5, we proposed that sensory modulation disorders occur along a continuum of sensory registration. At one end of the continuum is overresponsiveness or heightened awareness, manifested by such disorders as sensory defensiveness or gravitational insecurity. At the other end of the continuum is diminished responsiveness or failure to register sensory information. We refer to these as sensory modulation disorders since many clients' responses to sensory intake fluctuate between the two extremes. We already have discussed sensory modulation disorders characterized by heightened responsiveness. In this section, we will discuss diminished sensory registration.

Based in part on the work of Pribram (1975), we think of sensory registration as an "umbrella term" that involves at least three processes. These are (1) arousal, (2) orienting to the sensory stimulus (and evaluating it for significance), and (3) preparing for action (or ignoring the stimulus and returning to previous activity, if the stimulus is deemed irrelevant). The action that often follows sensory registration may be either an adaptive behavior or a fight-or-flight response.

Diminished sensory registration is manifest by significant delays in responding to sensory information (as in the case of Rebecca in Chapter 12) or in an apparent failure to notice sensory information at all (as with Rick in Chapter 5). Disorders of sensory registration often are most noticeable when affected individuals experience an incident that most people would find to be painful or very noxious; yet they are either delayed in responding to the stimulus or fail to respond to it at all. However, as with all sensory modulation disorders, we believe that difficulties with sensory registration also occur in relation to movement and to other forms of sensory information (e.g., visual/auditory).

Penny, a 7-year-old girl, demonstrated very poor registration of tactile information and pain. Her mother reported that Penny recently had received a black eye from being hit by a brick that she was attempting to throw over a fence. Penny did not report feeling any pain from this blow; we interpreted this as an indication of extremely poor sensory registration. During Penny's first treatment session, she fell against the wall as she moved to pick up a ball. Her skin reddened and the therapist applied ice to prevent bruising; however, at no time did Penny appear to feel any pain. She also did not seem to be aware of the cold ice on her skin.

Clients who have poor sensory registration often are severely impaired in their ability to carry out daily life tasks and roles. Many of these clients are individuals who have mental retardation, autism, or other pervasive developmental disorders; however, we also have treated individuals whose sensory registration difficulties seem to be the result of severe sensory integrative dysfunction.

When a client has a decreased ability to register sensory information, he or she, understandably, also may lack the inner drive to be involved in some sensorimotor activities. Clients may fail to register one type of input, but overreact to (fail to modulate) another type of sensation. As with all types of sensory integrative dysfunction, clients who have deficits in sensory registration may vary in their responses depending on their mood, the time of day, and other environmental factors. Indeed, for clients whose deficits in sensory registration are associated with sensory integrative dysfunction, such fluctuations are common. Thus, the behavior of these clients can be very difficult to interpret; it often is necessary to evaluate these clients over several sessions, and chart their behaviors, in order to identify any consistencies that are related to time of day or environmental factors. It also is important to gather information, from those who know the client well, about the frequency and consistency of her or his reactions to sensory intake.

Ayres and Tickle (1980) devised an informal assessment tool for evaluating clients' responses to sensory input. This assessment enables the therapist to rate the client's responses to a variety of sensory experiences, on a 4-point scale ranging from Failure To Register to Hyperresponsivity To Input. It provides a systematic method of collecting information on a client's behavior when more formal assessment cannot be completed (as often is the case with more severely involved clients).

In treating the client who has diminished sensory registration, we use many of the same activities that we described above for the treatment of other sensory modulation problems. We emphasize activities that provide opportunities for the client to take in linear vestibular-proprioceptive and tactile information. Jumping up and down on the trampoline and brushing body parts with a wide paint brush have formed the basis for many successful activities with our clients.

Clients who fail to register sensory information can be particularly difficult to treat. It frequently is difficult to assist them to orient to, and focus their attention on, objects, people, or activities. They often ignore, or appear to automatically reject objects and activities in their environments. However, once they *do* become involved in an activity, they may tend to perseverate. If this behavior occurs during an activity that provides strong sensory experiences, such as orbiting in a dual swing, it can be difficult for the therapist to determine whether the client craves and is benefiting from taking in the sensory information or is perseverating.

We watch carefully for signs of sensory overload throughout treatment because the reactions of a client with diminished sensory registration sometimes vary from moment to moment. A client who seems slow to arouse, may become aroused to what appears to be an optimal state. However, after several moments, the client may begin to show pupil dilation, sweating, increased body movement, or other signs of over-arousal. We experiment with the type and amount of available sensory information, and carefully observe the client's responses in order to determine the best direction for treatment.

## Treating Disorders of Sensory Discrimination

Clients who have sensory integrative dysfunction have a poor ability to discriminate touch, movement, force, or information about the position of their bodies in space. Typically, these individuals have a meaningful cluster of indicators of diminished vestibular-proprioceptive processing (see Chapter 4) or depressed scores on a constellation of tests of tactile discrimination (see Chapter 5). In older clients, other evidence that they have diminished discriminative ability may be provided by such complaints as "I can't tell a penny from a dime in my pocket without looking." We even have had some adult clients tell us that they have learned to discriminate "up" from "down" only by knowing that "up" is where their heads are (see the case of Chris in Chapter 4).

When clients have decreased abilities to discriminate touch, movement, or body position, we interpret these signs as poor *central processing* of sensory information (rather than as failure to modulate the information as in tactile defensiveness, gravitational insecurity, aversive responses to movement, and diminished sensory registration). Unlike sensory modulation disorders, in which the symptoms often fluctuate from day-to-day or even hour-to-hour, disorders of sensory discrimination remain relatively stable over time (without intervention). These disorders of decreased sensory discrimination are thought to underlie a number of other sensory integrative disorders, including bilateral integration and sequencing deficits and somatodyspraxia (see Chapters 4 and 6).

In our experience, many individuals who have decreased ability to discriminate sensory information seem to crave that type of sensory experience. We will illustrate and discuss intervention for this apparently paradoxical condition when it occurs in relation to angular vestibular stimulation. As we do so, we remain cognizant that *craving and need are not synonymous*. Recall the beginning of Chapter 4, when we advised not to be too quick to assume that craving is a sign that the craved stimuli will be therapeutic. Further, not all clients who have decreased ability to discriminate sensory information crave the types of stimulation that they do not process effectively.

## DECREASED DISCRIMINATION OF VESTIBULAR-PROPRIOCEPTIVE INFORMATION

Because the different vestibular-proprioceptive receptors are sensitive to different kinds of input, it is not surprising that disorders of the ability to discriminate vestibular-proprioceptive information manifest themselves in different ways. Clients who have difficulty discriminating information received by the otoliths have trouble automatically determining the spatial orientation of their heads (e.g., upright from upside down). Clients who have difficulty discriminating information received by the muscle receptors have trouble determining the relative position or movements of their body, or body parts, in space; they often have difficulty judging the amount of force or effort they are exerting. Moreover, they often are described as having a poor body scheme. Clients who have difficulty discriminating information received by the semicircular canals may have trouble distinguishing small, rapid movements (we speculate that this disorder frequently may be misinterpreted by therapists as poor equilibrium, since clients who are unable to discriminate small or rapid movements also would fail to respond effectively to those movements). Disorders of discrimination related to the semicircular canals also *may* be associated with diminished postrotary nystagmus.

When treating clients who have a decreased ability to discriminate the movements or positions of their bodies, we create activities that provide opportunities to take in enhanced vestibular-proprioceptive information. As with all interventions based on the principles of sensory integration theory, the *active participation* of the client in *meaningful tasks* is important. We will discuss separately interventions for each of the manifestations of decreased ability to discriminate vestibular-proprioceptive information. However, it is important to realize that they rarely occur in isolation.

**Disorders Related to the Otolith Organs.** For clients whose difficulty with discriminating vestibular-proprioceptive information manifests itself as a decreased ability to distinguish head orientation in space, we emphasize activities designed to provide the client with opportunities to take in linear vestibular stimulation. The activities used to treat this disorder are similar to those described for the treatment of gravitational insecurity and aversive responses to movement. However, since the client is not apt to fear movement or to have an aversive reaction to it (unless, as sometimes happens, the client has more than one type of vestibular-proprioceptive disorder), we usually are able to incorporate more movement and larger excursions.

We design activities that can be done in a variety of body positions (e.g., prone, sitting, quadruped, standing). We emphasize the use of suspended equipment. It is easiest to provide linear movement on swings when the swings are suspended from two points. A trampoline or bounce pad and scooter boards also provide the basis for activities that provide opportunities for the client to take in enhanced linear vestibular stimulation.

Although it is relatively rare for individuals to be unable to distinguish automatically between head-upright and upside-down positions, we have seen such individuals. We also believe that difficulty discriminating spatial orientation of the head occurs in more subtle forms. When this disorder is present in our clients, it is one of the first areas we address in treatment, because we believe that the ability to automatically determine one's spatial orientation provides an important foundation for many aspects of development.

**Disorders Related to the Muscle Receptors.** For clients whose difficulty with discriminating vestibular-proprioceptive information manifests itself as a decreased ability to distinguish the relative position or movement of the body or body parts, or judging the appropriate amount of muscle force to exert, we emphasize activities designed to provide resistance to *active movement.* Very commonly, this is done in the context of activities such as those described in the section above, since resistance to body movements is provided automatically (by gravity or the weight of the client's body) when the client propels a swing or scooter board independently, and as he or she lands on the surface of the trampoline. As was discussed in Chapter 4, it is the resistance to extension, rather than joint compression, that provides the most critical source of proprioception when jumping on a trampoline. Active movement against enhanced resistance, whether the client is squirting a squirt gun or jumping on a trampoline, provides clients with the added proprioceptive feedback needed to learn to calibrate the appropriate amount of force or judge the extent of their efforts.

**Disorders Related to the Semicircular Canals.** For clients whose difficulty with discriminating vestibular-proprioceptive information manifests itself as a decreased ability to distinguish rapid or small movements (or in depressed postrotary nystagmus), we emphasize activities designed to provide the client with opportunities to take in rapid or angular (rotary) movements. However, we do this with caution (see Chapter 4 and the section on Precautions, below). Further, we believe that increasing the duration of postrotary nystagmus should *never* be a stated objective of intervention. If duration of nystagmus "normalizes," so be it; but depressed postrotary nystagmus, in and of itself, never interfered with anyone's ability to carry out his or her life roles and tasks!

It is easiest to provide opportunities for the client to take in angular vestibular-proprioceptive input when swings are hung from a single suspension point. We have successfully used a variety of swings in this way, including the net swing, dual swing, T-swing, bolster swing, platform swing, frog swing, and others that are commercially available (see the Appendix 10–A for a list of vendors). Swings suspended from two points also can be used successfully to provide input to the semicircular canals when the client is involved in activities that incorporate *relatively* fast swinging.

Because it is during periods of acceleration and deceleration that the hair cells of the semicircular canals are stimulated, activities should include frequent starts and stops, changes in direction, and changes in speed. Activities that require clients to bat at suspended objects or pick up beanbags or balls from the mat as they swing by, also inherently require them to vary their head position. In turn, the stimuli to the vestibular mechanism are varied without the need to stop the swing or change the direction of the movement. Activities of this type also challenge clients' bilateral skills and abilities to perform projected movement sequences.

**The Paradox: Client Can't Discriminate, but Craves Input.** We often are confronted in the clinic with clients who have little or no response to spinning (e.g., diminished duration of postrotary nystagmus, absence of dizziness) and yet crave vestibular-proprioceptive (particularly fast or rotary) input. Often this is a child whose mother says, "He never gets tired of swinging. The other kids have left the playground long ago and he just wants to stay and swing." When a client like this is in the clinic, the child often expresses preference for spinning or for "swings that go hard and fast." What often gets interpreted as craving, in fact, *may* just reflect an absence of the normal response that would ordinarily limit the individual's tolerance.

As the client's sensory integration improves, and he or she is better able to discriminate sensory input that is derived from movement, the client usually shows less craving for the input. However, as this change begins to occur, the client may not readily interpret the body's signs that he or she has had enough stimulation and should stop doing the activity. We have known some clients who express displeasure when they begin to get dizzy as a result of spinning. They had seen their "increased tolerance" as a strength, and now need reassurance that it is normal to get dizzy after spinning.

**Some Precautions.** While we recognize the client's desire to take in a considerable amount of sensory input, we also are somewhat cautious about his or her doing so, since rapid rotary stimulation is extremely powerful. Further, negative reactions to this powerful stimulation sometimes do not become apparent for several hours after the treatment session has ended (Fisher & Bundy, 1989). After being involved in a number of activities that provide opportunities to take in enhanced vestibular-proprioceptive information during a treatment session, a client may later feel nauseated or complain that his or her body feels "funny" (see Chapter 4 for a discussion of sensory disorganization) even though he or she enjoyed the session immensely and had no signs of a negative reaction during, or immediately following, treatment. We remain cognizant that an inability to discriminate certain types of sensory input may include an inability to interpret the body's signs that the individual has had enough stimulation. Again, we emphasize the need to communicate regularly with the client and with the client's caregivers; in this way we can become aware of any negative effects from treatment.

If signs of sensory overload (pupil dilation, sweaty palms, changes in the rate of respiration, flushing or pallor) or sensory disorganization (distortions of body scheme) *are* observed or reported, we alter the amount and type of sensory information a client receives during his or her treatment. We do this by emphasizing activities that incorporate slow, and primarily linear, movement and that provide considerable resistance to the client's movements. Many clients who have described sensory disorganization as a sequela to treatment have indicated that deep touch-pressure helps to lessen some of the symptoms (see Chapter 4).

## TREATING DECREASED DISCRIMINATION OF TACTILE INFORMATION

As with stimulation to the vestibular-proprioceptive systems, some individuals with sensory integrative dysfunction seem to have a decreased ability to discriminate information processed by the tactile system. Ayres (1972) described this as an apparent problem with processing the spatial and temporal aspects of information gained through touch. Thus, these individuals seem to have difficulty knowing both where they have been touched and about the properties of an object they have touched. Often these individuals constantly touch and manipulate objects in their environments, seemingly unaware that they are doing this.

This problem is rarely, if ever, encountered in isolation. Usually, we discover through interview or from a client's scores on tactile testing that he or she has decreased ability to discriminate tactile input. However, most often, that individual was already being evaluated—for suspected somatodyspraxia. Therefore, the treat-

ment of tactile discrimination deficits usually is done *in conjunction with the treatment of deficits in motor planning that seem to have their basis in the tactile system.*

In treatment of tactile discrimination deficits, we have found that activities that provide deep touch-pressure often are beneficial. Although tactile discrimination deficits are thought to underlie somatodyspraxia, and thus have an affect on the client's ability to use the entire body, they seem to have considerable influence on hand skill and the ability to manipulate objects. Hence, we create activities that provide touch-pressure to the total body, but we pay particular attention to the hands.

As we described in the section on the treatment of tactile defensiveness, the therapist may provide opportunities for the client to brush the skin, rub the skin with various textures, use the vibrator, or hide body parts underneath the balls in a bubble ball bath, under heavy cushions, or in a mixture of rice and dried beans. As the client seems increasingly able to process tactile information, we begin to challenge the client's tactile discriminative abilities by having him or her search for objects in mixtures of dried macaroni, beans, corn, lentils, or rice. Finally, shape recognition games can be played in which the client is challenged to identify objects of different shapes without looking.

Nathan, a 6-year-old who had significant difficulty with tactile discrimination, constantly manipulated objects and ran his hand along the wall as he walked down the hall in school. Nathan also had poor hand skill development and other problems associated with somatodyspraxia. Initially in treatment, he showed great pleasure when he played in the bean mixture. He shoved his hands deep into the mixture and poured it over his arms. We placed 3-inch-long plastic animals into the mixture for him to find. Although he also was allowed to look, he often had difficulty locating the objects. When he finally "graduated" to finding the animals without looking, he was at first unable to describe the animal in his hand, despite his more than adequate verbal skills.

After several months of intervention, Nathan was better able to discriminate the animals and other similarly sized shapes. Eventually, he was able to find small objects, such as pennies and monopoly pieces, in a box of dried rice, peas, and popcorn. This required finer tactile discriminations and improved ability to manipulate the objects in his hands, and we interpreted his developing abilities as improvements in both. Also, Nathan's teacher reported that Nathan no longer inappropriately touched and manipulated objects within his reach.

## SIMULTANEOUS DISORDERS OF SENSORY MODULATION AND DISCRIMINATION

In some cases, a client may have both a decreased ability to discriminate some types of sensory input and a disorder of modulating other types of input. For example, Marianne, a 4-year-old girl, was very gravitationally insecure when she began treatment. During her initial evaluation, she refused the Postrotary Nystagmus Test. After 6 months of intervention, in which we emphasized activities involving controlled opportunities for her to take in enhanced proprioceptive and linear vestibular input, her gravitational insecurity seemed greatly diminished. She readily climbed onto equipment 4 or 5 feet off the ground and jumped off onto mats below (Fig. 10–13). She enjoyed performing somersaults and other activities requiring change of head position and angular stimulation. In fact, she also began to express a craving for angular input; she spun herself happily on the Sit 'N' Spin at home and on the swings in the clinic. When she was able to tolerate the Postrotary Nystagmus

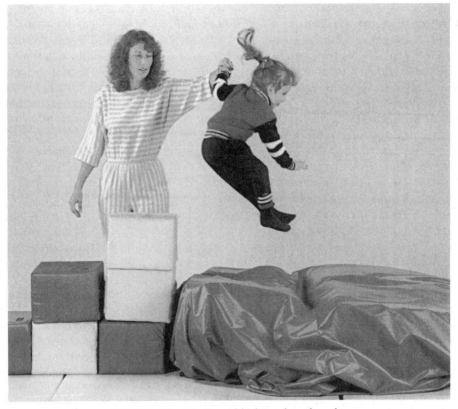

FIGURE 10-13. Foam blocks and crash pad.

Test, she had a *decreased* duration of nystagmus. Presumably, Marianne's decreased discrimination of vestibular-proprioceptive information (seen in her decreased postrotary nystagmus) had been "masked" by her sensory modulation problems (gravitational insecurity, aversive responses to movement) during her initial evaluation. As these problems diminished, her difficulties with discrimination became more apparent.

## AN IMPORTANT ASIDE

Our immediate reaction to clients who seem to have both decreased discriminative ability and a craving for certain types of sensory input may be to provide them with many opportunities to take in the enhanced sensory stimulation they seem to need and want. However, this paradox is not necessarily easily interpreted.

Some clients who fit the description of having both decreased discrimination of, and increased craving for, sensory information also exhibit frequent bursts of boisterous or uncontrolled behavior (which we may, in some cases, interpret as signs of overarousal). These individuals may need to engage *both* in activities that provide opportunities to take in enhanced sensory stimulation *and* in activities that are calming, in an intervention session. Otherwise, they could become so overaroused in treatment that their behavior actually deteriorates.

Even the above interpretation of a client's behavior, as complex as it is, may be too simplistic. Some clients who manifest decreased sensory discrimination, in-

creased craving, *and* frequent bursts of boisterous behavior actually become more active when we involve them in "calming" activities. It is as though those clients are running around to keep themselves awake. When we further decrease their levels of arousal, they must compensate by becoming more and more active. For these clients, opportunities to take in enhanced sensory information may serve the dual purpose of increasing their levels of arousal (and thereby diminishing the need for increased activity) and providing them with needed and wanted sensory input.

Kagan, Reznick, Snidman, and Garcia-Coll (1984) have observed a similar incongruity in their research with "inhibited" children that may have implications for our intervention. They found evidence suggesting that inhibited children may have lower thresholds for arousal than do uninhibited children. We should be aware that some of the quiet, shy, and apparently withdrawn children that we treat may become easily overaroused. We should be particularly alert to signs of sensory overload in these children.

## Treating Postural-Ocular Movement Disorders

In order to act effectively on objects in the environment, we must be able to assume and maintain stable positions and to move out of those positions without losing our balance. That is, we must have adequate postural control to support our movements.

Sensory integrative dysfunction often is manifest as a postural-ocular movement disorder (e.g., hypotonia of extensor muscles, poor postural stability, poor righting or equilibrium reactions, difficulty assuming and maintaining prone extension) or in poor tonic flexion (associated with somatodyspraxia). Because of their difficulties in assuming, maintaining, and regaining postures, clients often have difficulties acting effectively and efficiently on the objects in their environments. For example, one adult client we treated described that, each time she dropped her pencil at work, she had to get out of her chair, turn around, bend down, pick up the pencil, and then reverse the procedure to return to her chair. She lacked the postural control simply to lean down and retrieve her pencil while remaining seated.

When a client demonstrates both poor processing of vestibular-proprioceptive input and postural-ocular deficits, we hypothesize that poor sensory processing is interfering with the development of posture. Similarly, when a client demonstrates both poor flexor tone and a decreased ability to process somatosensory information, we hypothesize that poor sensory processing is interfering with the development of both flexion and praxis. In either case, we emphasize activities that provide controlled opportunities for the client to take in enhanced sensory information and that simultaneously challenge posture. We will discuss intervention to develop six aspects of postural-ocular control that we commonly address in treatment. These include: (1) tonic postural extension, (2) tonic flexion, (3) postural stability (balancing flexion and extension), (4) lateral flexion and rotation, (5) righting and equilibrium reactions, and (6) ocular control.

### DEVELOPING TONIC POSTURAL EXTENSION

In developing a client's ability to maintain extension against gravity, we emphasize activities that provide opportunities for the client to take in enhanced linear vestibular and proprioceptive information. These activities can incorporate movement in either the horizontal plane (such as swinging on a platform glider swing) or the vertical plane (such as jumping on a trampoline). Further, they can be done in any body position, although the prone position demands the greatest amount of extension. To enhance proprioceptive processing, we create activities that involve movement against resistance (including the resistance of gravity); we carefully grade the amount of resistance so that the client is able to perform the activity successfully.

For a client who is very hypotonic, we may need to begin our intervention with activities that provide challenges primarily to neck and upper back extensors (such as is required while swinging prone over a frog swing) without demanding total extension of the body (as would be required while riding prone in the dual swing). Similarly, we may create activities for the client to do in the prone-on-elbows position, which requires some upper body stability. One example of such an activity is to have the client assume a prone-on-elbows position on the platform glider swing and blow cotton balls off raised mats placed in front of the glider as it swings to and fro. We watch carefully to be sure that the client maintains a good body position in which the extensor muscles are active. That is, we ensure that (a) the head is not hyperextended, (b) the upper chest is raised off the surface, and (c) the upper arms are perpendicular to the surface.

Activities that require weight shifting while in the prone-on-elbows position, such as throwing at a target while riding prone on the platform glider swing, are slightly harder. Activities that require weight bearing on extended arms, such as lying prone on a barrel and "walking" it forward with the hands or placing objects on a magnetic board (Fig. 10–14), or that demand assumption of the prone extension posture, such as riding prone in a net while catching and throwing a beach ball at a target, provide an even greater challenge.

Finally, activities that require the client to extend fully against gravity and demand that the client support his or her own body weight (for example, lying in the dual swing while "climbing" hand-over-hand up a rope suspended from a corner of the room, and then letting go and swinging) provide the greatest kinds of challenges to a client's tonic postural extensor muscles. Another example of an activity that demands considerable extension against gravity is "net basketball." In this activity, the therapist (or another client) is prone in one net and the client is prone in another net; the two nets are suspended at least 6 feet apart. Each player attempts to throw beanbags onto the back of the other player. This activity also provides deep touch-

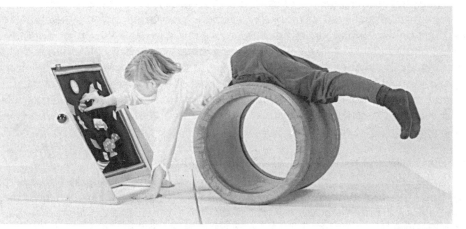

FIGURE 10–14. Barrel and magnetic board.

pressure from the weight of the beanbags and challenges the client's abilities to plan and perform projected action sequences with his or her arms.

## DEVELOPING TONIC FLEXION

Whereas difficulties with postural extension and neck flexion have been associated with the vestibular-proprioceptive systems, difficulties with tonic postural flexion, in general, seem to be related to the somatosensory system and to praxis (see Chapter 6). Thus, it is not unusual for clients to have relatively better postural extension than flexion, or vice versa.

When treating clients who have difficulties with tonic flexion, we create activities that provide resistance to movements into flexion and that require sustained postural flexion. As with extension, we carefully grade the amount of resistance and the amount of flexion required.

It is often possible to create activities that simultaneously incorporate opportunities to take in enhanced vestibular-proprioceptive information and require the client to flex his or her neck against gravity. In the course of those activities, "chaining responses" (Peiper, 1963) may assist the client to bring the rest of his or her body into positions of antigravity flexion. Similarly, activities that initially require flexion only of the legs and lower trunk sometimes seem to facilitate flexion of the neck. One activity of this type requires that the client lay on his or her back either on the platform glider swing or on the floor; if needed, a small wedge is placed under the clients' head. The therapist throws a large lightweight ball to the client who flexes his or her knees and hips and kicks it back to the therapist. Initially, the client's head may be fully supported. However, as the activity continues, the client usually begins to lift his or her head spontaneously in order to see the ball better.

For clients who have very hypotonic flexor muscles (especially neck and abdominal muscles), it may be necessary to begin treatment with activities that require modified flexion postures (head and upper trunk) rather than the assumption and maintenance of a full antigravity position. In one such activity, the client lies on a wedge and flexes the neck and head to blow bubbles from a wand held in position by the therapist. The therapist can facilitate the client's moving into flexion by placing his or her hand on the client's upper chest and exerting gentle pressure in a caudal direction.

We also have found that swings suspended from a vertical stimulation device (several lengths of bungy cord) are particularly useful for facilitating flexion. Riding on a disc swing (Fig. 10–15), which provides a stable base of support while simultaneously requiring flexion of the limbs around a central post, may initially challenge a client who has very hypotonic flexor muscles. Gradually, as the client develops sufficient flexion to be able to withstand greater resistance to flexion, swings such as the T-swing may be incorporated into direct intervention. Because the T-swing has a smaller base of support than the disc swing, it provides a greater challenge to maintaining tonic flexion. Activities such as sitting and swinging in a dual swing (which provides only minimal support) and kicking (with both feet) a ball that is suspended at an appropriate height in front of the client provide the next level of challenge to flexion.

As the client's flexion improves, activities such as holding on to the hotdog (Fig. 10–16), lying on top of a bolster swing while the therapist moves the swing rapidly back and forth, or going for a "rough ride" while straddling and hugging a large suspended inner tube offer even greater challenges to flexion. While activities such as the hotdog require fairly constant force from the flexors, both the bolster and

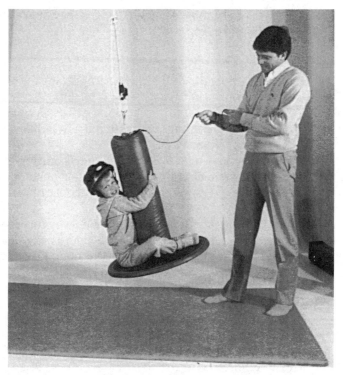

FIGURE 10-15. Disc swing.

large inner tube can be used in such a way as to require subtle adjustments to flexion. Some of the most popular activities on the bolster and inner tube require that the individual adjust his or her hold enough to slide around to the side of, and then underneath, the piece of equipment as it moves (Fig. 10-17).

The greatest challenges to postural flexion are provided in activities that require the client to maintain flexion against both resistance and the full force of gravity. Activities of this type include having the client lie in the supine flexion position on a scooter board and pull him- or herself the length of a room, using hand-over-hand motions on a rope suspended from both walls, approximately 2 feet above the floor. Activities on the trapeze that require the client to *maintain* a flexed position while swinging over obstacles also provide a very significant challenge to flexion.

Ayres (1977) found that once clients have developed adequate flexion, they often exhibit strong preferences for activities that include falling, such as releasing one's grasp while hanging underneath the bolster swing and falling onto crash pads below. In activities where falling is involved, the client uses flexion to pull him- or herself into a protected position while falling. Ayres believed that there was considerable affect and enthusiasm associated with the achievement of reliable flexion against gravity.

Jeanne, an 11-year-old who was totally unable to assume the supine flexion position when she began therapy, wanted to invite her parents and teachers to watch her when she mastered hanging on underneath the bolster swing. Although she had mastered many challenges during the course of her 2 years of therapy, apparently none of them was as salient to her as her mastery of postural flexion.

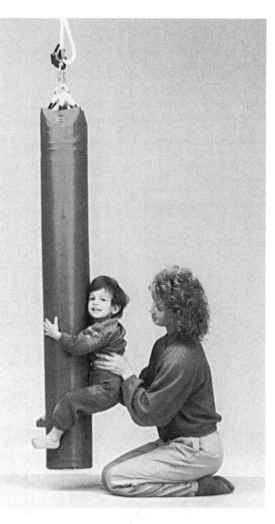

FIGURE 10–16. Hotdog.

## COMBINING FLEXION AND EXTENSION: DEVELOPING LATERAL FLEXION AND ROTATION

As antigravity flexion and extension develop, lateral flexion and rotation also emerge (Bly, 1983). Rotation, in particular, allows the client to move in ways that are efficient and that look smooth and fluid. Clients who have postural-ocular movement disorders frequently move with little rotation. Thus, creating activities that encourage the development of rotation can assist many of our clients to move more effectively and efficiently.

Unlike the development of postural flexion and extension, which are facilitated by engaging the client in activities that require symmetrical movements, the development of lateral flexion and rotation require movement into asymmetrical patterns. Perhaps the simplest means of encouraging rotation is by involving the client in an activity that includes rolling in an inflatable barrel (Fig. 10–18) across a mat. Many children enjoy "steam rolling" letters or shapes created from Theraplast or Silly Putty. Lateral flexion and rotation also can be elicited by having a client who is seated on a dual swing (Fig. 10–19) or in a net reach, as he or she swings by, for balls or beanbags on the mat, and then sit up and throw them at a target.

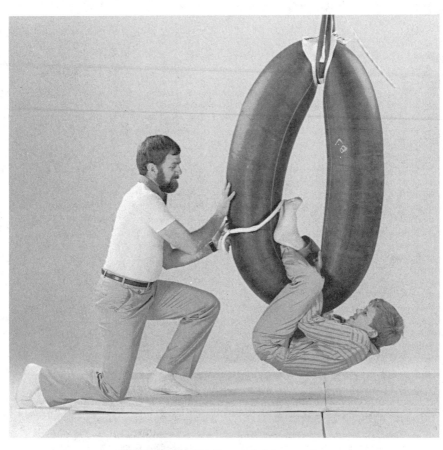

FIGURE 10–17. Suspended inner tube.

Another activity that we have found to be successful for encouraging rotation involves having a client swing on a trapeze from one landing pad to another, each time turning around to swing back while continuing to hold onto the trapeze with both hands. A variation on this idea involves suspending two ropes from the ceiling, in the middle of the room, approximately 6 feet apart. The client, who is seated on a scooter board in line with and facing the ropes, pulls on one rope to propel him- or herself toward the second rope. Reaching the second rope, the client lets go of the first rope and grabs the second. He or she continues to roll as far forward as possible and then uses the second rope to turn him- or herself and the scooter board around. If the client has rolled far enough, he or she can now pull on the second rope to propel him- or herself back to the starting position. If the client is able to maintain contact with both hands on the rope as he or she turns, rotation will happen during the turning.

## BALANCING FLEXION AND EXTENSION: DEVELOPING ALTERNATING MOVEMENTS

As flexion and extension develop, it is both possible and desirable to provide activities that require postural movements that alternate between flexion and extension. Having a client involved in an activity in which he or she is seated on a swing,

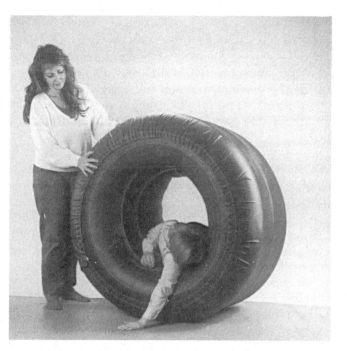

FIGURE 10–18. Inflatable barrel.

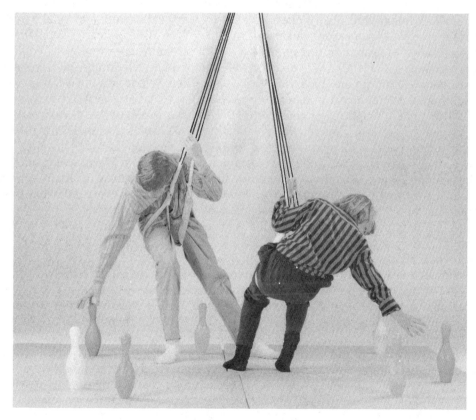

FIGURE 10–19. Dual swing.

propelling it by pumping, encourages a balance of postural flexion and extension. However, it is possible for the client to move a swing merely by pushing or pulling on the ropes, relying predominantly on one muscle group of the arms. It is important with all treatment activities that we carefully observe the type of postural patterns the client is using to accomplish the specified task. In this case, we are interested in having the client propel the swing by moving his or her arms, legs, trunk, *and* head into alternating patterns of flexion and extension. If that is not the response we observe, we may want to adapt the activity.

## DEVELOPING RIGHTING AND EQUILIBRIUM REACTIONS

Righting reactions provide the background for our movements between body positions. They also become a part of equilibrium reactions, where they enable us to maintain the head in an upright position and the body in line with the head. That is, righting reactions enable us to assume or regain a body position; equilibrium reactions enable us to maintain a body position when it has been threatened by perturbations to the body or the support surface (Bly, 1983; Weisz, 1938).

Clients with sensory integrative dysfunction who have postural-ocular movement disorders almost always have impaired equilibrium; this is the most complex of the postural responses and one of the first to be compromised by central nervous system dysfunction. Clients who have impaired equilibrium may or may not have subtle deficits in righting, as righting commonly develops before equilibrium. When deficits in righting *are* present, they may become a primary focus of our early intervention since they are fundamental to both movement and posture.

Sensory integration theory offers us little by way of description of what a good righting or equilibrium response should look like. Thus, we commonly supplement our knowledge of sensory integration theory with our knowledge of normal equilibrium reactions (cf., Fisher, 1989; Weisz, 1938) and of neurodevelopmental treatment (cf., Bobath, 1985; Boehme, 1988; Howison, 1988) when we address the development of righting and equilibrium reactions.

When a client's righting or equilibrium reactions are delayed, we develop activities to elicit those reactions in whatever positions are necessary, including prone, sitting, quadruped, kneeling, or standing. Initially, we develop activities in which we incorporate relatively small and slow movements on a platform glider swing, bolster swing, or tilt board. *Small* movements ensure that the client can adapt to the movement without falling, whereas *slow* movements allow the client sufficient time to react to the stimulus. Gradually, faster movements can be introduced.

In our daily lives, most of the equilibrium responses we use are very subtle and occur in response to relatively small perturbations. Thus, we should try to create treatment activities that require subtle adaptations to posture. This can be accomplished using virtually any piece of equipment we have in the clinic. However, since the responses we are seeking are subtle responses, it is not necessary (or even desirable) that we always elicit a full-blown equilibrium reaction in response to movement. Our goal is to create activities that challenge our clients' equilibrium, but that the clients can accomplish using automatic, fluid responses.

Bill, a 5-year-old, had significant delays in the development of righting and equilibrium reactions. He was first able to show signs of maintained righting of his head and upper body in prone when riding back and forth on a platform glider swing while pretending he was riding a boat. As his postural reactions improved, we pretended that whales (therapy balls) were coming to swim beneath his boat, hoping

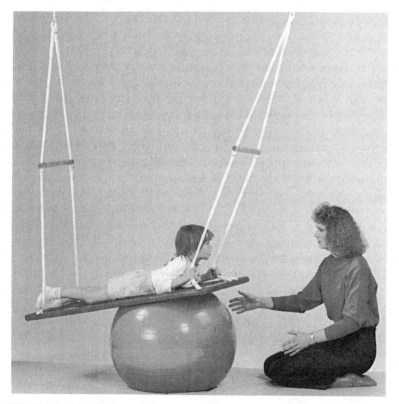

FIGURE 10–20. Platform glider swing "boat" and large therapy ball "whale."

to bump him into the water so that they could play with him (Fig. 10–20). As Bill moved back and forth, we initially pushed a small therapy ball underneath the swing, which caused it to tilt as it swung back and forth. Bill yelled with delight that he wasn't going in for a swim; he pumped the swing and automatically maintained an upright position on the swing. Occasionally, we had the bigger whales (larger therapy balls) swim under his boat, causing him to be tilted enough to elicit a full-blown equilibrium reaction. Periodically, he lost his balance and fell into the water, enjoying a playful and calming moment with the whales as we rolled the therapy balls over his back and legs. This activity provided Bill with an opportunity to take in enhanced vestibular-proprioceptive information and facilitated tonic extension, righting, and equilibrium reactions. In addition, the activity provided opportunities for him to take in deep touch-pressure to address his tactile defensiveness.

## A NOTE ON DEVELOPING CONTROL OF OCULAR MOVEMENTS

We have used the term "postural-ocular movement disorders" to refer to a constellation of signs frequently present in clients who have disorders of processing of vestibular-proprioceptive information. In this context, ocular refers to *compensatory* eye movements (specifically, to compensatory eye movements as measured by the Postrotary Nystagmus Test [Ayres, 1975]) that are initiated by the vestibular system in an attempt to maintain a stable visual field (see Chapter 4). We have differentiated between compensatory eye movements and eye movements used for tracking moving objects (smooth pursuits) or looking around the room (saccades) that are *under the control of the visual system.*

Sensory integration theory offers us very little in terms of understanding, assessing, or treating visually controlled eye movements. However, we have noted that our clients who have sensory integrative dysfunction often have difficulty with dissociating movements of their eyes from movements of their heads and the rest of their bodies. That is, they move their heads, and sometimes their bodies, in response to visual stimuli, rather than moving only their eyes. When "forced" to keep their heads still and move only their eyes, as is the case when we cursorily examine such functions as eye tracking (smooth pursuits), convergence, and quick localization (saccades), they frequently have difficulty producing these visually controlled ocular movements.

Visually controlled ocular movements are outside the realm of sensory integration theory. Some ophthalmologists and optometrists specialize in this area (referral of some clients to these professionals may be warranted). However, within our interventions, we often develop activities that, in addition to their primary purposes, provide challenges to the client's abilities to produce visually controlled ocular movements (such as tracking and quick localization) and to separate head and eye movements. Having the client throw beanbags at stationary or moving targets (such as plastic bottles disguised as "alien space ships"), while swinging, is an example of such an activity.

## Treating Practic Disorders

Ayres (1985) identified three processes that are a part of praxis: (a) ideation, or the ability to conceptualize an action; (b) planning and programming actions; and (c) executing the action. Clients with sensory integrative dysfunction have difficulty primarily with planning and programming movements. Thus, their movements appear to be awkward or poorly executed; however, their difficulties with motor execution are thought to be secondary to their problems with motor planning. More severely involved clients also may have impaired ideation; that is, they may have difficulty knowing what to do with objects in their environments.

In this section, we will emphasize the intervention for three types of problems commonly encountered in clients who have practic disorders associated with sensory integrative dysfunction. These disorders of planning and producing adaptive behaviors include (a) activities that require the coordinated use of two sides of the body (*bilateral integration*) and of the arms and legs, (b) *feedforward-dependent projected action sequences,* and (c) *feedback-dependent movements.* We also will address briefly intervention with clients who have disorders of ideation.

Disorders of bilateral integration and of planning and producing projected action sequences are typical of clients who have vestibular-proprioceptive processing deficits (see Chapter 4) while difficulties with planning and producing feedback-dependent movements have been associated with somatosensory processing (Ayres, 1989). Thus, clients who have somatodyspraxia, because they often have deficits in processing information from both systems, may manifest all three practic disorders simultaneously (see Chapter 6).

When we intervene with a client who has developmental dyspraxia using intervention procedures based on sensory integration theory, we develop activities that provide opportunities for the client to take in enhanced sensory information and to respond adaptively to practic challenges. More specifically, for the client who has deficits in bilateral integration and in the planning and production of projected limb movements, enhanced sensory information usually is vestibular-proprioceptive in nature. For the client who has a disorder in planning and producing feedback-dependent movements, enhanced sensory information should be polymodal.

To simplify the discussion, we will examine separately intervention for deficits in bilateral integration, projected action sequences, and feedback-dependent actions. However, these deficits rarely occur in isolation.

## DEVELOPING COORDINATED USE OF TWO SIDES OF THE BODY

There is scant research describing the development of coordinated limb usage that we can use as a guide for our planning intervention. As Williams (1983) and Keogh and Sugden (1985) have suggested, the ability to use a lead hand and an assistive hand together effectively (functional asymmetry) when acting on objects in the environment (in any spatial orientation with respect to the body) is the culmination of the development of bilateral motor coordination. Clearly, the newborn infant, who is unable even to bring his or her hands reliably and consistently to midline, must develop considerable ability and skill before we can expect him or her to draw, cut with scissors, or open a jar.

Further, in addition to bilateral integration, many tasks that require the use of two sides of the body in a well-coordinated fashion also require the ability to plan and produce projected action sequences (e.g., catching a ball). That is, the individual must anticipate future events in the environment and adjust his or her actions to meet those future conditions (see Chapter 4). In this section, however, we will confine our discussion to certain considerations for intervention related to the bilateral aspects of movement. While we will emphasize the motor demands to the limbs, it is important to realize that bilateral coordination refers to the use of *two sides of the body*, including the trunk.

When we test clients using the Bilateral Motor Coordination test of the SIPT (Ayres, 1989), we test only the ability of the client to produce sequences of alternating arm or foot movements. Developmentally, these represent relatively difficult bilateral movements (Keogh & Sugden, 1985). Thus, while we may learn that a client has difficulty with bilateral motor coordination, we have little knowledge of where on the developmental continuum the client first experiences difficulty. We know that he or she is unable to perform difficult bilateral tasks, but we do not know which of the easier tasks he or she is able to perform. Therefore, we need additional information before we can proceed with precise plans for intervention.

We often must begin intervention with tasks that represent developmentally earlier bilateral skills. In the course of intervention, we must observe the client's relative abilities and grade the bilateral demands of tasks so that they reflect these abilities. We create these activities based on our knowledge of the individual's development of bilateral skill.

This knowledge is drawn from the work of researchers (cf., Keogh & Sugden, 1985; Williams, 1983) who have described motor skill development in young children. Because these authors have provided us with important information regarding the development of certain aspects of bilateral coordination which we can use when creating and adapting activities used in direct intervention, we summarize their findings here. However, there remain significant gaps in knowledge about the development of bilateral motor coordination. For example, little is known about the ages by which the various aspects of bilateral performance usually are mastered.

**Discrete versus Sequenced Bilateral Movements.** Children seem to develop control of discrete bilateral movements before they develop the ability to produce sequences of bilateral movements. Short sequences of bilateral movements clearly are easier to produce than long sequences.

**Symmetrical versus Alternating Bilateral Movements.** Sequences of movements performed symmetrically are easier than sequences of alternating movements. However, clients do not *master* symmetrical movements before they begin to develop skill at performing alternating movements. Building on this knowledge, we propose that the activities shown in Table 10–1 form two hierarchical sequences from easiest to hardest. The first sequence refers to the development of bilateral symmetrical movements, the second to the development of bilateral alternating movements.

**An Aside on the Coordinated Bilateral Use of Arms and Legs.** Coordinated movements of both arms develop before coordinated movements of both legs (Williams, 1983). Thus, from a purely bilateral perspective, having a client kick a large ball suspended from the ceiling as he or she swings in the net might be harder than pushing that same ball away with both arms.

While, in general, coordinated bilateral upper extremity movements are easier than bilateral lower extremity movements, certain aspects, even of simultaneous

TABLE 10–1. TWO PROPOSED HIERARCHIES OF DIFFICULTY OF
BILATERAL ACTIVITIES

| Task Requirements | Activity Examples |
|---|---|
| **Bilateral Symmetrical** | |
| a. Hold on, move passively forward and backward with swing. | Client prone on glider; therapist pushes glider to and fro while client looks for pretend obstacles up ahead; client's arms move passively into flexion and extension as the ropes move. |
| b. Hold on, actively move equipment forward and backward using ropes that suspend the swing. | Client prone on glider; client actively moves glider to and fro by alternately flexing and extending arms. |
| c. Hold on, actively propel self forward and backward using a stable object. | Client prone in net; therapist holds stick or hula hoop between outstretched hands; client places hands between therapist's on stick and actively flexes arms to pull self closer to stick, then lets go and swings. |
| d. Hold on, actively propel self forward and backward using an unstable object. | Client prone in net. Two ropes with handles are suspended from wall opposite client (6 ft away); client holds handles and pulls rhythmically on them to propel self to and fro. |
| **Bilateral Alternating** | |
| a. Hold on, move passively with equipment side-to-side. | Client seated on platform swing; therapist pushes swing side-to-side while client looks for pretend obstacles on either side; client's arms move passively into alternating flexion and extension as the ropes move. |
| b. Hold on, actively propel self using ropes that suspend the swing. | Client seated sideways on glider, holding on to glider ropes; client actively propels self side-to-side by alternately flexing first one arm, then the other. |
| c. Hold on, actively propel self side-to-side using an unstable object. | Client seated in large inner tube suspended from ceiling; two handles are suspended freely by ropes from ceiling on either side of the tube. Client grasps handles and pulls self side-to-side. |

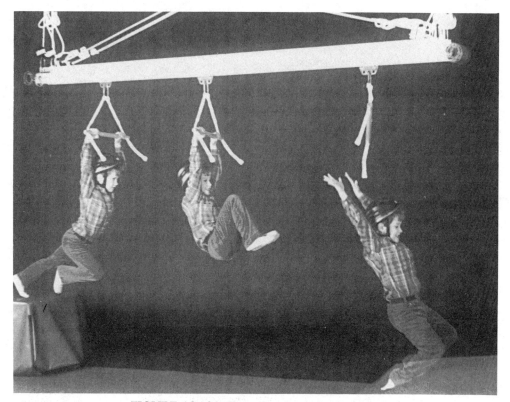

FIGURE 10–21. Trapeze with overhead trolley.

bilateral upper extremity movements, are considered to be relatively difficult. One such aspect is *bilateral symmetrical release* (Keogh & Sugden, 1985). Thus, creating an activity in which the client lets go of a trapeze with both hands simultaneously (Fig. 10–21) might be particularly difficult. Similarly, the bilateral demands of letting go with both arms and legs simultaneously when "falling" from the underneath of the bolster swing onto a crash pad also seem to be very great. Clearly, coordinated, *simultaneous use of all four limbs* is more difficult than using either arms or legs separately (Williams, 1983).

Little has been written about development of the ability to simultaneously flex the arms and extend the legs, or vice versa, as one might do while swinging from a trapeze to jump through an inner tube suspended from the ceiling (Fig. 10–22). In our experience, this is a particularly difficult aspect of coordinated limb usage. It may be even more difficult to swing holding onto the trapeze and *maintain* flexion of the arms and hands while simultaneously extending the legs and feet to kick a suspended ball.

**Inhibition of Movement.** In one or more extremities, inhibition of movement seems to develop relatively later than do many other aspects of coordinated limb usage. In fact, associated movements (i.e., movements of body parts not involved in the activity, such as the tongue or the opposite hand) are commonly observed in normal adolescents who are involved in difficult activities (Keogh & Sugden, 1985).

**Crossing the Midline.** The ability to cross the midline also seems to be related to coordinated bilateral upper extremity usage in daily activity. Moreover, in our

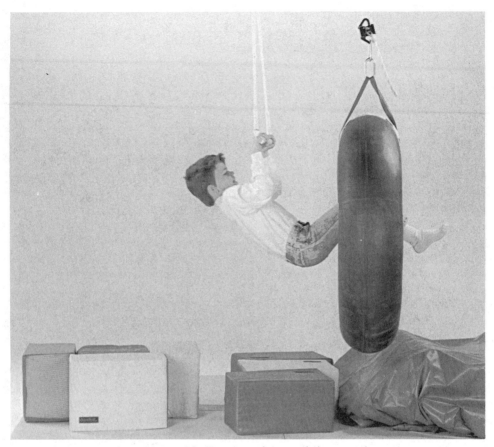

FIGURE 10–22. Trapeze and suspended inner tube.

experience, crossing the body midline seems to occur in conjunction with weight shifting and rotation of the trunk as an individual reaches for an object that is positioned in body space contralateral to the reaching hand. This seems to enable economy of movement, since the individual can pick up the object with the hand that will be used to stabilize it (assistive hand), and begin to act on it immediately with the lead hand. Simultaneous trunk rotation and crossing of the body midline also occur when an individual reaches with two hands for a large object that is slightly out of reach. In addition, combined trunk rotation and midline crossing are a part of mature throwing patterns (Keogh & Sugden, 1985; Williams, 1983).

Clearly, it is not *necessary* to rotate the trunk in order to cross the body midline, especially if the object to be obtained is within easy reach. Stilwell (1981) attempted to correlate body-righting reactions (rotation) with the Space Visualization Contralateral Use Test score (midline crossing) and failed to find a statistically significant relationship. However, we believe that trunk rotation facilitates midline crossing when objects are slightly beyond immediate reach, as they often are in real life. Further, we have observed that individuals who have difficulty crossing the midline often have difficulty rotating (and vice versa). When they attempt to obtain objects beyond their immediate reach, their movements look awkward and inefficient because they move their entire bodies or must transfer an object to the assistive hand before they can act on it with the preferred hand.

In interventions with clients who have difficulty with rotation and crossing the midline, we create a lot of activities that combine these two requirements. For example, activities such as picking up beanbags while swinging seated in the dual swing or net encourage trunk rotation because the client must hold on with one hand and reach toward the mats with the other hand. When the client throws the beanbags at targets located on the side of space contralateral to the throwing arm, crossing the body midline is required. We also commonly use squirt guns in activities designed to elicit rotation and crossing of the midline. When the client propels him- or herself in the swing, it is very likely that the swing will begin to rotate. Thus, if the client is to aim at a specific target while shooting the gun, trunk rotation and midline crossing are easily elicited. We find that squirt guns, however messy, are highly motivating to clients.

When creating activities that require trunk rotation and crossing the body midline, it is important that the activities not be contrived, that is, they should require trunk rotation and crossing the midline naturally, rather than because the therapist instructed the client to perform the task in a particular way. Unless the movement is natural, it is very unlikely that trunk rotation or crossing the body midline will generalize to everyday usage. Of course, some clients, particularly young children, may need to be reminded to use their preferred hands to throw or to shoot the squirt gun. We must be certain, however, that the client realizes that this request should help him or her to perform the activity more successfully, since, presumably, the client will be more accurate with the preferred hand.

## DEVELOPING THE PLANNING AND PRODUCTION OF PROJECTED ACTION SEQUENCES

Virtually every client who has sensory integrative dysfunction has difficulty planning and producing projected movements (see Chapters 4 and 6). That is, the client cannot plan and initiate effective movements in response to events in the environment that are changing or have not yet happened. This practic disorder is seen in the client's difficulties with such activities as catching or kicking a ball, riding a bicycle around obstacles, jumping rope, or walking through a crowded room without bumping into anything, to name just a few. That the disorder is so common is not surprising since, as Keogh and Sugden (1985) indicated, "children first must have sufficient control of their own movements before they can move in relation to external environmental conditions" (p. 101).

Many of the activities that we create during interventions based on the principles of sensory integration theory require that the client plan and produce projected action sequences. For example, the client must anticipate a point of interception between his or her feet and the ball that has just been rolled. The client must begin moving his or her feet toward the point of interception *before* the ball arrives there in order to kick it.

Because they require anticipation of future events, projected movement sequences are more feedforward- than feedback-dependent. Of course, this is a relative statement since feedforward and feedback may be considered to be two ends of a continuum that describe the sensory control of movement. As we have shown in Figure 10–23, the relative contributions of feedback and feedforward control are determined by the extent and speed of movement of both the client and the target.

This information is important to us since feedforward-dependent and feedback-dependent movements are associated with different types of sensory integrative dysfunction. Specifically, clients who have deficits in bilateral integration and se-

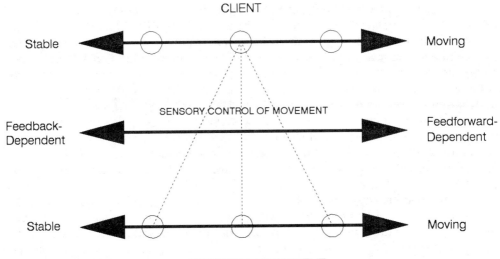

**FIGURE 10-23.** Relationship among client's movement, movement of target, and degree of feedback-, feedforward-dependence of movement. (Adapted from Keogh and Sugden, 1985.)

quencing have difficulty primarily in the planning and production of feedforward-dependent movements, whereas clients with somatodyspraxia generally have difficulty with performing *both* feedback- and feedforward-dependent movements.

Thus, clients who have bilateral integration and sequencing deficits may be able to perform quite well in activities in which both the client and the target are relatively stationary (e.g., throwing a ball at a target on the wall), whereas they may have greater difficulty either when they are moving (e.g., letting go of the trapeze as they swing over a pile of pillows) or when the target is moving (e.g., catching a ball). When both are moving (e.g., running to kick a rolling ball), the challenge is even greater. The degree of difficulty of the activity reflects the combined demands of the extent and speed of movement of both the client and the target.

In addition to issues related to feedforward control, activities performed when the client or the target (or both) are moving have spatial and temporal requirements that also help to determine their relative difficulty. In response to the temporal and spatial demands of the activity, the client must time the initiation of the movement appropriately and adjust its force and direction. Within an activity, however, the source of spatial demands is slightly different from the source of temporal demands. Spatial accuracy is required *whenever the client moves,*

> because the whole body or certain body parts must be moved to a particular spatial location and sometimes along a particular spatial path. The whole body or body parts also must be moved in an appropriate direction and for an appropriate distance, often with an appropriate amount of force and speed. (Keogh & Sugden, 1985, p. 106)

Keogh and Sugden (1985) have indicated that by age 6 most normal children are well on their way toward mastering the general movement problems associated with the spatial accuracy requirements of play-game skills (e.g., batting, throwing). They have listed five such general movement problems that we can observe and address by developing appropriate intervention activities. These include (a) controlling the sequence of limb segment movements while simultaneously controlling posture; (b) moving the limb in a direction and path that will contact the object in the desired position, or reach the desired release point; (c) coordinating the sequence of limb segment movements to finish at the time of contact or release; (d) modulating the force generated in the limb movement and imparted to the object; and (e) navigating in relation to stationary objects or other persons.

Temporal accuracy means "coinciding the self with objects and other people to stay in unison or to intercept or avoid them" (Keogh & Sugden, p. 111). Whereas requirements for spatial accuracy are related to the client's movements, external requirements for temporal accuracy arise *when the target moves or when the client moves rapidly (or both)*. Thus, tasks in which the client moves slowly and the target remains stable (e.g., swinging slowly back and forth while throwing a ball at a stationary target) demand primarily spatial accuracy; tasks in which both the client and the target move demand spatial *and* temporal accuracy.

In Figure 10–24, a number of activities commonly used in treatment are listed according to whether the client and the target are stationary or moving when the activity is performed. As was the case with feedforward and feedback, "stationary" and "moving" represent ends of a continuum. Clients who are moving very slowly or over very small distances are *relatively* stable. Also depicted in Figure 10–24 are the relative spatial and spatial-temporal demands of these activities.

According to sensory integration theory, difficulty with planning and producing projected action sequences is one sequela to a disorder of processing vestibular-proprioceptive input. Thus, we typically create interventions that are designed both to improve a client's ability to plan and produce projected action sequences and to provide opportunities for the client to take in enhanced vestibular-proprioceptive information. If the need arises to adapt an activity, we do so by modifying its spatial and temporal demands.

Recall Melanie, the 5-year-old child we presented earlier in this chapter when discussing decisions about where to begin intervention. Melanie has deficits in processing both vestibular-proprioceptive and tactile information. Among her many sequelae to these processing deficits, she has extraordinary difficulty planning and producing projected action sequences. We represent Melanie now to illustrate how we modify the spatial-temporal demands of an activity to alter the degree of challenge.

Early in her treatment, when Melanie was swinging prone in the frog swing, we asked her to "feed the fish" by throwing "fish food" (beanbags) into the "fish pond" (inner tube). This activity seemed to us to require a relatively simple response. Because the inner tube was stationary, the demands were primarily spatial. The only temporal requirement was that Melanie release the beanbag at the proper time; since the inner tube was quite large, neither the spatial nor the temporal demands were very great. However, Melanie refused.

We quickly modified the activity to require a simpler response; we requested that Melanie use both hands to push a stationary "boulder" (large therapy ball) out of her way as she swung past it. Because the boulder was large and directly in the path of Melanie's swing, this activity made even fewer spatial demands and essentially no temporal demands. However, Melanie also refused this activity, saying "I *just* want to swing!"

At that point, we complied with Melanie's request, interpreting her refusals as a statement that even the simplest projected action sequence presented too great a challenge for her (or that she believed they did). For the rest of that session and

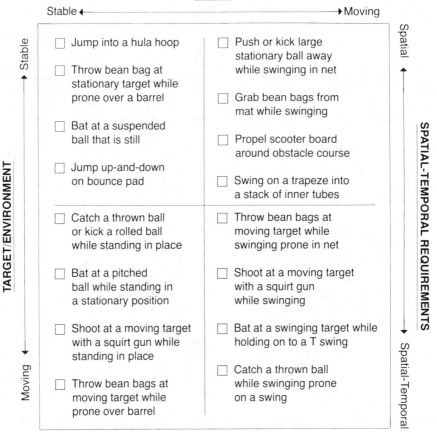

FIGURE 10–24. Common treatment activities, by category, according to their spatial-temporal requirements. (Adapted from Keogh and Sugden, 1985.)

several subsequent sessions, we emphasized, separately, activities that provided opportunities for her to take in enhanced vestibular-proprioceptive information (e.g., just swinging in the frog) and activities that involved limb movements that she did while stationary (e.g., tossing Velcro balls at a large stationary target).

Several sessions later, we reintroduced the "boulder" game. This time, Melanie eagerly pushed the ball. Apparently, it then represented the just right challenge. Either her ability, or her perception of her ability, or both had increased. After several more sessions, Melanie was able to meet the challenge of repeatedly throwing the beanbags into the inner tube, delightedly "feeding the fish."

Because we emphasize the use of suspended equipment in treatment, there are endless possible combinations of activities that can be used to facilitate a client's ability to plan and produce projected action sequences. By making simple modifications to these activities, we easily can alter the spatial-temporal demands of the activities to make them more or less challenging. We can vary the speed and extent of movement of the client or the target or both; we can vary the size of both the objects used and the targets.

One activity that we have found to be highly motivating to young clients is a game we call "bumper cars." To set up the activity, we suspend two large tractor inner tubes vertically from the ceiling, 6 to 8 feet apart. The client and therapist each straddle one of the tubes. They pull the tubes as far apart as the suspension ropes will allow and prepare to "take off" and smash into one another. The object of the game is to "bump" the "opponent" out of his or her tube. Because both the client and the "target" are moving, this game has both temporal and spatial requirements. If the force of the bump is to be hard enough to knock the therapist out of the tube, the client's movements must be timed, sequenced, and directed precisely. Bumper cars can be made more challenging by propelling the tubes with handles, especially if the tubes are high enough off the ground that feet don't touch. This also increases the postural demands of the activity.

We sometimes play a more challenging game of "tag" that is set up similarly to bumper cars. The object of this game, as in conventional tag, is not to be caught. For this game, the therapist and the client each are seated in net swings suspended 6 to 8 feet apart. Between the nets, we place a large tractor inner tube with a large therapy ball inside it. The therapist and the client begin by bracing their feet against the tube. They push off from the tube and whoever is "it" tries to tag his or her opponent. The opponent must time, sequence, and direct his or her movements in order not to get caught. "It," however, must time, sequence, and direct his or her movements to catch the opponent. The tire is a free space, but players can remain there for only 10 seconds at a time.

Tag is both challenging and highly motivating for older clients, but we recommend that it not be played by two clients together, since it is important that at least one of the players be skillful at timing and directing movements so that neither player gets hurt.

A more commonly used intervention activity that also has significant spatial and temporal demands consists of having two clients, both in seated positions, orbit one another in the dual swing. In order to accomplish this, the two clients must begin moving at the same time, in the appropriate direction, and at the same speed. They run for a few steps and then, on cue, simultaneously lift their feet and orbit.

**An Aside on Activities to Promote Sequencing.** When the term "sequencing" is used in sensory integration theory, it refers to *projected action sequences*, such as we have described above. However, we frequently read intervention plans in which the activity most commonly specified for clients who have difficulties with sequencing is an obstacle course. We wish to emphasize that sequencing occurs in nearly every activity of the type we have discussed above. Obstacle courses, because they usually contain several activities, *represent sequences of sequences.* Therefore, they are quite difficult. The best type of obstacle course for addressing difficulties with sequencing requires smooth transitions between several different kinds of projected action sequences. For example, have the client swing by a trapeze bar from a raised surface, jump off through a moving suspended inner tube onto a mat, lean down to pick up beanbags, turn around and throw them through the swinging tube, run back to the raised surface through a maze created with large plastic cones, catch the trapeze, and begin again.

## TREATING CLIENTS WITH SOMATODYSPRAXIA

In addition to the deficits in bilateral integration and in the planning and production of feedforward-dependent projected action sequences, clients with somatodyspraxia also have difficulties with the planning and production of feedback-dependent movements. Thus, while all the activities we have presented for use in the intervention for practic disorders may be used, at some point, in the intervention

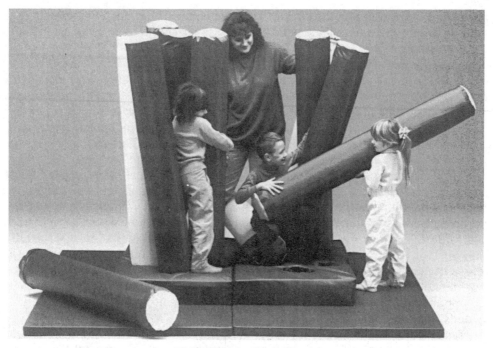

FIGURE 10-25. Forest.

with the client with somatodyspraxia, many of them may initially present too great a challenge. Further, some of the suggestions given below may be incorporated successfully into the intervention with clients with bilateral integration and sequencing difficulties.

We often need to begin our intervention by focusing on activities that require whole-body actions. Activities such as going down a scooter board on a ramp and knocking down a tower of large foam blocks, or lying on top of a bolster swing and hugging it tightly with both arms and legs, or moving through the forest (Fig. 10-25), can be particularly useful.

With some clients with severe dyspraxia we begin with very simple cause-and-effect tasks, such as blowing a whistle or jumping from a raised surface onto a pillow or mat below. Gradually, we increase the complexity of the activities. We might have the client blow a whistle a certain number of times to indicate that he or she is stopping, starting, or changing the speed of his or her movement on a swing. Another example of an activity requiring a simple motor plan is to pretend to be riding a train (a platform glider swing), getting on and off at each stop to retrieve a package (large, heavy beanbags or containers).

We progress in intervention from activities that require (a) simple, discrete movements to those that require more complex movement sequences, (b) whole-body movements to those that require movement of specific body parts and inhibition of others, and (c) relatively more feedback-dependent actions to those that require relatively more feedforward-dependent actions. Since clients with somatodyspraxia frequently have deficits in the processing of both vestibular-proprioceptive and tactile information, we incorporate opportunities for the client to take in enhanced polymodal information in the context of the intervention activities (see Chapter 6). We particularly emphasize having the client perform active movements against resistance to assist them in developing improved body schemes as a foundation for improving the planning of their movements.

We give considerable verbal instruction and feedback and physical cues to clients as they perform intervention activities. In play, children without deficits in praxis commonly use singing and counting to organize themselves. This ability to use verbal mediation to organize behavior may not naturally occur for the child with somatodyspraxia. We sometimes begin activities by saying "one, two, three, go" or by using songs or rhymes to help the child establish and maintain the rhythm of an activity.

We give brief instructions and talk about the quality of the movements clients have performed. In some cases (as with Kerry, whose attempts at performing a flip on the trapeze were described earlier in this chapter), we verbally label the clients' movements for them. We do this because we have become increasingly aware that, at least for these children, much of the learning of new skills happens first "cortically." Only when a skill is mastered does it become automatic. However, we also are cautious not to "talk too much." Sometimes clients pause before initiating a movement as though they were consciously planning it. It is important not to distract the client from this process.

We also have found that it can be helpful to have the client verbalize his or her motor plans; some clients can use their language skills to help organize and understand their actions. At first, the client may be able only to describe a plan that he or she has just completed. Later, the client can be asked to verbalize while executing the plan. Finally, clients may be able to verbalize a plan before they execute it.

Sometimes, however, we find that dyspraxic clients are able to successfully verbalize a plan for moving, but are unable to execute the plan. Jerry, a 7-year-old with somatodyspraxia, described a complicated sequence of movements needed for an obstacle course involving four pieces of suspended equipment. When we asked him to demonstrate the plan, he walked by each piece of equipment and pushed it while verbally describing the actions he would have *liked* to do. He was unable to figure out how to make his body do what his mind had conceptualized. Clients like Jerry, at least initially, may benefit more from *our instructions* and *our physical cues* than from their own verbalizations of a plan.

Because clients who have somatodyspraxia seem to have difficulty learning new motor skills (Ayres, 1972, 1979, 1985; Cermak, 1985), we incorporate novel tasks into our interventions. However, we also must incorporate ample time for practice into our sessions. An activity has not been mastered until the client can perform it automatically and without conscious effort; activities, thus, retain a degree of novelty for a long time. For clients with somatodyspraxia, mastery may require considerable practice.

Novelty also can be produced by slightly altering the way in which a familiar piece of equipment is used. For example, we can suspend a platform glider swing from only one point, rather than two. In so doing, we change the nature of the postural adjustments and movements the client must make when performing even very familiar tasks. Further, it is in the nature of some of the tasks that we use frequently in intervention that they always require new motor responses. For example, because a ball rarely is thrown in precisely the same spot in relation to the body, activities that incorporate catching or kicking remain novel for a long time. The same is true of any task in which either the target or the client is moving.

Clients who have somatodyspraxia usually have difficulty generalizing a motor plan to a different activity, even if that activity is similar to an activity with which they are familiar. When treating these clients, we help them to generalize the skills they are learning. We do this in at least two ways. First, we create activities that require similar, but slightly different, motor behaviors. For example, we may create an activity where the client jumps off a pile of mats into a large inner tube during one session, and then, during another session, have the client jump off the same pile of mats onto a pile of pillows. Or we might vary the first activity by having the child jump from the rungs of a jungle gym into a large inner tube.

Second, we point out the similarities between the requirements of a current activity and those of similar activities, both those that have been previously mastered in the therapeutic setting and those that the client must do in his or her daily life. We point these out so that clients become more aware of activities they can independently perform outside of the treatment area. For example, clients use similar movements when they sit in the net swing and propel it by pumping with their legs and trunk and when they propel a playground swing.

## DEVELOPING IDEATION

Clients who have poor ideation may not be capable of self-directed or self-initiated actions because of their difficulty in knowing what to do with the objects in their environment (Ayres, 1985). Initially in intervention, we select activities and objects that are very responsive to the smallest actions of the client. As Ayres (1985) indicated, "if the child can be only partially successful, the therapist should help the child to be completely successful. If the child leaves a task with a feeling of failure, he or she will probably not want to return to it" (pp. 67–68).

Sometimes typical sensory integrative equipment may be too far removed from the client's experience for him or her to be able to develop an idea about what to do with it. The client may need, initially, to use equipment that is very similar to playground swings or familiar riding toys. For Peter, a 4-year-old client, figuring out how to walk up and down a carpeted incline was an appropriate initial challenge.

Wehman (1977) described an instructional intervention hierarchy that we use when treating clients who have poor ideation. We begin our intervention by providing physical guidance to the client, as needed, when he or she attempts an activity. As soon as we can, we withdraw the physical cues and begin to model activities for the client. When less modelling is needed (and when a client's verbal receptive ability is adequate), we begin to provide specific instructions. We then attempt to fade those instructions into verbal prompting.

As the client begins to gain the ability to formulate ideas about what to do with objects in the environment, he or she may begin to respond more spontaneously in carefully arranged familiar environments (i.e., the clinic, home, or classroom). Only later can we expect the client to respond spontaneously in less familiar environments. Many clients whose dysfunction is so pervasive that they have significant deficits in ideation may never reach these higher functional levels (e.g., some clients with mental retardation or severe learning disabilities). We need to be particularly careful that we help these clients to generalize their newly acquired skills to home and school.

## PRACTICAL CONSIDERATIONS FOR PROVIDING SAFE AND EFFECTIVE INTERVENTION

As we make recommendations to our clients, and their caregivers, about intervention, we continually are confronted with a number of important issues that we must think about and discuss. These include issues such as (a) whether or not the age of the client is a significant factor, (b) how frequently and for how long intervention should be administered in order to be effective, and (c) whether or not sensory integrative procedures can be administered effectively to more than one client simultaneously.

Similarly, when we decide, as trained occupational therapists, to provide intervention based on the principles of sensory integration theory, in our own practices, that decision has important implications for the resources we will need. These include such issues as (a) designing and obtaining appropriate space and equipment and (b) acquiring sources of reimbursement for our services.

## Factors Important to Individual Client Recommendations

### AGE OF THE CLIENT

Because she believed that the plasticity of the central nervous system decreased after age 9, Ayres (1972) felt that younger children would respond more readily to intervention than would older children or adults. However, there is increasing evidence that plasticity exists *even in mature organisms.* A number of adults whom we have treated express that intervention has been very beneficial to them, because they have developed greater ease of performing motor skills, and, more importantly, because they feel better about themselves psychologically, and are thus better able to interact effectively in social situations. For older children and adults, the keys to success in treatment seem to be the clients' beliefs that intervention can make their lives easier and their willingness to be involved in the intervention activities. The adults and older children who have been referred to us have suffered a great deal in their daily lives as a result of their sensory integrative dysfunction. They usually are highly motivated to engage in therapy.

Paul, a 12-year-old, wistfully stated that he had dreamed of a place like our clinic since he was 5 years old. It was clear to us from watching his reactions to the equipment and activities that he had a strong inner drive to be involved in the intervention process. His inner drive was not manifested as obvious playfulness, but rather as a strong investment in working hard and succeeding at each activity.

### DIRECT INTERVENTION: HOW LONG AND HOW OFTEN

The length and frequency of individual sessions are important variables to consider when making recommendations regarding direct intervention. We have found that individual sessions that are between 45 and 60 minutes in length seem to be more beneficial than are short sessions, even if the shorter sessions occur more frequently and, thus, the total intervention time each week is the same. In longer sessions, we can allow intervention to unfold logically and successfully and come to its own natural conclusion; this seems to be particularly true for older clients and for those who may need periodic "breaks" in the session to become calmer or more organized.

Ayres (personal communication, April 14, 1984) felt that the frequency of intervention was very important. In her own private practice, she recommended that children receive direct intervention two to three times per week and occasionally more frequently. However, because of time and financial constraints, clients rarely can receive direct intervention more than once or twice a week. If, however, a child might need services for 2 to 3 years, and during that time might develop a number of secondary emotional problems, it might be more effective to provide services relatively more frequently over a 1-year period than to provide the same total amount of services spread out during a 2- to 3-year period. While this idea has intuitive appeal, research is needed to examine whether increased frequency of intervention, over a shorter period of time, actually is as effective, or more effective, than intervention provided less often over a longer period of time. Thus far, the limited research in this area has not supported the premise of increased frequency with any intervention approach used in pediatric occupational or physical therapy (cf. Harris, 1988).

## THERAPIST-TO-CLIENT RATIO

In our experience, we have found that it is very difficult, if not impossible, to provide truly effective sensory integrative direct intervention to more than one client at a time. If two or more clients are treated simultaneously, the therapist frequently is in the position of selecting only activities that are appropriate for intervention with both clients; this may greatly limit the number and scope of available activities.

Further, two clients doubles the observational demands on the therapist and the need for adaptation of the activities. Sometimes the adaptations required to address one client's particular difficulties are not appropriate for the other client. Children who have experienced severe rejection from their peers or adults in their lives may develop an unhealthy competition among themselves for the therapist's attention. If a therapist must intervene with groups of clients, we believe it is best to embrace a sensorimotor approach to treatment, even though the therapist uses his or her knowledge of sensory integration theory to create the group activities (see Chapter 13).

If a treatment space is large enough to accommodate several children *and* therapists at the same time, the interactions that can be facilitated are often very beneficial. Interaction among the children may result in improvements in social skills and the development of friendships. Further, the children are exposed to new activities and challenges that they create and that improve their sensory integration and motor abilities. However, because one therapist is working with each child, each therapist can modify his or her client's activities as needed, and each therapist-client team is free to do something with, or different from, other therapist-client teams.

## Implications for Resources

### DESIGNING ADEQUATE SPACE AND A SUSPENSION SYSTEM

The suspension system is critical to the provision of sensory integrative procedures; without it, the direct intervention cannot be considered to be based on the principles of sensory integration theory (Bonder & Fisher, 1989; Clark, Mailloux, & Parham, 1989). Further, unless (a) the suspension system is correctly installed, (b) there is adequate space to use the equipment suspended from it, and (c) the floors of the space are fully covered by mats, we cannot be certain that our clients will be safe during direct intervention.

To use suspended equipment effectively, it is necessary to have a room that is a minimum of 12 feet square. We prefer to work in a room that is at least 14 feet square (14' × 20' is ideal), since that amount of space allows clients to make full orbits and arcs on suspended pieces of equipment without any danger of crashing into a wall.

While one point of suspension is required to administer sensory integrative procedures, many pieces of equipment (e.g., bolster swing, platform glider swing) are best used when hung from two points of suspension. In our experience, at least three successive points of suspension, centered in the ceiling and spaced 3 feet apart, are optimal. This enables the therapist to combine equipment and to provide progressively greater challenges to the client (e.g., swinging on a trapeze to jump through two suspended inner tubes).

The use of suspended equipment requires a suspension system that will sustain a *minimum* working load of 1000 pounds. Although many clients are children who weigh less than 100 pounds, when they bounce and swing on a piece of suspended equipment, the *shearing forces* on the suspension system are tremendous.

It is critical that all suspension systems be installed properly. Southpaw Enterprises (see Appendix 10–A for a list of vendors) publishes a *Ceiling Support Manual* that illustrates a number of safe ways to install a suspension system. We have found that when installing a suspension system, it usually is advisable to employ a consultant (such as an engineer or a contractor) who has a background in design. However, we also have found that we must explain clearly the necessity for having a suspension system that supports such a large working load. Frequently, consultants assume that a structure similar to an outdoor swing set is sufficient; that is *not* the case.

When installing eye bolts or other similar pieces of hardware through support beams or the ceiling, all bolts *must be* locked securely with a nut and washers. It *never* is safe to put bolts directly into the ceiling, even if the bolts are lag bolts or bolts that expand as they are tightened. Only bolts that go all the way through a part of the ceiling structure (through-bolts) and are locked on the other side can safely support the strong shearing forces generated during direct intervention.

If a therapist cannot, or decides not to, install a suspension system through a beam in the ceiling, free-standing suspension systems are commercially available. However, many of the lightweight, portable systems have a working load that is less than 1000 pounds. These lightweight systems limit the types of activity that can be done on them. Larger, heavier, nonportable systems, that provide a working load of at least 1000 pounds, also are commercially available; they are preferred in situations where it is not possible to mount the suspension system to ceiling structures (Koomar, 1990) (see Appendix 10–A for a list of vendors).

## ESTABLISHING PROGRAMS BASED ON SENSORY INTEGRATION THEORY

Occupational therapists work in a variety of settings including hospitals, clinics, schools, private practices, and homes. Each setting provides different sorts of difficulties when a therapist attempts to establish an intervention program based on the principles of sensory integration theory. Because of the costs associated with establishing such a program, significant negotiations often are required before the program can be initiated. In our experience, it may be easier to begin an intervention program based on sensory integration theory in a hospital setting (where a wide variety of technical equipment is used routinely) than in a school setting, where the equipment (and even the theory itself) may be difficult for administrators to associate with educational purposes.

An occupational therapy private practice setting may be the easiest place to develop an intervention program based on the principles of sensory integration theory. In a private practice setting, the therapists are free to rent, buy, or design a clinic that has the necessary space, equipment, and ceiling structure (to support the suspension system). Again, other therapists who previously have developed such a practice are the best sources of the information when beginning such a venture.

Obtaining permission to begin an intervention program in hospitals or schools requires a multilayered process of negotiation. The therapists first must gain approval from their immediate supervisors for use of sensory integrative procedures. When the immediate supervisor has approved the program, permission must be sought from agency administrators. The following hints apply for negotiation with administration at all levels.

We have found that it often is beneficial to provide in-service training to administrators to provide them with an understanding of sensory integration theory and the hypothesized benefits of intervention with clients, as well as information on the number of clients who can be expected to seek such services. Therapists may need to provide several sessions of in-service training over a period of months or years before their administrators are willing to support the use of sensory integrative treatment procedures.

Sometimes therapists hit "roadblocks" in their attempts to establish a program because an administrator has reservations about the use of sensory integrative procedures. It is important that therapists are prepared to discuss, in a convincing, logical, and realistic fashion, current research that supports, and also research that refutes, the use of sensory integrative procedures.

Some administrators have been convinced to support further development of intervention programs based on sensory integration theory when the therapists have been willing to systematically measure effectiveness of intervention with their clients. Single-case, or small-group design, studies seem to be the most feasible in these cases. Providing an administrator with both supportive research results, and anecdotal remarks of progress from parents, teachers, or other staff can provide a very powerful impetus for continuing, and further developing, an intervention program.

However, in our zeal to begin a new program, we should not promise more than we can deliver. Research requires time and resources if it is to be conducted effectively. Further, although negative results in a study *may* suggest that the procedures are ineffective, they also may mean that we failed to measure the proper constructs, or to measure them in an appropriate way (Bundy, 1990). The results of one study neither proves nor disproves the theory or the effectiveness of the procedures associated with it (see Chapter 14). The "bottom line" here is that we feel that tying the establishment of a program to the outcomes of studies that have yet to be planned or implemented *may* be unwise.

Along with support for the concept of a program based on the principles of sensory integration theory, we must receive approval for funds to be allocated for the design and installation of a suspension system and for purchasing (or making) equipment for direct intervention. In a hospital setting, the approval of funds often is tied to whether or not the therapists can logically project that the program will make a profit. We will discuss third-party reimbursement below. Other therapists who have begun similar programs can assist us by providing estimates of start-up costs and helping to project the rate of income growth.

In a school setting, the approval of funds is much more likely to be tied to the availability of money. School personnel often work on very tight budgets and the incidence of students who actually will be enrolled in direct intervention is quite low (considering the total population of special education students).

## THIRD-PARTY REIMBURSEMENT FOR SERVICES

Obtaining reimbursement for services always is a concern when establishing an intervention program in a hospital or private practice. Third-party reimbursement for occupational therapy varies greatly from state to state. In general, hospitals are more frequently reimbursed by third-party payers for occupational therapy services than are private practices.

When seeking reimbursement, it is important to use proper codes on documentation. *The International Classification of Disease Codes* (US Department of Health and Human Services, 1989) is useful for establishing diagnoses. Two codes that we have found to be appropriate for clients with sensory integrative dysfunction (who do not have any other medical diagnosis) are Dyspraxia Syndrome (315.4) and Coordination Disturbance (781.3); the latter includes apraxia as a subcategory.

*The Physician's Current Procedural Terminology* (CPT-4) (American Medical Association, 1989) provides codes for evaluation and treatment procedures. We have found the following codes to be most closely related to elements of sensory integrative evaluation: Developmental Testing (95881) and Physical Strength, Dexterity, Stamina (97720-21). Similarly, the following codes are related to elements of sensory integrative intervention: Therapeutic Exercise (97110), Neuromuscular Re-Education (97112), Functional Activities (97114); ADL-Not Diversional (97540-41). It is important to use the most current versions of the diagnostic codes and procedural terminology codes for billing; these manuals are revised periodically.

On occasion, we have found it useful to specify that sensory integrative intervention procedures are being used, especially with insurance companies that provide reimbursement only when specialized evaluation or intervention procedures are documented. However, we describe the goals of intervention in "traditional" occupational therapy terms, such as *specific* improvement in activities of daily living, and avoid discussing sensory processing difficulties, since these terms usually are unfamiliar to the insurance company personnel who process the claims and because our goals are to improve a client's occupational performance.

## Continuing Education

Sensory integration theory is a complex, and continually changing, body of knowledge. In order to provide effective, state-of-the-art intervention based on the principles of sensory integration theory, it is important to acquire a sound understanding of the theory and to update our knowledge continually.

The staff at Sensory Integration International (1987/1988), a private, not-for-profit organization whose mission is to promote sensory integration theory and practice, has developed an official statement suggesting that therapists who use sensory integrative procedures have a minimum of 3 months of supervision from a therapist knowledgeable in sensory integration theory and experienced with the procedures used in intervention. In addition, they recommend ongoing participation in continuing education courses that specifically address recent advances in sensory integration theory and practice and neurobiological theory. It is also recommended that therapists keep abreast of current research and developments of the theory that are published in professional journals.

## CONCLUSIONS

Providing intervention based on the principles of sensory integration theory is both a complex and an exciting process. It requires that the therapist be able to combine a working knowledge of sensory integration theory with an intuitive ability to engender a client's trust and create the just right challenge.

The ultimate goal of intervention is to facilitate a client's development, self-actualization, and occupational performance. To do this, several critical elements must be present in the therapist's direct intervention with the client. First, after setting *specific objectives*, the therapist is guided by the client to *create an environment* that invites the client's interaction and provides realistic challenges to the client. The environment includes both the physical layout of the clinic space (including the available equipment) and the kinds of interactions that occur between the client and the therapist. The therapist tailors the environment to meet the needs of the client and provides encouragement and feedback regarding the client's progress.

Second, the therapist and the client *design and create activities* that (a) are motivating to the client, (b) provide controlled opportunities for the client to take in appropriate types and amounts of enhanced sensory information, (c) involve active participation on the part of the client, and (d) require that the client respond adaptively to the just right challenge. The ability to participate and guide the client in creating treatment activities is based on the therapist's knowledge of sensory integration theory, his or her understanding of the client's needs and interests, and the objectives that the client and therapist have established together.

Third, the therapist *observes* the client's responses to the treatment activities and process, and *adapts* both ever so slightly to enable the client to attain the maximum benefit from intervention. This requires that the therapist (a) communicate regularly with the client and his or her caregivers, (b) vigilantly observe the client's cues, (c) thoroughly understand the purpose of each aspect of an intervention activity, (d) anticipate the best course of action, and (e) skillfully alter the activities (without disruption to the overall flow of the session). The therapist also helps the client, and his or her caregivers, to *understand* the effects that sensory integrative dysfunction has on the client's daily life and to *develop strategies* that minimize or eliminate those negative effects.

Finally, the therapist, together with the client and his or her caregivers, continuously *monitors the client's progress* toward meeting the specified objectives and the degree to which direct intervention has helped the client to meet the demands of his or her daily life more easily. An important part of this monitoring is discovering whether or not the client has generalized the skills he or she has gained in the clinic to everyday life. Based on the results of these assessments, the therapist adapts the intervention program and recommends a time when direct intervention should be *discontinued.*

In this chapter, we have focussed on the provision of direct intervention based on the principles of sensory integration theory. We have discussed elements of the art of therapy and the ways in which art is intimately intertwined with science in the creation of intervention activities. We have outlined activities that we have used successfully with clients who have a number of different sequelae to sensory integrative dysfunction. We have discussed practical considerations both for establishing direct intervention with individual clients and for developing programs within occupational therapy departments in a number of different kinds of settings.

We believe that direct intervention is a powerful tool for effecting changes in the lives of individuals who have sensory integrative dysfunction. Because direct intervention based on the principles of sensory integration theory is a complex and difficult process, we have devoted this entire chapter to discussing its provision.

However, we wish to emphasize two points. First, direct intervention is *only one means* for treating individuals who have sensory integrative dysfunction. We believe that direct intervention rarely should be provided (especially with children) unless the therapist also provides consultation to the client's caregivers.

Second, we believe that the most effective direct intervention is rarely, if ever, comprised only of sensory integrative procedures. Because individual clients have a variety of needs with regard to their daily lives, an integrated approach to intervention generally is both the most effective and the most efficient.

# REFERENCES

American Medical Association (1989). *Physician's current procedural terminology* (4th ed.). Chicago: Author.

Ayres, A. J. (1972). *Sensory integration and learning disorders.* Los Angeles: Western Psychological Services.

Ayres, A. J. (1975). *Southern California Postrotary Nystagmus Test.* Los Angeles: Western Psychological Services.

Ayres, A. J. (1977, March). Developmental dyspraxia. Symposium conducted in Dayton, Ohio.

Ayres, A. J. (1979). *Sensory integration and the child.* Los Angeles: Western Psychological Services.

Ayres, A. J. (1985). *Developmental dyspraxia and adult-onset apraxia.* Torrance, CA: Sensory Integration International.

Ayres, A. J. (1989). *Sensory Integration and Praxis Tests.* Los Angeles: Western Psychological Services.

Ayres, A. J., & Tickle, L. S. (1980). Hyper-responsivity to touch and vestibular stimuli as a predictor of positive response to sensory integration procedures by autistic children. *American Journal of Occupational Therapy, 34,* 375–381.

Bly, L. (1983). *The components of normal movement during the first year of life and abnormal motor development.* Birmingham, AL: Pathway Press.

Bobath, B. (1985). *Abnormal postural reflex activity caused by brain lesions* (3rd ed.). Rockville, MD: Aspen Systems.

Boehme, R. (1988). *Improving upper body control.* Tucson, AZ: Therapy Skill Builders.

Bonder, B. R., & Fisher, A. G. (1989). Sensory integration and treatment of the elderly. *Gerontology Special Interest Section News, 12* (1), 2–4.

Bundy, A. C. (1990). The challenge of functional outcomes: Framing the problem. *Neuro-Developmental Treatment Association Newsletter.*

Cermak, S. A. (1985). Developmental dyspraxia. In E. A. Roy (Ed.), *Neuropsychological studies of apraxia and related disorders* (pp. 225–250). New York: Elsevier.

Clark, F., Mailloux, Z., & Parham, D. (1989). Sensory integration and children with learning disabilities. In P. N. Pratt and A. S. Allen (Eds.), *Occupational therapy for children* (2nd ed., pp. 457–507). St. Louis: C. V. Mosby.

Fisher, A. G. (1989). Objective assessment of the quality of response during two equilibrium tests. *Physical and Occupational Therapy in Pediatrics, 9*(3), 57–78.

Fisher, A. G., & Bundy, A. C. (1989). Vestibular stimulation in the treatment of postural and related disorders. In O. D. Payton, R. P. DiFabio, S. V. Paris, E. J. Protas, & A. G. Van Sant (Eds.), *Manual of Physical Therapy Techniques* (pp. 239–258). New York: Churchill Livingstone.

Fisher, A. G., & Dunn, W. (1983). Tactile defensiveness: Historical perspectives, new research: A theory grows. *Sensory Integration Special Interest Section Newsletter, 6*(2), 1–2.

Harris, S. R. (1988). Early intervention: Does developmental therapy make a difference? *Topics in Early Childhood Special Education, 7,* 20–32.

Howison, M. V. (1988). Cerebral palsy. In H. L. Hopkins and H. D. Smith (Eds.), *Willard and Spackman's occupational therapy* (7th ed., pp. 675–706). Philadelphia: J.B. Lippincott.

Kagan, J., Reznick, J., Snidman, N., & Garcia-Coll, C. (1984). The biology and psychology of behavioral inhibition in young children. *Child Development, 55,* 2212–2225.

Keogh, J., & Sugden, D. (1985). *Movement skill development.* New York: Macmillan.

Koomar, J. (1990). *Providing sensory integration therapy as an itinerant therapist. Environment: Implications for occupational therapy practice. A sensory integrative approach.* Rockville, MD: American Occupational Therapy Association.

Luria, A. (1961). *The role of speech in the regulation of normal and abnormal behavior.* New York: Liveright.

May, T. (1988). *Identifying gravitational insecurity in children with sensory integrative dysfunction.* Unpublished master's thesis, Boston University, Boston.

Peiper, A. (1963). *Cerebral function in infancy and childhood.* New York: Consultant's Bureau.

Pribram, K. (1975). Arousal, activation and effort in the control of attention. *Psychological Review, 82,* 116–149.

Schaefer, C. E., & Reid, S. E. (1986). *Game play: Therapeutic use of childhood games.* New York: John Wiley & Sons.

Schumaker, E. F. (1977). *A guide for the perplexed.* New York: Harper & Row.

Standards of practice for the evaluation and treatment of sensory integrative dysfunction. Sensory Integration International (1987/1988). Vol. 6–8.

Smith, S., & Scardina, V. (1980). *Ethical intervention.* Torrance, CA: Center for the Study of Sensory Integrative Dysfunction, *4*, 1–2.

Stilwell, J. (1981). Relationship between development of the body-righting reaction and manual midline crossing behavior in the learning disabled. *American Journal of Occupational Therapy, 35*, 391–398.

US Department of Health and Human Services (1989). *The international classification of diseases, (9th revision), Clinical Modification.* DHHS No. (PHS) 89–1260. Washington, D.C.: US Government Printing Office.

Wehman, P. (1977). *Helping the mentally retarded acquire play skills: A behavioral approach.* Springfield, IL: Charles C. Thomas.

Weisz, S. (1938). Studies in equilibrium reactions. *Journal of Nervous and Mental Disease, 88*, 150–162.

Wilbarger, P. (1988). Sensory Defensiveness. Paper presented at the Annual Interdisciplinary Doctoral Conference, Boston University, Department of Occupational Therapy, Boston.

Williams, H. G. (1983). *Perceptual and motor development.* Englewood Cliffs, NJ: Prentice Hall.

# APPENDIX 10 – A

---

# List of Vendors by Type of Equipment*

---

## Floor Equipment

Air Matresses
Achievement Products; Flaghouse; JA Preston; Southpaw
Balance Beams/Boards
Achievement Products; Childcraft; Community Playthings; Flaghouse; Fred Sammons; J. A. Preston
Balance Stools
Equipment Shop; Flaghouse; J. A. Preston
Balls
Achievement Products; Best Priced Products; Childcraft; Equipment Shop; Flaghouse; Fred Sammons; JA Preston; PDP Products; Southpaw
Ball Baths
Flaghouse; Fred Sammons; JA Preston
Bounce Pads
Achievement Products; Flaghouse; Southpaw
Bubble Ball Bath (See Ball Baths)
Climbing Structures
Childcraft; Community Playthings; Southpaw
Equilibrium Boards/Boats
Achievement Products; Community Playthings; Flaghouse; Fred Sammons; JA Preston
Foam Play Pools
Southpaw Enterprises

Foam Ramps
Childcraft; Community Playthings; Flaghouse; Southpaw
Foam Steps
Flaghouse; Southpaw
Inner Tubes (stackable)
Fred Sammons; Southpaw
Mats
Best Priced Products; Childcraft; Community Playthings; Equipment Shop; Flaghouse; JA Preston
Nested Benches/Stools
Best Priced Products; Flaghouse; Southpaw; Tramble
Pon Pon Balls (Large balls w/handles)
Equipment Shop; Flaghouse; Southpaw; Best Priced Products; Equipment Shop; Fred Sammons; JA Preston; Southpaw; Tramble
Rocker Boards (see equilibrium board)
Tractor Crawler (flexible barrel)
Achievement Products; Flaghouse
Trampolines (also see bounce pad)
Achievement Products; Community Playthings; Flaghouse
Vestibular Boards (see Equilibrium)
Vestibular Bowls/Discs
Childcraft; Equipment Shop; Flaghouse; Southpaw

## Wheeled Floor Equipment

Roller Racer
Childcraft; Flaghouse; Southpaw
Scooter Boards
Achievement Products; Best Priced Products; Community Playthings; Equipment Shop; Flaghouse; Fred Sammons; JA Preston; Southpaw; Tramble

Sit 'N' Spin (by Kenner)
Southpaw
Tilt N' Whirl (by Wham-O)
Southpaw
Turtle (see roller racer)
Whiz Wheel (by Marx Toys)
Equipment Shop; JA Preston; Southpaw

## Obstacle Course Equipment

Barrels
  Best Priced Products; Flaghouse; Fred
  Sammons; JA Preston; Southpaw
Bolsters
  Best Priced Products; Community Playthings;
  Flaghouse; J. A. Preston; Southpaw; Therapy
  Skill Builders
Foam Animals
  Flaghouse; Southpaw
Foam Blocks
  Childcraft; Community Playthings; Flaghouse;
  Southpaw

Foam Shapes
  Flaghouse
Tunnels
  Achievement Products; Childcraft; Flaghouse;
  Fred Sammons; JA Preston; Just for Kids;
  Southpaw
Wedges
  Best Priced Products; Childcraft; Community
  Playthings; Flaghouse; Fred Sammons; JA
  Preston; Southpaw; Therapy Skill Builders

## Suspended Equipment

Bolster Swings
  Community Playthings; Flaghouse; Southpaw
Biorbital Accelerator (See Dual Swings)
Disc Swing (see Flexion Disc Swing)
Dual Swings
  Flaghouse; Southpaw
Flexion Disc Swings
  Flaghouse; J. A. Preston; Southpaw
Frog Swings
  Southpaw
Gliders
  Childcraft; Just For Kids; Southpaw
"Helipcopter" (see Dual Swings)
Inner Tube Swings
  Flaghouse; Southpaw

Ladders (suspended)
  Southpaw
Nets and Net Swings
  Achievement Products; Community Playthings;
  Flaghouse; Fred Sammons; JA Preston; Southpaw
Platform Swings
  Achievement Products; Community Playthings;
  Flaghouse; JA Preston; Southpaw
"Surfboard" (rectangular platform swing)
  Flaghouse; Southpaw
Tire Swings
  Flaghouse; Southpaw
Trapeze
  Flaghouse; Southpaw

## Miscellaneous Equipment

Ceiling Supports
  Flaghouse; Southpaw
Free Standing Supports
  Community Playthings; Flaghouse; Fred
  Sammons; JA Preston; Southpaw
Hug Machine
  Tramble Co.
Helmets
  Flaghouse; Fred Sammons; JA Preston, Corp.;
  Southpaw
Inflators/Air Pumps
  Equipment Shop; Flaghouse; Fred Sammons,
  Inc.; JA Preston; Southpaw

Oral Motor Activity Supplies
  PDP Products; Southpaw
Shock or "Bungy" cord
  Airport or Boat Supply Stores
Stopwatches
  Feldmar; Forbes and Stillman; Meylan; Western
  Psychological Svs.
Tactile Activity Supplies
  Fred Sammons; JA Preston; PDP Products;
  Sensory Integration International; Southpaw

## Sources

Achievement Products
P.O. Box 547, Mineola, NY 11501
(516)747-8899

Best Priced Products
P.O. Box 1174, White Plains, NY 10602
(800)824-2939

Childcraft
20 Kilmer Road, Edison, NJ 08818
(800)631-5657

Community Playthings/Rifton Equipment
Route 213, Rifton, NY 12471
(914)658-3141

J.A. Preston Corp.
60 Page Road, Clifton, NJ 07012
(201)777-2700

Just for Kids
75 Paterson Street, P.O. Box 15006
New Brunswick, NJ 08906-5006
(800)654-6963

Meylan Corporation
264 West 40th Street, New York, NY 10018
(212)391-9150

PDP Products
12015 N. July Ave.,
Hugo, MN 55038

The Equipment Shop
P.O. Box 33, Bedford, MA 01730
(617)275-7681

The Feldmar Company
9000 West Pico Blvd., Los Angeles, CA 90035
(213)272-1196

Flaghouse, Inc.
150 N. MacQuesten Parkway, Mt. Vernon, NY 10550
(800)221-5185, NY (914)699-1900

Forbes and Stillman Company
6 North Michigan Avenue, Chicago, IL 60602
(312)332-2875

Fred Sammons, Inc.
P.O. Box 32, Brookfield, IL 60513
(800)323-5547

Sensory Integration International
1402 Cravens Avenue, Torrance, CA 90501
(213)533-8338

Southpaw Enterprises, Inc.
800 West Third Street, Dayton, OH 45407
(800)228-1698

The Tramble Company
894 St. Andrews Way, Frankfort, IL 60423
(815)469-2938

Therapy Skill Builders
3830 E. Bellevue, Dept. C, Tucson, AZ 85716
(602)323-7500

Western Psychological Services
12031 Wilshire Blvd., Los Angeles, CA 90025
(800)222-2670, CA (800)423-7863

*Source:* SI equipment: Where to find it. Sensory Integration International (1990). *Sensory Integration Quarterly, 18*(1), pp. 6 – 7. Copyright 1990 by author. Adapted by permission.

# CHAPTER 11

# Consultation and Sensory Integration Theory

Anita C. Bundy, ScD, OTR

*The utilization of interpretive models for the treatment of individual [clients] is a basic characteristic of all clinical practice, whether the clinician is an [occupational therapist], internist, psychiatrist, spiritualist healer, Chinese shaman or Iranian prayer writer.*

*Good & Good, 1981, p. 177*

Often, when we think of intervention based on sensory integration theory, we think of intervention administered to individual clients in treatment areas equipped with swings, suspension systems, and other equipment that can be used readily to provide the client with opportunities for enhanced sensory intake; that is, we think of *direct intervention.* However, direct intervention is not the only, or even the most important, means by which occupational therapy is provided. In this chapter, we will discuss the application of the principles of sensory integration to another, equally important type of service provision, *consultation.*

Consultation occurs in the context of a partnership established between the therapist-consultant and the consultee (parent, teacher, etc.). The problems addressed are those identified by the consultee. In the process, both partners have equal voice in developing the strategies for intervention; however, the consultee implements the strategies. Both share equal responsibility for evaluating the effectiveness of the strategies and for the outcome.

The expected outcome of consultation is that the environment (both human and non-human) will better "fit" the needs of the client. Said another way, consultation enables the client to succeed in his or her environment despite the limitations imposed by the sensory integrative dysfunction. Because of the importance of this expected outcome, we believe that consultation should almost always be used with clients who have sensory integrative dysfunction (except in the most extraordinary of circumstances), whether or not they are simultaneously receiving direct intervention.

---

The author wishes to acknowledge the contributions of Phyllis Hindery, Lee Ann Lilly, and Linda Silber to the case examples in this chapter.

## PURPOSE AND SCOPE

In this chapter, we will define consultation and discuss the various stages and phases associated with the provision of consultation. We also will address problems we commonly encounter as we try to establish an effective consultative partnership. We will illustrate through case examples the stages of consultation, the problems associated with it, and possible solutions to those problems.

## WHAT IS CONSULTATION?

When we use the term *consultation*, we refer to a collaborative process by which we use occupational therapy theories (in this case, sensory integration) to help consultees to (a) understand the client in a new way, and (b) develop new, and more effective, strategies for interacting with the client. That is, we provide others with access to theoretical explanations of the client's behavior (that they otherwise would have no reason to know), and we serve as catalysts to enable the parent to become a better parent or the teacher to become a better teacher (Bundy, unpublished manuscript; Niehues, Bundy, Mattingly, & Lawlor, in press). In the course of consulting, we often suggest specific activities or materials to use; however, *our primary purpose is to address, and minimize, the problems encountered by the parent or teacher as they try to effectively parent or teach the client.*

## Reframing

We refer to the process of enabling others to understand the client's behavior in a different way, or to view the behavior from a new perspective, as "reframing the behavior." We speak of reframing, rather than "setting the frame" (Schön, 1983, 1987), because we find that invariably, parents, teachers, and others already have set a frame for the client's behavior. Setting the frame only is necessary when someone has no prior view or interpretation of the client's behavior. This is rarely the case with parents and teachers who know a client well.

Moreover, in the case of the client with sensory integrative dysfunction, often the frame that parents or teachers have used to explain behavior is negative. Because the client behaves in the ways he or she does, parents, teachers, and others may view him or her as poorly disciplined, immature, destructive, careless, rigid, or overreactive.

The frame that parents, teachers, and others have for viewing the client's behavior determines how they will react to that behavior, that is, the strategies they will use for parenting or teaching the child. By using sensory integrative theory to change the frame for viewing the client's behavior, we provide the parent or teacher with the basis for developing different kinds of strategies for interacting with the client. In turn, these strategies often result in a dramatic lessening of problem behaviors because situations or activities that are apt to be difficult for the client can be avoided or made easier.

Rebecca is a 5-year-old child with sensory integrative dysfunction. Rebecca exhibits extreme hypersensitivity to touch and to minor pain. However, Rebecca's reaction to pain is delayed; often 5 or more minutes pass after a minor incident, such as bumping her elbow, before Rebecca erupts in tears and screams of agony: "This is gonna hurt me forever!" Rebecca's parents and the other children and adults in her life view Rebecca's reactions as melodramatic. "After all, if she really were hurt, wouldn't she begin to cry immediately?" asked her parents. Believing that Rebecca was only "acting" to get attention, Rebecca's parents tried ignoring her wails and telling her that she was not hurt and was "acting silly." However, both responses only resulted in Rebecca's screaming more loudly.

During a conference following Rebecca's evaluation, we told her parents about the extent of Rebecca's difficulties registering and interpreting sensory information. They discussed her reactions to pain with us and we helped them to see how this behavior might be explained by her sensory integrative dysfunction. "Perhaps," we reasoned, "Rebecca's sensory integrative dysfunction results in its taking longer for sensory information to register. When it *does* register, Rebecca interprets stimuli that others would think of as nonaversive as being painful."

The result was that Rebecca's parents came to view this very problematic behavior in a different way. Rather than seeing her behavior as melodramatic, they understood that Rebecca's intense, but delayed reaction to pain was the result of her difficulty registering and processing sensory information. The frame was changed.

## Developing New Strategies

Reframing is one of the therapist-consultant's most important tools. However, the role of the consultant usually does not end with reframing. Rather, reframing provides the basis on which further consultation is built. Once the new frame has been established, the therapist helps the parent or teacher to develop new strategies for enabling the client to succeed in performing his or her daily life tasks and roles more effectively and efficiently.

The story of Rebecca provides us with a good example of successful strategies built on a new frame. With our help, Rebecca's parents used their newfound knowledge to develop different strategies for responding to her outbursts. They began to acknowledge that what Rebecca felt *was* pain and that they understood that *she* felt as though it would "hurt her forever." They asked to see the hurt place and applied deep touch-pressure and firm rubbing to the area. Using these strategies, they found that Rebecca was much easier to console. Although her reaction to minor pain remained intense and delayed, she screamed less and was more easily distracted from her pain.

Rebecca's parents felt much better also. As they became more skilled at using their new strategies, they no longer dreaded taking Rebecca to their friends' homes. They stopped feeling that they had to apologize for Rebecca's "overreactions." When it seemed appropriate, they explained the source of Rebecca's discomfort. Otherwise, they used their new strategies to avert "disaster" and behaved as though nothing out of the ordinary had occurred. Other adults picked up on this new strategy and also began to implement it. The result was that everyone became more comfortable with Rebecca, including herself.

With the story of Rebecca, we have illustrated an example of effective consultation with parents. However, consultation also can be provided effectively with teachers. For example, the teacher who believes that a child constantly gets into fistfights while standing in line because he or she is poorly disciplined behaves entirely differently toward that child than does the teacher who understands that the child is tactually defensive, interprets touch poorly, and probably was jostled accidentally from behind. In the latter case, the child may be allowed to stand at the back of the line where he or she can avoid unexpected touch. In the former case, the child is likely to be kept near the front of the line, under the teacher's watchful eye, but also an easy target for more accidental jostling. The likely result is more fistfights. Thus, the child is apt to be punished repeatedly for circumstances beyond his or her control. Because the teacher does not understand the real basis of the problem, his or her solution is likely to make the problem worse.

The concept of consultation is deceptively simple. The process, however, may prove much more difficult.

## PROVIDING CONSULTATION: A CASE EXAMPLE

In the following case example, we illustrate the consultation process that occurred between an occupational therapist-consultant and a teacher during the course of a school year. We then will use that case as the basis for a discussion of the stages of consultation.

Charlie is an 11-year-old boy of average intelligence, who has been placed in a self-contained classroom for students with learning disabilities. His teacher, Mrs. R, having attempted unsuccessfully for 2 years to teach Charlie to write in cursive, has reached her "level of tolerance." She has referred Charlie to Lily, the occupational therapist, for evaluation and possible treatment.

Upon questioning Mrs. R about the instructional methods she had tried with Charlie, Lily learned that Mrs. R had attempted numerous strategies, and that she was currently using a "multisensory approach" to teach handwriting. When asked to describe the multisensory approach, Mrs. R indicated that she showed Charlie the formation of a letter, then asked him to practice making that letter in, or with, various media. These media included sand, rice, fingerpaint, chalk, markers, and others. When asked about the problems Charlie had reproducing letters with a pen or pencil, Mrs. R showed Lily copies of some of Charlie's papers. The letters were poorly formed and so light that they were barely legible.

Lily spent some time in the classroom watching Charlie form letters with the various media his teacher had described. As she watched, Lily realized that, rather than practicing the same letter formation over and over, Charlie was actually performing new motor patterns as he moved from one medium to another. When he formed the letter in fingerpaint, he used finger motions; but when he wrote on the chalkboard, he used whole arm movements. Both of these were different from the motor patterns he used when he attempted to write the letter on paper with a pencil.

In addition to observation of Charlie in his classroom and interviews with his teacher, Lily's evaluation consisted of clinical observations of neuromotor behavior, the sensory portions of the Luria Nebraska Test (Golden, 1987) and the Bruininks-Oseretsky Test of Motor Proficiency (Bruininks, 1978). Charlie had deficits on all of these measures.

After gathering all the data, Lily concluded that (a) Charlie was dyspraxic; his dyspraxia seemed to stem from decreased processing of tactile and vestibular-proprioceptive input; and (b) Charlie's dyspraxia seemed to be interfering with his ability to learn cursive handwriting skills. Having determined that much, Lily was faced with the important decision of what type of intervention to recommend to the educational team.

Lily believed that Charlie probably would benefit from occupational therapy intervention. However, rather than recommending direct intervention, Lily suggested to the team that she provide occupational therapy intervention through consultation with Mrs. R.

This recommendation was based on a number of factors. First, Charlie's inability to learn cursive writing seemed to be caused by dyspraxia. However, Lily reasoned that it would take months, perhaps years, of direct intervention before his deficits could be remediated sufficiently for him to learn handwriting through the methods Mrs. R was using. At 11, Charlie already was significantly behind his peers in learning to write. He could not afford for another year to pass before he mastered this basic skill.

Second, Charlie's primary difficulty in his classroom seemed to be with learning handwriting. Mrs. R was instructing Charlie *daily* in handwriting. While Lily could have developed a direct intervention program that targeted improvements in handwriting, she could only have provided intervention once or twice a week. Further, Lily knew very little about teaching proper letter formation, but that was one of Mrs. R's areas of expertise.

Third, although he is of average intelligence, and in spite of his good auditory learning skills, Charlie had difficulty keeping up in school. If he heard information and instructions, he could remember them, but it was difficult for him to learn by reading. Therefore, it was important that Charlie be present for, and attend to, his teacher's instructions. He could not afford time out of class for therapy because he would probably fall further behind in school. Even if Lily elected to provide direct intervention in his classroom, it was very likely that Charlie would miss some important information during that time.

Finally, Mrs. R's openness to working with Lily was an important factor in her recommendation to engage in consultation with Mrs. R. Mrs. R was a skilled teacher who had invested a lot of time and effort in teaching Charlie to write. However, nothing she tried had worked. She knew that his problems required the input of another professional and she was eager to accept help from someone who could explain Charlie's problems to her. Although Mrs. R was a master teacher, and had taught letter formation for years, her knowledge of dyspraxia was limited. As a result, she unknowingly developed a method to teach Charlie to form letters that "played to his weaknesses." This method, while creative and motivating for Charlie, resulted in his having to formulate several different motor responses for each new letter he learned. Because forming new motor responses was his greatest deficit, Charlie had not learned to write by this method.

When Lily presented her recommendation to the special education team, including Charlie's parents and teachers, they agreed with Lily's recommendation for consultation. In fact, Lily's presentation of Charlie's motor planning difficulties and the benefits of consultation was so clear and convincing that the gym teacher also requested consultation with her.

Shortly thereafter, Lily began consulting with Mrs. R. She began by listening carefully to Mrs. R's concerns and reframing the problem for her. Lily again explained about Charlie's extraordinary difficulty with planning new movements. She told Mrs. R that Charlie's difficulties were the result of poor feedback he received from his body when he moved. She also showed Mrs. R that each of the media that Charlie was using to learn letter formation required that he plan a new way of moving. That simple reframing was all that Mrs. R needed to help her to understand the problem. She had already known that Charlie was poorly coordinated and that he seemed not to know how his body moved. Therefore, she had reasoned that providing him with a lot of sensory input might help him to learn to write better. However, she had not recognized that, with each new medium, Charlie had to formulate a new plan for moving.

"I guess that means that I should pick one medium to use to teach him and stick with it," Mrs. R stated. Lily agreed. She and Mrs. R agreed that, at age 11, Charlie needed to concentrate on learning to write with a pen or pencil. They discussed Charlie's difficulties both with forming the letters and with pressing hard enough on the paper that the letters could be seen. Lily knew that Charlie was not getting adequate feedback from his body as he wrote with his pencil, and she believed that the deficit in feedback was contributing to his poor letter formation. She suggested that Charlie write with a grease pencil because its increased resistance would provide him with more feedback. Mrs. R agreed that the grease pencil might work. She and Lily made arrangements to meet again the next week to discuss Charlie's progress.

The following week, Mrs. R reported that the grease pencil did not seem to be working; she was still concerned that Charlie did not press down hard enough to make his handwriting legible. Lily and Mrs. R then devised a plan for Charlie to use carbon paper between two sheets of paper when he wrote with a pencil. Mrs. R taught Charlie to lift the carbon periodically to see whether or not he had been pressing down hard enough for his writing to come through.

Charlie responded very well to the changes in his handwriting program. Within a few weeks, Charlie had learned to write much more legibly and to press harder with his pencil. After about 6 weeks, Mrs. R and Lily decided that the carbon paper might no longer be necessary. Mrs. R prepared Charlie for the change by trying to make him conscious of the amount of pressure he used when he wrote successfully using the carbon paper. She gradually withdrew the carbon paper by giving him more papers each day that did not have carbons attached to them.

An important part of consultation was that Lily continued to meet regularly with Mrs. R. They worked together to solve a number of difficulties that Charlie had in the classroom. As Mrs. R came to better understand Charlie's difficulties with formulating new motor programs, she began to devise her own alternative strategies for teaching Charlie. Initially, she liked to discuss her plans with Lily before implementing them, to be sure she was on the right track. However, as she began to succeed, she needed less and less input from Lily. During one of their sessions, about 3 months into the consultation process, Mrs. R remarked to Lily, "You know, this all was once so new to me; now it seems so logical. I know that I will look at other students' problems differently from now on."

Lily did a similar type of consultation with the gym teacher that also was highly successful. Charlie's gym class focused on physical fitness. The students spent the majority of their time doing calisthenics. Mr. S, the gym teacher, led the students in various routines comprised of jumping jacks, push ups, sit ups, running in place, and other basic skills. Although the exercises were always the same, he varied their order.

Charlie's coordination was not very good, but if he concentrated intensely, he could perform some of the exercises passably. However, this required inordinate effort on his part and he often chose to stand and watch the others rather than to participate. When Lily talked with Mr. S, she learned that it was Charlie's "standing around" that bothered Mr. S the most.

In her consultation with Mr. S, Lily recommended some very simple adaptations to the way the class was run, which resulted in Charlie's participating more frequently and more effectively. Lily explained to Mr. S that Charlie would be able to do the exercises better if there were set routines. He could then memorize them and would not have to think so hard about what was coming next. Further, she explained that Charlie's strongest channel for learning was his auditory channel. Thus, she suggested to Mr. S that it might be helpful to Charlie if Mr. S always called out the next exercise shortly before it changed and again at the time of the change. Lily also recommended that Mr. S stand near Charlie and perform the exercises with the class. In that way, Charlie would always hear the instructions and he also would have a visual model for each exercise.

Lily was able to use her knowledge of sensory integrative theory to help Mrs. R and Mr. S to understand Charlie's motor planning difficulties. In so doing, she helped them to see why their teaching methods had failed and to develop new strategies that worked. When Mrs. R's knowledge of proper letter formation was combined with Lily's cognizance of Charlie's motor planning deficits, the result was the development of strategies that allowed Charlie to learn cursive writing. Initially, Charlie did not participate in Mr. S's gym class. With a few simple modifications, however, Charlie became an active member of the class. None of these professionals could have accomplished their goals alone in such a short time period; together they succeeded.

## STAGES OF CONSULTATION

The general goals that guide our consultation are to use our practice theories to reframe a client's behavior for our consultees and, based on that reframing, to help our consultees develop new and more effective strategies for interacting and working with the client. We believe that there are four stages to the consultation process. These are: (a) formulating expectations, (b) establishing the partnership, (c) planning strategies, and (d) implementing and assessing the plan. The relationship of these stages to one another is shown schematically in Figure 11–1.

STAGES OF CONSULTATION

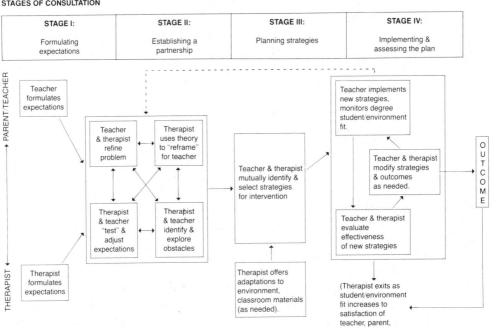

| STAGE I: | STAGE II: | STAGE III: | STAGE IV: |
|---|---|---|---|
| Formulating expectations | Establishing a partnership | Planning strategies | Implementing & assessing the plan |

FIGURE 11–1. Stages of consultation.

Each of the four stages is equally important to the process. In certain instances (and in all of the examples we have used), some of the stages seem to be accomplished very easily, almost automatically, and the therapist-consultant and the consultee are able to make rapid progress. Thus, an observer to this process might have been unaware that some of the stages had occurred. In instances where the process does not go so smoothly, we attempt to trace backward through the stages to find out where the process went awry. In so doing, we are able to determine where to begin again to facilitate the consultation process.

The therapist-consultant and the consultee participate as equals in all four stages of the process. However, it is the therapist's responsibility to facilitate and examine the process, and to change its course if the process does not seem to be working.

Now let us look at each of the stages of the consulting process in more depth. We will use the case of Lily and Mrs. R as an example to illustrate how partners pass through these stages. We also will describe one therapist's attempt at developing a consultative partnership that did not begin smoothly. We will discuss some strategies that therapists used to facilitate the development of the relationship. Although parents frequently are our partners in the consultative process, we will simplify our discussion in the next section by referring to the consultee as the teacher.

## Stage I: Formulating Expectations

This first stage of the process occurs before the therapist and the teacher have begun to work together in the consultative relationship. In preparation for beginning the process, both the teacher and the therapist, consciously or unconsciously, formulate expectations of what will happen during, and as a result of, intervention.

Mattingly (1989) suggested that these expectations take the form of real or imagined stories that the individuals create, using information from a number of sources. These sources may include information that the teacher and therapist have because they have worked together before; information shared with one of them by a colleague or the child's parent; past experiences that they have had working with, or observing, other therapists or teachers; or their own imaginations. The creation of expectations enables us to prepare for intervention. When we understand that we begin the process with expectations that may be based in "fiction," we are prepared to seek new information and to alter the stories we have created in response to our actual situation as we begin working with the teacher.

In instances where the teacher and the therapist have worked together before, as with Mrs. R and Lily, the stories or expectations that the two create may be very similar to what actually happens when they begin working together. However, in situations where a therapist and teacher have not worked together, one or both of them may have created stories, or set expectations, that impede the development of the relationship.

## Stage II: Establishing a Partnership

This second stage of the process is comprised of four very important phases (see Fig. 11–1). Because it is a preliminary stage (in that the partners are not yet ready to develop strategies), we may minimize its importance and "gloss over" it in favor of moving on to the "more important business" that lies ahead. However, if we move on too quickly at this stage and attempt to offer solutions or strategies to the teacher before we have established an equal partnership with him or her, we may give the impression that we "know all the answers" and are not interested in the teacher's contributions to the process. Clearly, perceived inequality in the relationship will hamper both the development of a partnership and the effectiveness of the process. This is particularly true of therapist-teacher teams when they have not worked together before or one of the team members has considerably less experience than the other. Thus, it is not surprising that consultative relationships that go awry often do so at this stage.

There are many valid reasons why a teacher may be hesitant to enter into a consultative partnership. The teacher may feel that the therapist is "invading" or interrupting the important business of the classroom. He or she may think that since teaching is a full-time job, taking on additional work just is not possible. The teacher may never have worked with a therapist who was interested in consulting before. Based on past experience, he or she may perceive that therapy is a somewhat mysterious process carried on somewhere other than the classroom. Some teachers may even be concerned that the therapist will be judging his or her teaching ability, and may feel threatened.

We must be prepared for whatever reaction the teacher may have. We must realize that there are *real* reasons why the reaction is occurring. Further, we must enter the process knowing that intervention is most successful when the teacher is willing and able to add his or her valuable knowledge and skills to the process. We must do whatever it takes to facilitate the development of a consultative partnership with the teacher. Above all, we must realize that the formation of this relationship can take a great deal of time. However, the benefits to the client, and to future students in the teacher's classroom, are well worth the time and energy invested.

Therapists, also, are sometimes hesitant to enter into a true consultative partnership. Many have told us that they feel that being a consultant requires that they be experts in a particular problem area, and that often they don't feel like experts. Others have felt that teaching is the teacher's business and that they have a separate role, which is to provide therapy. Others have expressed that "real therapy" involves "putting their hands on a client" and that working with the teacher, while it is important, is a secondary concern (Niehues, et al., in press). Still others have become confused by their perceptions that particular parents or teachers are demanding that a child's intervention be provided one-on-one. We believe that many of these fears and beliefs arise from therapists' misconceptions about consultation. Historically, occupational therapists have not been trained to be consultants. Further, very little literature exists in our field to assist us in developing these skills. Because we have not understood consultation clearly nor envisioned ourselves in a primary role as consultants, we have not been able to explain effectively the benefits of consultation to the parents and teachers with whom we work. As we have said earlier, we believe that the importance of the outcomes associated with consultation necessitates that we develop our skills in this area, and that we take a proactive stance with regard to consultation for our clients.

The phases of stage II are somewhat circular. That is, there is no particular order in which they must be accomplished. Rather, each "feeds into" the others. For the sake of simplicity we will begin with the phase in Figure 11–1 labeled "teacher and therapist test and adjust expectations"; we will discuss each phase as it appears in Figure 11–1, moving in a clockwise fashion.

## TESTING AND ADJUSTING EXPECTATIONS

It is not until the teacher and the therapist begin working together that they can begin to "test" and adjust their expectations of one another. That is, they begin to compare the stories they have created about the other individual with the "real" individual they are encountering. Expectations often are created about (a) the person with whom we will work, (b) the form the intervention will take, and (c) the anticipated outcomes of the intervention. As much as possible, we try to uncover the teacher's expectations as he or she enters into the consultation process. We use our skills to elicit the teacher's expectations in a non-threatening manner and we share some of our own expectations (Lilly & Silber, unpublished manuscript).

While learning about the teacher's expectations for consultation and the partnership, we listen and observe carefully to try to discern the teacher's preferred styles of thinking and interacting. We remain cognizant of our own typical styles and alter them as needed (DeBoer, 1986).

If the style and expectations of the teacher are somewhat similar to our own, we can move forward in building our relationship. However, what happens when, for example, the teacher's expectations for intervention do not include *any* relationship between the teacher and the therapist? In the following story, this is precisely what happened. Unlike Lily's experiences with Mrs. R and Mr. S, Lynn, the therapist in this story, never really felt that she was able to develop a true consultative relationship with Ms. M, the teacher. While Lynn did not attempt to pressure Ms. M into receiving consultation she didn't want, Lynn used several strategies that resulted in Ms. M's seeking consultation the following school year.

Kelly is a 7-year-old child with sensory integrative dysfunction manifested in somatodyspraxia and significant visuomotor and form and space deficits; she was mainstreamed in a regular first grade classroom. Because she had extreme difficulty with any classroom task that required motor output, Kelly qualified for occupational therapy services at school.

Kelly's individual educational program (IEP) called for her to receive occupational therapy twice weekly. Lynn was new to the district. When she went to see Kelly for the first time, she mentioned to Ms. M that she would like to provide direct intervention to Kelly once a week and spend the second period consulting with Ms. M. Ms. M responded immediately that she had understood that Lynn would remove Kelly from the classroom for both periods each week. Ms. M's "story" of therapy did not include any interaction between herself and the therapist. Ms. M hadn't realized that she would have to participate in any way and she did not leave Lynn with many choices.

Lynn decided to move very slowly; she responded by providing direct intervention to Kelly twice a week. However, each time she arrived at the classroom to get Kelly, she asked Ms. M what Kelly was having trouble with that she might address in therapy. She frequently took math papers to work on, adapting them so that Kelly could figure out where to place the answers. Each time she returned Kelly to the classroom, Lynn spent a few minutes telling Ms. M what they had accomplished, and sharing the adaptations she had tried to allow Kelly to complete a particular assignment.

One day when Lynn arrived, Ms. M handed her a math assignment and told her she would like to have it done when Kelly came back. Lynn responded by telling Ms. M, again, how she had been using the papers to work on Kelly's form and space abilities, in a functional way, and that she did not feel qualified to teach her math. Ms. M seemed a little offended, but the next time Lynn arrived Ms. M shared with her that Kelly was having a lot of trouble with phonics. She asked if Lynn could incorporate phonics into her occupational therapy treatment activities. Lynn said that she could. She and Kelly spent time doing an eye-hand coordination activity in which Kelly used a magnetized fishing pole to "fish" for different letter sounds. When she and Kelly returned to the classroom, they both excitedly told Ms. M about what they had done.

Ms. M began to think of other concepts that could be incorporated into Kelly's therapy. Gradually, she began to ask Lynn's advice about various classroom activities, such as cutting with scissors. This was the breakthrough for which Lynn had been hoping. She responded by coming into the classroom during several art activities. She took the opportunity to work with Kelly, but she also adapted the task for several other students who seemed to be having difficulty.

The following school year, Lynn treated another student in Ms. M's class. When Lynn approached Ms. M about the schedule, *Ms. M suggested* that maybe a part of the time devoted to this student's therapy could be spent consulting with her.

Clearly, Ms. M's expectations of occupational therapy changed markedly because of her interactions with Lynn and Kelly. The process of changing those expectations took a considerable amount of time, but by the beginning of the second year, Ms. M and Lynn were well on the way to establishing a real partnership. Initially, Lynn had been able to recognize that she could not implement the consulting program she had envisioned for Kelly. However, she still devoted a few minutes each week to telling Ms. M about occupational therapy as it related to Kelly. Lynn went out of her way to find out how she might tailor her therapy to meet Kelly's needs in the classroom. By viewing the situation as a challenge and by being assertive, she won Ms. M over. Ms. M learned a great deal about occupational therapy; she gained new respect for Lynn; and she learned something about how Lynn's training in occupational therapy could help her to change the classroom environment so that it better met the needs of her students.

## REFINING THE PROBLEM

Another important part of Stage II involves our eliciting from the teacher as much detail as we can about the problem the teacher is experiencing in attempting to teach the student. That is, we refine the problem. We keep asking questions and making observations until we can pinpoint a solvable problem, and until we know whether it is a problem we can "explain" by our theories and that together we have the expertise to solve. We want to find out as much as we can about how the student's sensory integrative dysfunction is impairing his or her ability to benefit fully from the educational experience, and in what ways the student is able to compensate for his or her difficulties. We also begin to explore what resources we will need.

In this phase, we must use caution not to insinuate that anyone is responsible for the problem. We must be mindful of the fact that the source of a child's difficulties is hard to pinpoint.

## REFRAMING THE PROBLEM

Also, in this stage, we use sensory integration (or another) theory to reframe the problem that the teacher has described. We have described reframing in some detail above. However, to reiterate, it is important that we listen carefully to the difficulties the teacher is describing and address our comments to these difficulties. In the above example of Lily and Mrs. R, Lily listened carefully to Mrs. R's problem teaching Charlie to write cursive letters. She observed Charlie in his classroom and interpreted the results of his testing in light of what she saw and heard. Lily then explained Charlie's dyspraxia as it applied to handwriting. She did not attempt to give too much detail by explaining the neuroanatomy of the tactile or vestibular-proprioceptive systems. Rather, Lily made it clear that there is a *hypothesized* causal relationship between sensory feedback from the body as it moves and the child's ability to learn new motor tasks. She told Mrs. R that the tests Charlie took revealed that he had difficulty processing information about touch and body movement. Lily then went on to show Mrs. R that the handwriting tasks she had created for Charlie required many new motor plans rather than just one for each letter. With the frame shifted in this way, Mrs. R saw Charlie's problems in a new light. This new frame also suggested possible strategies for Mrs. R and Lily to explore together.

## IDENTIFYING OBSTACLES

The final phase of the second stage of consultation requires that the teacher and therapist identify the obstacles that may interfere with their effecting a change. Scheduling sufficient time to meet together when the teacher is not worried about what is going on in her classroom, or the therapist thinking about traveling to the next school, is a commonly encountered obstacle. We must remember that the decision to provide consultation was a team decision, and the team has the responsibility to provide, within reason, the resources needed for the consultation to be effective. Thus, we must ask for the resources that will be needed.

If it is not possible to schedule uninterrupted time before or after school, or during lunch breaks, it may be necessary for the principal or some other adult to take responsibility for the teacher's class while we consult with him or her. This is the strategy Lily and Mrs. R used when they found that it was impossible to be free at the same time. Lily explained to the building principal what she hoped to accomplish and why she needed a particular block of time. The principal agreed that he, or another adult, would be free during that time period.

The principal was willing to provide support to Mrs. R and Lily once he had been informed of the problem. Had Lily not gone to talk with him, he probably would have remained unaware that there was a problem and Lily and Mrs. R might have compromised their plans for consultation needlessly. Further, it was Lily's, rather than Mrs. R's, responsibility to approach the principal since it is our responsibility to insure that we have the necessary resources to conduct intervention. Lily did so, however, with Mrs. R's knowledge and approval.

Bundy, Lawlor, Kielhofner, and Knecht (1989) recently reported the results of a large national survey of special-education administrators. When asked what one thing therapists could do to improve their effectiveness in public schools, these administrators commonly answered, "Be more assertive." We should not take this suggestion lightly. In order to provide high-quality consultation to teachers, we need the support of the educational team and the administration. Unless we make our needs known, they will not be met.

## SUMMARY

Four phases comprise Stage II (Establishing a Partnership) of the consultation process. The formation of the consultative partnership is, perhaps, the most crucial phase in the consultation process. To be effective at this stage, we must strive to demonstrate our respect for our educator colleagues and their knowledge and skills, our willingness to respect the constraints of their positions, and our ability to share what we know in a way that is meaningful to them (Bundy et al., 1989). Sometimes this stage flows so smoothly that we are hardly aware that we have passed through it. However, when we become aware that the consultation process feels uncomfortable or is not yielding the strategies we had hoped for, we should examine the phases associated with this stage to determine where the process went awry.

## Stage III: Planning Strategies

In Stage III of the consultation process, the therapist-teacher partners use the new frame together to examine and select strategies for the teacher to use in intervening with the student. If the groundwork has been laid well in the previous stages (that is, the underlying problems have been identified correctly and the partnership firmly established), and the therapist has access to a repertoire of strategies for addressing the difficulties commonly encountered by students with sensory integrative dysfunction, it should be *relatively* easy to develop strategies to address these difficulties.

In the above example, Lily, having explained that Charlie was not getting adequate feedback from his body as he wrote, suggested a different kind of writing implement. When the problem of Charlie's not pressing down hard enough with his pencil persisted, Lily and Mrs. R decided he should use carbon paper when he wrote. Without it, Charlie did not seem to get enough feedback from his body or from the paper he was writing on to determine how hard was "hard enough." By giving him the carbon paper, "hard enough" became defined as hard enough to make the marks appear on the paper underneath. This was the kind of feedback from which Charlie could benefit. He was able to lift the carbon paper periodically by himself to make sure that he was writing "hard enough." Consequently, Mrs. R was freed from having to continually stand over him and give him verbal feedback.

This mutually developed strategy was agreeable to everyone. While, ideally, all strategies would be mutually developed and agreeable to both the therapist and the teacher, we must keep in mind that the problems we are addressing are problems *the teacher* feels need to be corrected. Moreover, the teacher is the one who must implement the strategies. In cases where the teacher and the therapist cannot come to a mutually agreeable solution, *the needs and wishes of the teacher should take precedence.*

As part of her role in the partnership, Lily provided alternative writing utensils and paper. These materials were not really "adaptive equipment," per se. However, we may find that one important role we play in the planning stage is to provide the teacher and student with adaptive or alternative devices and materials. This is an important tool of consultation and a way of modifying the environment so that it better fits the needs of the student with sensory integrative dysfunction.

## Stage IV: Implementing and Assessing the Plan

In the final stage of the consultation process, the teacher implements the plan developed in consultation, and the teacher and therapist mutually evaluate its effectiveness and modify the plan as necessary. This stage is fairly self-explanatory. However, as in the previous stage, it is important to recognize that the teacher is responsible for implementing the plan; therefore, no matter how well *we* think something is working, *if the teacher is not comfortable with it, the plan must be modified.*

There are many reasons why a strategy may not feel comfortable to a particular teacher. Perhaps it does not reflect his or her teaching style or values. Perhaps the teacher just needs to practice the strategy until it becomes more "his or her own."

Perhaps the teacher needs to see someone "model" the strategy before implementing it him- or herself. Perhaps the strategy just isn't practical. It is important that the teacher and therapist try to uncover what is causing the teacher's discomfort with a strategy, so that the appropriate changes can be made. The solution to the problem when the teacher needs a model is very different from the solution when the problem is that the teacher just needs practice. We need to be careful not to give up on a strategy because it does not work the first time. However, we also need to be careful to work with the teacher to modify the strategy when it is clear that it is the wrong strategy.

## RESOURCES REQUIRED FOR CONSULTATION

All service provision requires resources; consultation is no exception. Without the proper resources, it is unlikely that consultation will be effective. Thus, to some extent, a discussion of the required resources also describes some of the limitations of consultation.

The success of consultation centers on the ability to build the relationship between the participants. This depends, in large part, on the skills and commitment of the individuals involved, and the time available to them. Because consultation requires a partnership, a relationship of equals, the skills needed to build and maintain it are particularly important. Each participant must respect the other's skills and knowledge, and demonstrate that respect openly. Participants must communicate regularly and the therapist must actively listen to the problems the consultee is experiencing (De Boer, 1986). The participants must believe that between them they have the skills and commitment to solve the problem. Both of the participants must feel comfortable with their own skills and professional identities; each must feel free to admit when he or she does not know an answer (Niehues et al., in press). Each must be willing to take risks and to credit the other for the contribution he or she makes to the improvement of the client. In addition, the therapist must be willing to ask for, and obtain, the administrative support required to facilitate the development of the consultative relationship.

If, as happens on rare occasions, it is impossible to form a partnership, then consultation cannot be effective and should not be implemented. However, we believe that this rarely occurs. Good consultation is designed to resolve problems that the *consultee*, not necessarily the therapist, is facing. The therapist may need to invest considerable time and energy to establish and maintain the consultative partnership, but usually it can be done.

## SUMMARY

In consultation, we offer others (e.g., parents, teachers) access to sensory integration theory as a way of understanding the client's behaviors differently. Once the client's behaviors have been "reframed," the therapist can assist the parent or teacher to develop new strategies for interacting effectively with the client.

The expected outcome of consultation is that the client's human and non-human environment changes such that it more closely reflects the needs of the client. In other words, consultation enables the client to succeed in his or her own environment despite the limitations imposed by the sensory integrative dysfunction.

# REFERENCES

American Occupational Therapy Association (1989). *Guidelines for occupational therapy services in school systems* (2nd ed.). Rockville, MD: Author.

Bundy, A. C. & Kielhofner, G. (1988, October). *A conceptual model of school system practice for occupational and physical therapists.* Paper presented at the US Department of Education, Office of Special Education and Rehabilitation Services, Washington, DC.

Bundy, A. C., Lawlor, M. C., Kielhofner, G., & Knecht, H. (1989, April). *Educational and therapeutic perceptions of school system practice.* Paper presented at the Annual Conference of the American Occupational Therapy Association, Baltimore, MD.

De Boer, A. L. (1986). *The art of consulting.* Chicago: Arcturus Books.

Dunn, W. (1989, April). *A comparison of service provision patterns in occupational therapy.* Paper presented at the annual conference of the American Occupational Therapy Association, Baltimore, MD.

Fisher, A. G., & Bundy, A. C. (1989). Vestibular stimulation in the treatment of postural and related disorders. In O. D. Payton, R. P. Fabio, S. V. Paris, E. J. Protas, & A. F. Van Sant (Eds.), *Manual of physical therapy techniques* (pp. 239–258). New York: Churchill Livingstone.

G. & C. Merriam Company. (1981). *Webster's new collegiate dictionary.* Springfield, MA: Author.

Golden, J. (1987). *Luria-Nebraska Neuropsychological Battery: Children's Revision.* Los Angeles: Western Psychological Services.

Good, B., & Good, M. D. (1981). The meaning of symptoms: A cultural hermeneutic model for clinical practice. In I. Eisenberg & A. Kleinman (Eds.), *The relevance of social science for medicine* (pp. 165–196). Boston: Reidel.

Mattingly, C. F. (1989). *Thinking with stories: Story and experience in a clinical practice.* Unpublished doctoral dissertation, Massachusetts Institute of Technology, Boston.

Niehues, A. N., Bundy, A. C., Mattingly, C. F., & Lawlor, M. C. (in press). Making a difference: Occupational therapy in public schools. *Occupational Therapy Journal of Research.*

Schön, D. (1983). *The reflective practitioner: How professionals think in action.* New York: Basic Books.

Schön, D. (1987). *Educating the reflective practitioner.* San Francisco: Jossey-Bass.

# CHAPTER 12

# The Process of Planning and Implementing Intervention

**Anita C. Bundy, ScD, OTR**

*"Would you tell me, please," [asked Alice,] "which way I ought to walk from here?"*
*That depends a good deal on where you want to get to," said the Cat.*
*"I don't much care where — " said Alice.*
*"Then it doesn't matter which way you walk," said the Cat.*
*"——so long as I get somewhere," Alice added as an explanation.*
*"Oh, you're sure to do that," said the Cat, "if you only walk long enough."*

*Carroll, 1923, p. 68*

The intervention process comprises two phases, planning and implementation. Each of these phases depends on the other for its effectiveness. That is, unless implementation is preceded by well-constructed plans, intervention becomes haphazard, at best, and chaotic or harmful, at worst. Similarly, unless planning is followed by skillful implementation, the plan dies.

Developing a plan to address the specific needs of a client with sensory integrative dysfunction is the *most essential component* of the intervention process. The intervention plan is comprised of three parts: (a) setting the goals and objectives, (b) determining the type, or types, of service delivery that will be used when providing the intervention (e.g., direct service, consultation), and (c) developing preliminary ideas about intervention. Having a plan ensures that intervention is carried out in (a) a way that is mutually agreeable to the therapist, the client, and, if the client is a child, to his or her caregivers; and (b) an orderly, efficient, and effective fashion.

While developing the plan, the therapist thinks in a logical, deductive manner (Rogers & Masagatani, 1982). Based on a synthesis of information gathered during the evaluation and knowledge of occupational therapy practice models, we collaborate with the client (and his or her caregivers) to set goals to minimize or eliminate the presenting problems. Having established general goals, we engage the client and his or her caregivers in a discussion to determine objectives representative of those goals. That is, we seek to learn, specifically, how the client would *behave* differently or what he or she would like to be able to *do*, following treatment, that he or she cannot currently do. Based on the goals and objectives formulated and on the realistic constraints of the system within which we work, we recommend an intervention plan to meet these goals. That is, we reason that certain goals can best be met by consultation, whereas others can be met better through direct service (Bundy, 1990).

Further, we develop a general idea about the kinds of activities that can be used to meet the goal, the desired physical layout for intervention, and the types of interactions we wish to foster. If, for example, a child has hypotonia and decreased postural stability from a vestibular-proprioceptive processing deficit, we may reason that we will incorporate activities that provide linear vestibular stimulation into direct intervention. If the same child also is distractible at school, we may reason that we should work with the teacher to modify the classroom environment to reduce the number of distractions. The client and his or her caregivers, having helped to shape each decision in the planning, then respond to our recommendations by stating their own constraints (e.g., finances, time). Together with the client, we modify the recommendations until a working plan is established.

Intervention proceeds in the manner suggested by the plan. While this idea may seem rather simplistic, the process of translating the plan into action requires a kind of reasoning quite different from that employed during the development of the plan.

That is, while the logic demanded by the planning process is fairly linear, the logic demanded when conducting the intervention can be described much better as dialogic reasoning, or a kind of ongoing "conversation" between the therapist and the client (Mattingly, 1989). To a great extent, this conversation is a non-verbal exchange. In this process, we set up the environment in such a way as to encourage the client to seek activities that will promote his or her own development (self-actualization). Then, guided by the client, we skillfully introduce particular activities and watch to see how the client responds. We modify the activities ever so slightly and examine the results, asking ourselves whether the changes produced the results desired. We reflect on our actions and those of the client *as they occur*; then, we modify the approach accordingly (Schön, 1983, 1987).

## PURPOSE AND SCOPE

In this chapter, we will illustrate the development of an intervention plan and its implementation with Steven, the child whose evaluation data we presented in Chapter 9. We will "walk through" each step and comment on the process. We will discuss not only those aspects of the intervention that went "according to plan," but also some of the difficulties we encountered as we attempted to translate our plan into action. In this process, we will demonstrate how the therapist both reflects-in-action and reflects-on-action (Schön, 1983, 1987). (See also Chapter 2 for more information about these different types of reflections.)

## STEVEN REVISITED

The reader will recall that Steven is a 6½-year-old boy who lives with his parents, brother, and two sisters; Steven is the second child. Steven's parents, Mr. and Mrs. P, are very sensitive to the subtle differences between Steven's behavior and that of his brother and sisters. His mother has provided us with a clear description of Steven and has described her concerns about him. She believes that Steven has two primary areas of difficulty, his distractible and overly active behavior and his motor incoordination. She thinks that these two problem areas have resulted in Steven's feeling bad about himself and having few friends. Steven's negative self-concept is Mrs. P's greatest concern.

For our part, we have evaluated Steven using the Sensory Integration and Praxis Tests (SIPT) (Ayres, 1989) and related clinical observations of neuromotor performance. We also have observed Steven at school. We have concluded that Steven's difficulties are based, at least in part, on sensory integrative dysfunction. More specifically, Steven appears to have a vestibular-proprioceptive processing disorder that is manifested by a postural-ocular movement disorder. In turn, his poor vestibular-proprioceptive processing appears to have resulted in a bilateral integration and sequencing disorder and in poor visuomotor skills, constructional abilities, and form and space perception. Further, Steven shows signs of tactile defensiveness and some difficulty with the modulation of auditory input; he also is highly distractible and overly active. We have explained our findings to Mrs. P and interpreted her concerns in light of these findings. (See Chapter 9 for additional information.)

When we completed our evaluation, we specified options for intervention and made certain *preliminary* recommendations to Mrs. P. For example, we recommended that Steven obtain direct intervention in a clinic setting and we encouraged Mrs. P to seek consultation services from the occupational therapist at Steven's school. Mr. and Mrs. P spent a couple of days thinking about our report and talking over our recommendations. They then made an appointment with us to discuss formulating goals and developing a specific plan.

## SETTING GOALS AND DEVELOPING OBJECTIVES

We began our meeting with Steven's parents by telling them that we wanted them to work with us to formulate the goals for Steven's intervention. In other words, we wanted to know what *specific* things they wanted Steven to be able to do, in order for all of us to know that Steven had made progress as a result of intervention. We set a 6-month time frame as a guide for these predictions.

We reiterated for Steven's parents those things that we thought they had expressed as their major concerns about Steven. We tried to explain the relationships between those concerns, as we understood them, and asked for confirmation, clarification, and correction of our perceptions.

We believed that his parents' major concern about Steven was that he did not feel very good about himself or his skills. They were worried about the effect that his negative sense of self would have as he grew older. We believed that there were two major areas contributing to Steven's negative beliefs about himself. These were (a) his poor motor coordination, which interfered with Steven's ability to perform the same kinds of skilled activities that his peers performed easily; and (b) his distractibility and the level of his activity, which resulted in Steven's being reprimanded more frequently than his peers or his brother and sisters. Mr. and Mrs. P agreed with this assessment. We all agreed that our goals should reflect each of these major areas of concern.

## Modifying Steven's Expectations About Himself

We believed that Steven's expectation that he would fail was both a cause of some of his difficulties and the result of others. Because Steven knew that he lacked many of the skills he needed, he avoided certain activities; in avoiding them, he deprived himself of the opportunity to develop and practice his skills. He fell further and further behind his peers and came to believe, even more firmly, that he was not equal to his peers. When he was forced to do activities that he knew he couldn't do well (such as handwriting), he became anxious about performing and his performance deteriorated. When he became anxious, he also became overaroused. Steven, who always had difficulty modulating incoming sensory information, became even more overwhelmed. His behavior further deteriorated, and he was reprimanded for behaving badly. As a result, he had more reason to believe that he was "bad," and that others also viewed him that way. (See also Chapter 2.)

Mr. and Mrs. P concurred with this line of reasoning. They punctuated our conversation with examples that illustrated our developing "theory" of Steven's beliefs and behavior.

Based on our jointly held perceptions, we proposed to Mr. and Mrs. P that one general goal for our intervention would be to help Steven to *develop a belief that he will succeed at activities that he values and that are appropriate for his age.* Steven's parents thought this was an important goal. However, we wanted to be sure that we could evaluate Steven's progress toward meeting that goal at the end of 6 months' time. That is, we needed to formulate specific objectives for intervention.

Thus, we asked Mr. and Mrs. P what kinds of things they thought Steven would *do* that would tell them that he had changed his perceptions of his skills. How would Steven *act* differently if he believed that he would succeed? What activities were both important to him and reflected skills appropriate to his age? We were unable to answer these questions fully by ourselves; only Mr. and Mrs. P could fill in the details that would make the goal both meaningful and measurable. We *did* suggest that we would set as one objective Steven's actively *selecting at least one activity that requires age-appropriate skills during each direct intervention session.* Mrs. P indicated that she would know that Steven felt better about his skills when *he willingly went off to play with other children in the neighborhood who are about his age, at least once a week.*

We all recognized that these objectives might be difficult to meet, but they exemplified for us how Steven would act as he began to feel better about himself. They were all things that we cared about. Further, we understood that objectives are a way of organizing our actions; they are predictions, not contracts. If Steven did not accomplish these objectives, we would reexamine them to determine whether it was our predictions that were out of line or our methodology that was ineffective. Because the objectives we specified were readily observable, all of us would be able to determine whether or not they had been met. We needed only to attend carefully to the evidence that he was or was not actively selecting a different kind of activity and playing more with his peers.

### AN ASIDE ABOUT DEFINING OBJECTIVES

The reader may not agree that the objectives of selecting an age-appropriate activity during treatment, and willingly going off with children his own age, adequately reflect the goal of Steven's developing a belief that he will succeed at activities that he values and that are appropriate for his age. It is not important that the objectives, developed to define achievement of a goal established by a team, necessarily be agreeable to individuals who were not members of that team. It *is* important, however, that *all members of the team agree* that the objectives are reflective of the goals they have established (Mager, 1972) and that they all are able to measure those objectives (Mager, 1975).

Further, we do not feel that it is important that we write objectives for *every* behavior related to self-concept (or any other function) that might change as a result of intervention. We feel that it is far more critical that we target *a few really meaningful objectives* and work toward those with all of our collective efforts. We then measure improvement in those areas as representative of the larger goal of improving his beliefs about his skills. Steven might well make other gains in this area, and they may be equally important, but they would not have objectives attached to them.

## Improving Steven's Motor Skills

Both of Steven's parents expressed very real concerns that Steven develop new motor skills that would enable him to complete his schoolwork more easily and to *enjoy* playing the kinds of games and activities that his peers clearly loved. We agreed that *improving Steven's motor skills* was an important general goal. However, once again, we were at a loss to create specific objectives without access to the important information that only Steven and his parents had. That is, what specific skills did Steven *most* need to develop? What should Steven be able to do better, in 6 months, that would enable all of us to say that he had made progress as a result of intervention? And, what would it *look like* if he performed a particular skill *better*?

We discussed this area for some time. His parents focused on such skills as riding his bicycle, pumping a swing, throwing a ball, catching a ball, handwriting, and buttoning. We talked about what seemed to be preventing him from doing each of those skills easily. We reiterated that we were interested in selecting only the one or two skills that everyone (most importantly, Steven) thought were most important. We felt certain that if Steven changed in the ways we specified, he also would develop other skills simultaneously. These would be equally important, but we viewed them as an added bonus.

Steven's parents indicated that Steven had, on numerous occasions, expressed a desire to be able to make the swing go, by himself. That way he could play on it as long as he wanted, rather than having to stop because his parents were tired of pushing him or had to do something else. Further, Steven loved swinging, but he was acutely aware that his 5-year-old sister, Laura, had learned some time ago to pump the swing by herself and his 4-year-old brother could nearly do it, too. Thus, we decided that our objective would be that Steven *independently propel a swing by pumping.*

### AN ASIDE ABOUT SPECIFYING CRITERIA FOR OBJECTIVES

The reader who is familiar with the parts of a behavioral objective (i.e., learner, behavior, condition, criterion) will notice that we have not defined a criterion for measuring this objective. That is, we have not specified how well Steven will have to propel his swing in order for us to say that he has met this objective (e.g., four out of five attempts). In our experience, the issue with pumping a swing is simply learning to do it. Once the child knows what it feels like to work *with* the swing, the child can swing until he or she tires of the activity. Thus, we did not feel that the specification of a criterion was necessary. Because no criterion is specified, we will assume that he will be able to do it whenever he wants. Since that really is our intent for Steven, the lack of a criterion does not present a problem.

Mrs. P also expressed particular concern about Steven's poor handwriting. She felt that the inordinate difficulty he had with writing caused him to be slow and messy when working at his desk in school. This, in turn, resulted in his being made to repeat his work or receiving negative feedback from his teacher. Many times he brought home papers with the word "messy" written across the top.

We agreed with Mrs. P that *improved handwriting* was an appropriate goal for Steven. Again, we began the process of discovering what *exactly* Mrs. P meant by this goal. Should Steven be able to write faster? If so, how fast? Should he be able to form letters more legibly? And, if so, what would constitute legibility? After discussing this, it became clear that Mrs. P actually hoped that Steven would improve in both areas; however, she recognized that he probably could not accomplish both within 6 months' time. We told her that, in our experience, a child who wrote quickly could learn to write more legibly. However, a child who became overly concerned with legibility often had a particularly difficult time learning to write more quickly. We all agreed that the more important immediate objective for Steven was to *complete at least three of four written assignments within the allotted class time.*

## Improving Steven's Behavior

Steven's behavior (his distractibility, level of activity, and tendency too lash out at other children who bumped into him inadvertently) was a major concern for his parents and teacher. Steven's behavior "got in his way" more obviously than did anything else; it was probably the greatest single reason for the negative feedback he got from the adults and children around him. Thus, we all readily agreed that *improving Steven's behavior* was an appropriate general goal.

We explored this difficulty more fully with Mr. and Mrs. P so that we could formulate the most relevant objectives. We asked them to tell us about circumstances when Steven's behavior was most problematic (e.g., circumstances that occurred particularly frequently, were unavoidable, or in which his behavior was especially intolerable to those around him). Again, we asked how Steven would *behave* differently, in the next 6 months, if he was making progress as a result of intervention?

Mr. and Mrs. P talked about Steven's behavior at some length. They mentioned the difficulties they had taking him to restaurants, shopping malls, and their friends' homes. In the end, Mr. and Mrs. P concluded that, although all of these circumstances created difficulties for them, they had learned to manage these situations. For example, when they anticipated that the situation would be particularly loud or crowded (such as a shopping mall during a holiday season), one of them either stayed home with Steven (and often one or more of the other children) or they left some or all of the children with a sitter. They tried to take "whole family outings" to places where they knew Steven would not be overstimulated or overwhelmed; they knew many such places that Steven really enjoyed.

Steven's parents were most concerned about his behavior at school. Nearly every week, Steven's teacher called, or sent a note home, about Steven's fighting or his inattention to his work. Thus, we created one objective that *Steven would not hit classmates who bumped into him accidentally at school.*

### ANOTHER ASIDE ON CRITERIA

The astute reader will note that the comments we made above pertaining to the lack of a specified criterion in the objective apply here also. Since we have not specified a criterion, we will assume that when Steven meets the objective, he will *never* hit a classmate who accidentally jostles him. This is precisely the criteria we have in mind. Although Mager (1975) indicated that perfect performance is rarely achievable, we believe that in this case it would be nonsensical to write an objective that said that Steven would only hit a classmate once a month or once a year. Hitting another child because he or she accidentally bumps into you is *never* an acceptable behavior. Further, Steven is not a child who has a serious problem with violent outbursts; his mother indicated that his fighting occurs about twice a month and is triggered by very predictable occurrences. Therefore, we believe that the objective, as specified, is attainable. We expect that Steven, like most other children, may occasionally "backslide." However, our objective for him is that he not respond to accidental touch by hitting.

Besides fighting, the other significant aspect of Steven's behavior at school that Mr. and Mrs. P had mentioned was his inattention to his work. When questioned about what exactly that meant, they indicated that Steven's teacher complained that he rarely got his work finished on time. We decided that the objective (already specified under the goal to improve his motor skills) that Steven would *complete at least three out of four written assignments within the allotted class time* also was a behavior that pertained equally well to the goal of improving his behavior. Thus, we listed it under this goal also.

## Summary

Together with Mr. and Mrs. P, we formulated five important objectives that will guide our intervention over the next 6 months. Although this process was difficult and time-consuming, it was well worth the effort. It helped all of us to clarify our thinking and to make explicit those things that were the most desirable outcomes of intervention. Mr. and Mrs. P also expressed that the process had assisted them in making decisions about the things on which to work hard with Steven during the next several months. They indicated that, prior to our discussion, they felt guilty if they didn't try to teach Steven to do something better or differently each time they interacted with him. Yet at the same time, they felt that he needed time to "just be himself." They were relieved to finally sit down and talk with someone who understood Steven and who could help them to make decisions and a plan about how to concentrate their efforts.

We want to emphasize that there is nothing magic about the number five with reference to the creation of objectives. In fact, we feel that five is *about the maximum number* of objectives that should be specified for a short time period such as 6 months. We feel that *a small number of representative and meaningful objectives* form the basis for a much more cohesive plan than would a large number of objectives that reflected the detailed sequence of development in which we expect Steven to progress.

Two points regarding objectives cannot be emphasized strongly enough. First, *objectives belong to the client*; unless they are meaningful, they are pointless. Second, *treatment is "driven" by objectives.* As the Cheshire Cat from *Alice in Wonderland* (Carroll, 1923) reminded us at the beginning of this chapter, if you're not sure where you're going, it doesn't matter how you get there. If you walk long enough, you're sure to get somewhere — but that somewhere might not be desirable, and surely a lot of time will be wasted on the journey. In our intervention, we care both about where we are going and how we are going to get there. We are interested in improving Steven's (and other clients') abilities to perform their daily roles and tasks in as effective and efficient a manner as possible. Thus, we must develop, and follow, a meaningful plan.

## DETERMINING TYPES OF SERVICE DELIVERY

Having formulated our objectives, we then went on to determine what types of service (i.e., consultation, direct intervention, indirect intervention) we would use to meet each objective. We explained to Steven's parents that direct service meant that the therapist intervened directly with Steven in order to change his skills. We said that consultation meant that the therapist intervened with them (his parents) or with the teacher in order to (a) help those individuals understand Steven's needs better and (b) develop more effective strategies for working with Steven. In indirect service, we explained, the therapist teaches the parent or teacher a simple procedure that they, in turn, conduct with Steven. (See Chapter 11.) We also explained that the same therapist could readily serve all three roles in order to meet the objectives in the most effective way.

Steven was fortunate in that he was eligible to receive occupational therapy services at school in addition to those that he would receive in our clinic. We recommended that Mr. and Mrs. P request that the occupational therapist at school serve a primary role as a consultant to Steven's teacher and a secondary role as a direct service provider (for the times when Steven needed to practice a new skill at school). We further recommended that Colleen, the therapist in our clinic, serve in a primary role as a direct service provider and secondarily as a consultant to the family and as an indirect service provider when she developed a home program. We explained that Colleen would remain in contact with the school therapist to assure that the services Steven received were complementary. We also explained that the therapist at school, along with the special education team, would undoubtedly set some additional objectives. However, we used the objectives we had developed together to demonstrate to Mr. and Mrs. P how the two therapists would serve complementary roles. The suggestions we presented to Mr. and Mrs. P are summarized in Table 12–1.

Mr. and Mrs. P agreed with our recommendations. They explained that Steven's Individualized Education Program (IEP) team meeting was in another week, and they were glad to have had an opportunity to participate in goal-setting before that meeting. They indicated that they would take the goals we had established together to the meeting and have them incorporated into Steven's Individualized Education Program.

## DEVELOPING PRELIMINARY IDEAS FOR USE IN INTERVENTION

In preparation for Steven's first treatment session, Colleen, the occupational therapist, thought about three things: (a) the types of activities that would best address his needs, (b) the physical layout of the equipment in the clinic, and (c) the types of interactions she hoped to have with Steven. In each case, she wanted to maximize Steven's participation in, and ability to benefit from, intervention. Although these aspects of Steven's direct intervention will become inextricably linked in the experience of the treatment session, each is important enough to be considered separately. Further, slightly different purposes are associated with each of

**TABLE 12–1. COMPARISON OF CONTRIBUTIONS OF CLINIC OT AND SCHOOL OT TO MEETING STEVEN'S OBJECTIVES**

| Goal | Objective | Clinic OT* | School OT† |
|------|-----------|------------|------------|
| Develop belief that he will succeed | Actively select at least one activity that requires age-appropriate skills, during each direct intervention session. | Set up environment; provide Steven with knowledge of available equipment and toys; facilitate and monitor choices; grade activities carefully so that Steven improves his skills; point out improvements to Steven. | |
| Develop belief that he will succeed | Willingly go off to play with other children in the neighborhood, who are about his age, at least once a week. | Work with Steven's mother to develop strategies for teaching Steven skills to enter a group of children; work with Steven's mother to identify activities in which one of Steven's peers could be included (consider including a peer in clinic sessions). | Work with Steven's teacher to develop strategies for teaching Steven skills to enter a group of children; work with Steven's teacher to develop activities in which Steven has a partner; work with Steven to develop particular skills he needs in play with other children. |
| Improve motor skills | Independently propel a swing by pumping. | *Improve bilateral integration and ability to plan and produce sequenced projected limb movements*; work on his ability to propel swings in the clinic; point out similarities between clinic swings and playground swings. | Encourage Steven's teacher to help Steven with this skill. |
| Improve motor skills (handwriting); Improve behavior | Complete at least three of four written assignments within the allotted class time. | *Improve postural stability* so his posture improves at his desk; *improve bilateral integration and ability to plan and produce sequenced projected limb movements; improve visuomotor skills; improve ability to modulate incoming sensory information;* design home program specifically addressing handwriting speed. | Work with Steven's teacher to rearrange the classroom so that Steven's workspace is in a quieter area; work with Steven's teacher to adapt assignments as needed; provide adaptive equipment as needed. |

*(continued)*

**TABLE 12-1. COMPARISON OF CONTRIBUTIONS OF CLINIC OT AND SCHOOL OT TO MEETING STEVEN'S OBJECTIVES** (*continued*)

| Goal | Objective | Clinic OT* | School OT† |
|------|-----------|------------|------------|
| Improve behavior | Not hit classmates who bump into him accidentally. | *Improve ability to modulate incoming sensory information;* explain tactile defensiveness and sensory modulation disorders to Steven and his parents in terms they understand; talk to Steven about strategies he might use when he is feeling "overwhelmed"; work with Steven's parents so that they can help Steven develop effective strategies. | Explain relationship between Steven's behavior, tactile defensiveness and sensory modulation disorders in educational terms; work with Steven's teacher to rearrange the classroom so that Steven's workspace is in an area with less traffic; work with Steven's teacher to explore and find alternatives to other circumstances when fighting is a problem (e.g., standing in line). |

*Primary role: direct intervention; secondary roles: consultant to family, indirect intervention.
†Primary role: consultant to teacher; secondary role: direct intervention.

these aspects of direct intervention, therefore, we will discuss each briefly before we illustrate how they are integrated into the treatment experience.

## Selecting Activities

In developing ideas about activities that she might use in Steven's treatment, Colleen was aware of the need to consider both the types of enhanced sensory stimulation that she would incorporate into the activity and the adaptive behaviors she was seeking. She planned to address four primary areas in Steven's direct intervention. These areas are italicized in Table 12-1 in the column describing the methods to be used by the clinic therapist. They include (a) postural stability, (b) bilateral integration and sequencing of projected limb movements, (c) visuomotor skill, and (d) modulation of sensory information.

Sensory integration theory suggests that Steven's difficulties with postural stability and bilateral integration and sequencing of projected limb movements should be addressed by activities that provide opportunities for him to take in enhanced vestibular-proprioceptive information. More specifically, the theory suggests that opportunities to take in linear vestibular-proprioceptive information in the context of activities that demand sustained postural control (in a variety of positions) and coordinated use of both sides of the body, will be most appropriate for Steven's treatment. (See Chapter 4.)

Although sensory integration theory indicates that difficulties with visuomotor skill may stem from difficulties in processing *any* type of sensory information, the results of Steven's evaluation suggested that his visuomotor difficulties also were sequelae to his poor processing of vestibular-proprioceptive information. Thus,

Colleen planned to build visuomotor demands into the activities she created for Steven's treatment.

Steven's difficulties with the modulation of sensory information presented Colleen with a dilemma about the direction she should take in his treatment. Steven is tactually defensive; he also shows some signs of defensiveness to auditory information. Sensory integration theory suggests that the most direct approach to remediating his tactile defensiveness is by providing opportunities for Steven to take in enhanced deep touch-pressure in the context of activities that require him to respond adaptively. Colleen might do this either by covering the surfaces of the swings and other equipment that Steven will use in the clinic, or by creating activities where Steven rubs his arms and legs firmly with a textured mitt or a paint brush. Since his difficulties with modulating incoming sensory information seem to cause particular difficulties for Steven in his everyday life, Colleen might even consider "imposing" (on a trial basis) some form of tactile scrubbing on him repeatedly during his day, following a program such as that recommended by Wilbarger and Royeen (1987) and described more fully in Chapters 5 and 10.

The "best solution" to the dilemma of addressing Steven's difficulties with the modulation of sensory information has not yet been clearly spelled out in sensory integration theory. Colleen therefore made her decision based on what she knew of Steven, and on what she has learned from other clients with problems similar to Steven's. She developed a working hypothesis about the best way to address this difficulty, and she created and implemented activities that reflected her hypothesis. As with all of her strategies for intervention, Colleen will carefully observe Steven's behavior and seek information from his parents that will enable her to determine whether or not her strategy is successful. If she does not have visible evidence within the first few weeks of treatment that Steven's tactile defensiveness is decreasing, she will develop an alternative working hypothesis and implement a plan that reflects her new hypothesis.

Colleen's "hunch" about Steven's tactile and auditory defensiveness is that it is the result of generalized overarousal and that it is not specific to the tactile or auditory systems. This belief is based on conversations with his parents and observations of his generally distractible behavior. If that is the case, then she should be able to address the level of his arousal through the vestibular-proprioceptive channel as well as through the tactile channel. Thus, she decided to see how Steven's tactile defensiveness would respond to activities that provide opportunities for him to take in controlled linear vestibular-proprioceptive information. In creating and implementing these activities, Colleen will emphasize use of equipment that is covered with a variety of textured materials.

Because Steven is easily overstimulated, which Colleen believed to be related to his tactile defensiveness, she thought about activities that she might create that would help to calm him and allow him to organize himself. She thought of a number of different activities she might introduce that would provide him with resistance to his movements and opportunities to take in enhanced linear vestibular-proprioceptive and deep touch-pressure information.

## Physical Layout of the Clinic

Having thought about some activities she might create with Steven, Colleen turned her attention to thinking about the physical layout of the clinic that would be most conducive to meeting the therapeutic goals. From her own observations, and from discussions with Mr. and Mrs. P, she knew that Steven was easily overstimulated and found it difficult to maintain his attention when there were a lot of distractions in the room. She also knew that Steven was exceedingly curious. If a lot of equipment was visible to him, he might choose to run from swing to swing in order to discover what they all do, rather than choose one swing, develop an activity with it, and then turn his attention to another swing and activity.

Therefore, Colleen's knowledge of Steven's distractibility suggested that she should minimize the amount of equipment in the room. In fact, she had as a major objective to try to help Steven's family and teacher create environments for Steven in which the number of distractions is reduced. However, at the same time, she had a second major objective for Steven to select equipment, help create activities, and begin to guide his own treatment.

In the creation of objectives to meet Steven's needs, Colleen has created a dilemma for herself, that is, how to structure the environment to help Steven focus his attention and also allow him to make choices in his treatment. She decided to resolve this dilemma by selecting three or four swings to leave in the clinic and putting the others out of sight. She will "rotate" the swings periodically, bringing out a "new" one and putting an "old" one away. Colleen believed that three or four swings was more than sufficient to give Steven choices about how to spend his time in treatment, but not so many as to result in his having difficulty focusing his attention.

In choosing the swings to introduce first to Steven, Colleen wanted to have two or three that could be suspended by two points, since her plan was to create activities that incorporate linear vestibular stimulation. Realizing that most of this equipment is new to Steven, she also wanted to be sure that at least some of the swings would look like equipment he had seen before, so that he easily could develop ideas of what to do with them. Thus, Colleen chose to keep the glider, the bolster swing, the net hammock, and the trapeze out for Steven's first visit.

Anticipating that she might need to engage Steven in activities in which he could organize himself, Colleen also wanted to ensure that the room was arranged such that it would be easy to create "small spaces" where Steven could go, and in which almost all distractions were eliminated. Thus, she made sure that a barrel and a few other pieces of equipment that he could climb into were readily available. She also thought about some activities that he might enjoy doing in a confined space and that could be used to further her goal of improved fine motor coordination. Colleen thought of activities such as blowing and breaking bubbles, fishing with a Velcro fishing rod for Velcro fish, and locating and picking up "bedbugs" (small objects) with a large pair of plastic tweezers.

## Thinking About Interactions

Recognizing that the therapist's interactions with Steven would be an important part of his intervention, Colleen thought about various things she wanted to incorporate into that aspect of her intervention program. She thought first of strategies for providing him with choices that would give him a sense of control in creating his activities. Colleen wanted to be sure that she had a repertoire of strategies available that she could draw on automatically.

Colleen wanted to develop strategies to afford Steven the opportunity to make choices that would result in activities that provided the just right challenge, but that would not overstimulate him. Colleen knew that she had begun to deal with this issue already in deciding which swings to leave in the room. She now began to think about ways for Steven to make choices while she controlled the level of challenge. For example, she could ask Steven to select the swing and she would decide on the activity, or vice versa. Colleen also thought that she could ask Steven to select a ball (or another toy) to use in an activity, then she would choose a bat that would maximize his chances of hitting the ball while still providing an adequate challenge (i.e., a bigger-diameter bat if he chose a small ball, a smaller-diameter bat if he chose a bigger ball).

Colleen also thought about ways to introduce discussion of Steven's sensory integrative dysfunction to him, to enable Steven to better understand its effect on his life and develop strategies for minimizing its everyday consequences. Colleen wanted to have these conversations with Steven when they would be most meaningful to him, rather than sitting down with him and discussing his problems out of context. She knew that at some time fairly early in his intervention, Steven was likely to become overstimulated in the clinic. Therefore, Colleen planned to direct Steven into a situation that would be calming. Once he had a chance to organize himself, she would use that opportunity to begin to create plans with him that he could use at other times in his life when he felt overwhelmed by all that was going on around him. For example, she might point out to him that when there was just too much going on, he could go to a quiet place for a little while, and that "getting away" might help him to concentrate better. Colleen knew that it might take many such conversations before he could actually use this information, and that she would have to "check out" any strategies she planned and recommended to Steven with his parents (and perhaps his teacher) ahead of time. She also thought about engaging Steven in similar discussions of his feelings about his poor motor coordination and his tactile defensiveness when the opportunities presented themselves.

Colleen recognized that asking a $6\frac{1}{2}$-year-old boy to engage in meaningful conversations about sensory integrative dysfunction was likely to be difficult. However, she felt that a very important part of her intervention was to help him to understand why he was unable to do some of the things that other people expected him to do, and to realize that he was neither "bad" nor "dumb" (words his mother had mentioned that he used frequently to refer to himself). Further, she believed that he must develop strategies for dealing with his own difficulties, and that these strategies also were an important part of her intervention with him. Colleen knew that Mr. and Mrs. P planned to spend time talking with Steven in a similar fashion. She planned to "touch base" with them frequently so that their efforts would be complementary.

## PROVIDING INTERVENTION

Now that all of the pieces of the plan were in place, Colleen was ready to intervene directly with Steven. We will describe a number of "snapshots," taken during the first 3 months of Steven's intervention program with Colleen. In so doing, we will illustrate how the plan for Steven's intervention was translated into action, and how Colleen resolved some of the difficulties she encountered in the process. We will demonstrate how Colleen reflected, both in-action and on-her-actions.

### The First Direct Intervention Session

We will look in on Steven and Colleen, for the first time, during their initial session together. Colleen had given Steven a tour of the clinic, pointing out several things that she thought might interest him.

Colleen had hung a net swing from a single point of suspension in the middle of the clinic; she had inserted a sheepskin rug into the met. After the tour, Colleen suggested that Steven might like to try "flying" in the net. She had several thoughts in mind. First, she knew that Steven, like many boys his age, was really "into" the superheroes. Many of Colleen's other clients enjoyed pretending they were Superman while "flying" in the net. Second, Colleen saw the net as a way of developing a fun activity for Steven that would provide him with an opportunity to take in enhanced vestibular-proprioceptive information, and also encourage him to maintain an extended position against gravity. She also knew that it would be easy to create activities in the net that required visuomotor skill, bilateral coordination, and the ability to plan and produce projected action sequences.

Steven was excited about trying the net. Anticipating that he might have difficulty getting into it, Colleen was ready to "talk him through it" at the first sign of failure. Indeed, on his first attempt, Steven ended up lying prone over a rolled up net. Colleen intervened immediately by saying, "I forgot to tell you how hard it was to get in, but I know a trick. Would you like to learn it?" Steven nodded, and Colleen helped him back into an upright position. She handed him the edge of the net that was farthest from his body and instructed him to use his arms to "stretch it out." Then she told him to put one knee into the side of the net that was closest to him and to lay down into it.

The second time, Steven succeeded. He immediately began to propel himself with his hands, and Colleen encouraged him to see how high he could go. Steven called out, "I'm flying like Superman!" He seemed delighted with his accomplishment and yelled out for his mother (who was observing from behind a one-way mirror) to watch him.

However, Colleen noted that, as Steven reached down and propelled himself, he tended to flex his entire body with the effort. Since she was looking for extension against gravity, and since Steven's flexion was becoming more and more pronounced, Colleen recognized that she must adapt the activity.

Colleen grabbed a long dowel rod from the shelf behind her, held it at either end between her two outstretched arms, and entered into Steven's game. "Hey, Superman!" she yelled, "Grab onto this branch and look in this window; I think there's someone who needs your help!" Steven reached up and grabbed the bar with his arms outstretched. "Hold on," yelled Colleen. "Pull hard so you can come a little closer." As Steven began to flex his arms, Colleen watched closely to make sure that his body and head remain extended. At the first sign of neck, hip, or knee flexion, she lowered the bar a little to reduce the amount of body weight he had to hold.

"What do you see?" asked Colleen. Steven replied, "There's a whole bunch of bad guys in there." Colleen suggested that maybe he'd better fly for help since there were too many bad guys for even Superman to take on alone. Steven let go of the bar and swung back and forth several times, calling for Batman and Superwoman to come help him.

Meanwhile, Colleen had pulled a cushion underneath Steven and laid several beanbags on top of the cushion. She hoped to arrange the beanbags so that they were high enough for Steven to reach down to get them as he flew by, and so that he would do so without using total body flexion. After several more "peeks through the window," Colleen suggested that the superheroes might want to use these special "bombs" (beanbags) to throw at the bad guys.

"I know," said Steven, "let's pretend that clown over there (pointing to an inflatable clown that tips when hit) is one of the bad guys. I'll hit him with these special bombs."

The game continued with Colleen gradually altering the demands on Steven and watching his responses. By the time it was over, Steven was pushing himself off the cushion with both hands, grabbing a beanbag or two on the way by and throwing them at the inflatable clown. Colleen was impressed with the accuracy of his throw and with the amount of extension he was able to maintain. She cheered as he knocked the clown over. Colleen also told Steven that this game would help him to have stronger muscles and that throwing the beanbags was good practice for learning to be better at throwing a ball when he played catch.

But as Steven began to fatigue, his accuracy at throwing decreased and Colleen noticed that he began to pull into flexion again. He complained that his neck hurt and that he wanted to sit up to throw the beanbags. Colleen helped him out of the net. It was time for the session to end anyway, and, as Steven put his shoes and socks back on, Colleen spoke briefly with Mrs. P. Steven was very excited to tell his mother about everything he had done, even though she had seen everything through the mirror.

## One Week Later

Having had such a successful first session with Steven, Colleen looked forward to repeating the same activity during Steven's second session. However, Steven announced, upon arriving for his second session of direct intervention, that he didn't want to lie down to do *anything*. He only wanted to *sit* on the swing because lying down hurt his neck. Mrs. P concurred that Steven had complained about sore neck muscles for 2 days after his initial session. However, she also said that she had told Steven that his muscles were sore because they were getting stronger.

Colleen had to think quickly. She knew that she had probably demanded too much of Steven in their last session and that she should have him spend less time in the prone position. However, she felt that he *needed* to work in prone because that was the best position to encourage maintained extension against gravity. While Colleen planned to create activities for Steven to do in sitting, she was afraid to create a lot of those activities at this point in his intervention because it might be difficult to get him to go back to prone when sitting demanded less from his postural muscles.

However, Colleen also knew that when children try throwing from a sitting position in the net, they often come to realize on their own that the prone position is easier. Thus, Colleen decided to follow Steven's lead. She and Steven set up the net swing, the cushion with the beanbags, and the clown, in much the same way she had set them up the week before. Steven sat in the swing and began pushing it with his feet. He soon found that it was difficult to reach the beanbags, and his throwing became very inaccurate because he had to throw around the sides of the net and hold on at the same time. After a few minutes, Steven told Colleen that he thought "it worked better when he was lying down."

Hoping that this would happen, Colleen agreed immediately. Steven got out of the net and, this time, was able to use the "trick" he'd learned the last time to lie down in it in prone, with very little assistance from Colleen. He seemed pleased with his accomplishment and quickly engaged in "bombing the bad guys."

Colleen could have insisted that Steven lie prone in the net if he wanted to do the activity. She could have explained to him that it wouldn't work so well in sitting. She also could have helped him to create an activity in sitting, using a different swing, that probably would have been successful. However, Colleen felt it was important to demonstrate to Steven that he had an active role in determining what he would do during his direct intervention sessions. She wanted to facilitate his learning that *he* could adapt situations to make them turn out better. Colleen knew, from her experience, that Steven probably would learn on his own that prone was a better position for doing that particular activity. Although the prone position was, in general, more difficult for Steven, Colleen believed that he would choose prone for this activity because he had enjoyed both the activity and the feelings he had when he succeeded at it.

Once Steven was busily engaged in the activity, Colleen watched the time and his reactions closely. After about 10 minutes, and well before Steven began to appear fatigued, she suggested that they "bomb the bad guys" from a different swung. This time she helped him to create an activity that he could do well while sitting on the glider.

As Colleen reflected on her sessions with Steven, she was surprised and quite pleased by some things that had happened. For example, Steven had been able to focus his attention remarkably well in the clinic. He did not exhibit much of the distractibility that she had observed in him during testing and at school. Thus, Colleen learned that, with the undivided attention of an adult, and when offered activities that he found highly motivating, Steven seemed able to pay attention to relevant stimuli and to screen out those that were irrelevant. While Colleen was pleased that this was the case, she also was not fooled into believing that Steven necessarily would be able to focus his attention in situations that he found more difficult, when he had less adult attention, or when there were many more sources of distraction. However, Colleen recognized that his had implications for the way in which she structured the environment. She felt that she might not have to be so careful to be sure that only certain swings remained in the room.

Colleen also knew that she was probably "buying time" with regard to Steven's willingness to work on the equipment in a prone position. She hoped that she would be able to develop activities, best done in prone, that were highly motivating for at least a few more sessions. If she was able to do that, Steven might begin to find that position easier to maintain and be less resistant to it. However, she knew that if he balked at doing things in the prone position, she probably would have to work primarily in a sitting position for a time, and then go back to prone as his postural stability improved.

## Six Weeks Later

Let us look in on Colleen and Steven again, 6 weeks later. As Colleen had anticipated, Steven had become more familiar with the various activities and tried to "steer clear" of activities that must be done in the prone position. She had been able to bargain with him a little, but as we entered the clinic, they were engaged in an activity where Steven is seated in the swing. Colleen had created an activity in which she hoped to work on the timing of his projected bilateral limb movements, as well as on his ability to flex his neck against gravity. She also was hoping that this activity would carry over directly into his being able to pump the swing independently.

Steven was standing on a pile of mats, the net swing slung around him. He was holding on to the net with both hands. Colleen was standing on the floor opposite Steven, far enough away that she wouldn't get hit as he swung. She was holding a large hula hoop between her outstretched arms. On cue, Steven jumped off the mats and extended his legs. The task was too lean back in the net and flex his knees around the hoop as he approached it. Colleen yelled "Now!" a fraction of a second before he should bend his knees. Once Steven had successfully "grabbed" the hoop with his legs, Colleen pulled him up a little higher, watching to see how far she could move him, not wanting him to lose control of his head and neck. Once she had attained the best possible position for Steven, Colleen moved the hoop from side to side and back and forth, making "roaring" noises as she did so.

"Let go! Let go!" Colleen says over and over. "You'll never capture me, you mean old monster!" Steven, fully involved in the activity, *did* let go after a few seconds, saying, "Okay, just one more chance to be good. But, if you do anything else bad, I'll be back to get you!" As soon as Steven landed back on his mats, Colleen did something to make Steven "attack" her again, and the game went on.

After a time, Colleen stopped telling Steven when to flex his legs in order to grab the hoop because Steven seemed no longer to require her assistance. Steven continued to be successful at the activity. In fact, she thought that Steven was doing so well that he might be able to shift to pumping the swing by himself. Colleen feigned tiredness. She said to Steven, "I need a break. Why don't you just swing by yourself for a few minutes?"

He continued to push off the mats, catching himself after each swing. Colleen watched for a while and then suggested he not stop so frequently. "You know," she said, "when Linda (Steven's older sister) pumps the swing, it's like she's leaning back and reaching out with her legs to catch an imaginary hoop. After she catches it, she pulls it back with her. Then she reaches out for a new hoop. And it just keeps going. Why don't you try that? Pretend I'm still standing there with that hoop."

Steven thought for a while. Then he tried it once. He leaned back with his trunk as he had when catching the hoop, but he flexed his knees too fast. Knowing that it hadn't worked, he caught himself on the mats. "Try again," Colleen urged, "but wait until I say 'now' to bend your legs."

Steven jumped off the mats and Colleen began to say quietly, "Now," just before he reached the full arc of the swing. At first, Steven had trouble coordinating his leg movements with his body movements, but gradually he began to coordinate the flexion and extension of his body with the flexion and extension of his legs. He did it very forcefully and his swinging was jerky, but his timing seemed to be better. "See if I can do it without you telling me when," Steven said. Colleen followed his lead and Steven was able to pump the swing himself, after a fashion. He practiced for a few minutes until it was time for the session to end.

Mrs. P had been watching intently behind the one-way mirror. She was beaming at Steven as he entered the observation room. "We'll have to hurry home so you can practice before it gets dark. Your father will be very excited when he sees what you've learned," Mrs. P said.

Two days later, Mrs. P called Colleen to say that Steven had mastered his first objective. "He's so excited," she said. "He spends every minute on the swing, practicing. His teacher sent a note home yesterday saying that he tried the swing at school for the first time by himself. That's the first positive note we've gotten all year."

Colleen also was excited. She talked for several minutes with Mrs. P, and they decided that the following week Steven's *individual* session would be only half as long. Mrs. P requested that she spend the other half of the session with Colleen so that they could begin working out a home program to address Steven's handwriting problem. Colleen made a note to call the occupational therapist who was seeing Steven at school.

## Indirect Intervention: Developing a Home Program

When Mrs. P and Colleen sat down together the following week, Mrs. P mentioned that she thought she could see progress in Steven's handwriting already. She had had only one note in the past month from Steven's teacher indicating that he failed to get his work done on time. Nonetheless, Mrs. P felt that a home program focusing specifically on handwriting would be helpful.

Colleen explained that the occupational therapist working with Steven at school had told her that she was working with the teacher to adapt Steven's assignments so that he had a little less written work to do. She had given Steven a device to put on his pencil that helped to encourage a better grasp, and had obtained a slant-top surface to encourage better posture. Also, as a result of her consultation, Steven's teacher had decided to move Steven's desk to a rear corner of the classroom, where his classmates rarely went. Both the therapist and Steven's teacher were encouraged by the results. However, they believed that a home program could be beneficial.

Colleen reminded Mrs. P that their objective for Steven was that he write more quickly and get his schoolwork done on time. Thus, she believed that the home program should concentrate on speed rather than on legibility or proper letter formation. She also told Mrs. P that she thought a home program should not be just "exercises" that they had to "cram" into their already busy schedules. Mrs. P agreed with all of these suggestions. With three other active children, she didn't have time to stand over Steven to make sure he did his home program. She continued to express the need to facilitate positive interactions with Steven, rather than setting up situations where he might need to be reprimanded for his performance.

Colleen wanted to ask Steven to write in a situation where he wouldn't worry about forming his letters perfectly. One idea she had was that Steven could practice quickly writing simple phrases on brown paper bags while he was watching television (Benbow, 1982). Mrs. P thought that Steven would love that idea. Steven and his brother and sister were allowed to watch only a minimum of television at home; they often protested this rule. If Steven's home program called for half an hour of television each night, all the children would be delighted.

Colleen had obtained, from the occupational therapist at school, lists of the letters that Steven should already know, those that Steven was currently working on, and the letters that he would be working on in the near future. She and Mrs. P constructed silly phrases, like "the duck barked," "the cat flew." The plan was that Steven would select one of those phrases each night and write it as many times as he could while he watched a half hour television show. Colleen asked Mrs. P to remind Steven that he should "just write" and not pay attention to each letter. He should only need to look down at his paper when he started a new line. It didn't matter if he made a mistake; he should just keep going.

When they told Steven of the plan, he thought it was a "great idea." He wanted to know if he could start that very night. He promised to bring his "bags" in each week to show Colleen.

In selecting an idea for an indirect intervention to be used with Steven, Colleen considered that one of Steven's problems was planning and producing projected action sequences. Writing phrases on a bag (because he was not copying them) involved the ability to plan in advance and write without feedback. As Steven practiced, Colleen hoped that he would develop a better "feel" for the way to make each letter and that his speed would improve as he did so. Further, she believed that the procedure should be fun and that it should increase the ease with which he wrote. That all the children in the family would be delighted with the "requirements" of Steven's therapy was an added bonus. Both Mrs. P and Colleen felt that the creation of this home program was an important part of Steven's intervention. Thus, there was no question that they should use some of Steven's intervention time to work on creating his home program. In fact, they scheduled a similar time for a month later when they agreed that they would talk about, and develop, strategies for helping Steven to enter a group of playing children successfully. They also would talk about having a friend of Steven's choice join Steven and Colleen in some of their sessions.

We felt that it was important to emphasize that, while the indirect intervention that Colleen created for Steven was guided by her knowledge of sensory integration theory, it was not a sensory integrative procedure. Rather, Colleen employed a type of skills training in her indirect intervention. She drew from her knowledge of several practice models to create the most effective intervention for Steven. This "integrated approach" to intervention is discussed more fully in Chapter 13.

## After 4 Months

Our final "snapshot" of Steven and Colleen was taken about 4 months after Steven began his intervention. Steven had, in fact, made a new friend named Jason. Jason had recently moved next door to Steven and was in his class at school. Steven had invited Jason to join him at his "special gym class." This was Jason's first visit to the clinic and the boys were very excited. Steven had just completed giving Jason a tour of all the swings. Colleen had asked Steven what he and Jason would like to do first. Steven responded that they would like to "fly" in the nets. "It's really neato. You're gonna like it," he told Jason. "It's just like being Superman."

In response to Steven's request, Colleen hung two nets from single suspension points 8 feet apart. She asked Steven if he would like to play the "hockey" game with Jason that she and Steven had devised together. Steven agreed.

The game consisted of both boys riding prone in the nets. Each had a long stick that they held at both ends. Off to each side, and slightly behind each boy, was a stack of cardboard blocks. The object of the game was to use the sticks to hit a large ball that was centered in a small hula hoop on the floor between them. Each boy was trying to use the ball to knock over the other's stacks of blocks. The game continued until one boy's blocks were completely knocked over.

Steven had played this game with Colleen. Colleen saw it as a means of providing him with an opportunity to take in vestibular-proprioceptive information, while demanding that he plan and produce bilateral projected action sequences. Steven had gotten to be fairly good at this activity and he took the lead with Jason, teaching him the rules and showing him how to get into the net.

The two boys were engaged for several minutes in the activity. However, with the competition, Steven had gotten very excited. He began to swing the stick with one hand and accidentally hit Jason quite hard. Jason was clearly upset and yelled at Steven, "Hey, that's too hard. We're just playing."

At this point, Colleen intervened. She indicated that the boys should get out of the nets and she directed them to a medium-sized box filled with lentils. They climbed in excitedly. Meanwhile, Colleen turned off the fluorescent lights and put flashlights in her pockets for each boy. Steven was still overstimulated. He immediately began to throw lentils at Jason. Colleen intervened again, before a full-blown lentil fight could develop. "Steven," she said, "lie down in the corner here and Jason and I will bury you, all but your head." Colleen knew, from past experience, that this was an activity that Steven found calming.

Colleen and Jason began dumping containers full of the lentils on top of Steven. When Steven moved too much, uncovering a limb, Jason reminded him to be very still. After Steven was completely covered, Colleen suggested that Jason lie down beside him and she buried Jason. She talked to the boys in hushed tones and Steven calmed down noticeably. Colleen gave each boy a flashlight and they played a modified game of "I Spy" for a while.

Colleen noticed that Steven's proximity to Jason in the lentil box suggested that his tactile defensiveness was somewhat reduced. Mrs. P also had observed this. In one of their conversations together, Mrs. P had told Colleen that Steven's fighting at school had almost been eliminated.

Colleen recognized that being in the lentil box provided a good opportunity to talk with Steven about developing strategies to use when he felt out of control. She began a discussion with the two boys about what it felt like to be buried under all those lentils. Jason indicated that it made him feel calm, kind of like he felt after he had just taken a bath. Colleen skillfully guided the conversation so that both boys contributed and so that Steven could see that even Jason sometimes felt over- whelmed by "too much stuff going on around him." Seeing that Steven was very intrigued by this knowledge, Colleen probed a little more. "What do you do when you feel like that"? she asked. Jason answered that sometimes he went to his room to be alone and sometimes he just put his head down on his desk. Steven did not contrib- ute much to that part of the conversation, but he listened intently. After a time, Colleen turned the lights back on and dumped some small plastic "bedbugs" into the lentil mixture. The boys spent the last few minutes of the session busily searching for them and picking them up with the large plastic tweezers Colleen had given them. Colleen had skillfully scattered the bedbugs so that it might be slightly easier for Steven to find them. By the end of the session, both boys had found an equal number of bedbugs. They climbed out of the box and got ready to go home, chatting about what they would do together the next time Jason accompanied Steven to the clinic. They planned that date for 3 weeks later.

## CONCLUSIONS

We have demonstrated how one expert therapist took the information she gathered in evaluation and applied that information, together with her knowledge of sensory integration theory, to the development and implementation of an effective plan for intervention. We have emphasized the importance of working with the client, and his or her caregivers, to formulate objectives for intervention. We have demon- strated the therapist's ability to reflect-in-action (Schön, 1983, 1987) and to modify her intervention based on her reflections.

In this chapter, we have highlighted the reasoning and roles of the clinical therapist, performing direct intervention and using the principles of sensory inte- gration theory. We have referred only briefly to the complementary roles of the school therapist and to the consultative and indirect service roles of the clinical therapist. We have done so, in part, because consultation and the role of the school therapist were emphasized in Chapter 11. We have *not* done so because we feel that the direct service role of the clinical therapist is any more important than the consultative role of the school therapist.

Direct intervention, conducted by a skilled occupational therapist, is a powerful approach to intervention for individuals who have sensory integrative dysfunction. However, it is only one avenue by which to address the difficulties that these individuals encounter in daily life. Further, intervention based on sensory integration theory alone often is not enough to eliminate these difficulties. We believe that the greatest benefits are attained when a team of individuals pools *all* of its relevant skills and knowledge, sets meaningful and achievable objectives, and implements an integrated approach to intervention.

## REFERENCES

Ayres, A. J. (1989). *Sensory Integration and Praxis Tests*. Los Angeles: Western Psychological Services.

Benbow, M. (1982, March). *Problems with handwriting*. Paper presented at Eunice Kennedy Shriver Center, Waltham, MA.

Bundy, A. C. (1990). *A conceptual model of school system practice for occupational and physical therapists*. Unpublished manuscript.

Mager, R. (1972). *Goal analysis*. Belmont, CA: Fearon.

Mager, R. (1975). *Preparing instructional objectives*. Belmont, CA: Fearon.

Mattingly, C. F. (1989). *Thinking with stories: Story and experience in a clinical practice*. Unpublished doctoral dissertation, Massachusetts Institute of Technology, Cambridge, MA.

Rogers, J. C., & Masagatani, G. (1982). Clinical reasoning of occupational therapists during the initial assessment of physically disabled patients. *Occupational Therapy Journal of Research, 2*, 195–219.

Schön, D. A. (1983). *The reflective practitioner: How professionals think in action*. New York: Basic Books.

Schön, D. A. (1987). *Educating the reflective practitioner*. San Francisco: Jossey-Bass.

Wilbarger, P., & Royeen, C. B. (1987, May). *Tactile defensiveness: Theory, applications, and treatment*. Paper presented at Annual Interdisciplinary Doctoral Conference, Boston University, Department of Occupational Therapy, Boston.

CHAPTER **13**

# Integrating Sensory Integration Theory and Practice with Other Intervention Approaches

**Elizabeth A. Murray, ScD, OTR**
**Marie E. Anzalone, MS, OTR**

*Integrating: forming, coordinating, or blending [parts] into a functioning or unified whole.*
*Eclectic: selecting what appears to be best in various [but not necessarily compatible] doctrines, methods, or styles.*

*Merriam-Webster, 1989*

Sensory integration theory is only one of the many models of practice used by occupational therapists in planning and implementing intervention. This text emphasizes the use of sensory integration theory for understanding behavior and implementing intervention. We need to remember, however, that as occupational therapists, our primary goal is to improve the function, or adaptive behavior, of our clients. In many instances, sensory integration may be used in combination with, or replaced by, other approaches in order to provide the most effective intervention.

An *integrated approach* to intervention is one in which the therapist uses his or her knowledge of various practice theories in order to gain a clearer picture of the client's problems and to plan and implement the most effective intervention program. In order to use sensory integration theory in an integrated approach to intervention, we need to examine its compatibility with other theories of practice as well as to recognize when it is *not* compatible with these other theories.

Let us return to Max, the 8-year-old child presented in Chapter 3. As you may remember, Max was a boy who had sensory integrative dysfunction. While his therapists, Linda and Jill, may have had several direct intervention goals for him, *Max's* goal was to play dodgeball. Catching and throwing with a Nerf ball were incorporated into Max's direct intervention, and Linda and Jill did notice improvement in ball skills within this setting. But Max was not meeting *his* goal; he still could not play dodgeball. It was at this point that Linda recognized the need to incorporate some specific skill training into Max's therapy, teaching him how to throw the ball and giving him practice in dodging when she threw it at him. Max learned some specific strategies that he could call on when he played dodgeball with other children. While Linda and Jill believed that sensory integration procedures would improve Max's underlying dysfunction, and that this would lead ultimately to a generalized improvement in motor skills, they wisely recognized that this process was too slow to meet Max's immediate goal. Further, they recognized that there was no conflict in combining sensory integration procedures with teaching specific skills. These two approaches are compatible.

Another factor in judging the usefulness of a practice theory to our profession is its applicability to the various disabilities commonly evaluated and treated by occupational therapists. As was discussed in Chapter 1, there are boundaries in the application of sensory integration theory, and we must be careful not to overstep them. For example, the child with Down syndrome often has a cluster of symptoms that suggest deficits in processing of vestibular-proprioceptive inputs. However, as was pointed out in Chapter 1, in the child with Down syndrome, these symptoms are more likely due to actual abnormalities of brain structure rather than merely to a problem in sensory processing. Similarly, a young child with muscular dystrophy may display difficulty with balance and low muscle tone. Here the problem is with the muscles themselves, not with sensory integration. Further, a child with mental retardation may perform poorly on the Sensory Integration and Praxis Tests (SIPT) (Ayres, 1989) because of difficulty with understanding the directions, or because the child's motor planning skills reflect his or her cognitive ability, rather than because of a problem with sensory integration. It is essential to realize that sensory integrative dysfunction is not the *only* explanation for behaviors such as poor balance, low muscle tone, poor motor planning, or even decreased SIPT scores.

We also need to recognize when it may be appropriate to apply concepts derived from sensory integration theory to children with diagnoses other than learning disabilities. For example, a child with mental retardation also may demonstrate tactile defensiveness. In this situation, the therapist could use sensory integration theory to guide that aspect of treatment that relates to decreasing the tactile defensiveness.

Finally, sensory integration intervention procedures, in some cases, may be a useful part of direct intervention even when deficits are not thought to be due to sensory integrative dysfunction. A child with low muscle tone and problems with balance, for whatever reason, may benefit from the varied types of movement activities, on suspended equipment, that challenge balance and require maintenance of a stable posture. Additionally, since the vestibular system has synaptic connections with extensor muscles (especially of the neck and trunk; see Chapter 4) activities that stimulate the vestibular sytem may help to facilitate these muscles (Fisher & Bundy, 1989).

Sensory integration procedures have the added benefit of being fun and, therefore, highly motivating. Generally, children are easily engaged in activities incorporating sensory integration procedures. A child may be more likely to practice specific skills, such as throwing and catching a ball, when the procedure is incorporated into these enjoyable activities.

There are times when we are unsure whether (a) a client we have evaluated has sensory integrative dysfunction, (b) the behaviors we observe are the result of other factors, or (c) both sensory integrative dysfunction and other factors are present.

For example, Eric is a 6-year-old boy who suffered a mild head injury at age 3. Recent cognitive testing found him to be of average on tests both of praxis and of tactile discrimination. Although we *might interpret* these findings as indicating that Eric had somatodyspraxia, with a sensory integrative basis to his problems, we also need to consider that his dyspraxia and poor tactile discrimination are likely to be at least partly a result of his previous head injury. In this situation, we might wish to use sensory integration procedures for a trial period, carefully monitoring Eric's behavior for improvement in motor planning. Direct intervention would be part of an ongoing diagnostic process.

## PURPOSE AND SCOPE

The purpose of this chapter, then, is to re-present sensory integration within the context of an integrated approach to intervention. We will review briefly several other approaches commonly used by occupational therapists and discuss their compatibility with sensory integration. Then, through the use of case studies, we will demonstrate how sensory integration theory can be combined with other approaches, both in intervention with children who have learning disabilities, for whom it was originally developed, and with clients who have other disabilities.

## OTHER APPROACHES TO INTERVENTION USED IN OCCUPATIONAL THERAPY

In order to understand how sensory integration theory can be combined with other approaches, we need to review some of the basic concepts of these other interventions. As principles of normal development are incorporated into most direct intervention approaches that are used with children, including sensory integration, we will begin with a discussion of the developmental approaches. Selected approaches that are based on sensorimotor principles also will be reviewed. These include perceptual-motor approaches, as well as neurodevelopmental treatment. Sensorimotor approaches, then, will be contrasted with sensory stimulation. Finally, we will describe behavioral or learning theory, showing how it is used both to influence the behavior of a child and to analyze tasks for the teaching of specific skills.

We need to make it *very* clear that we are presenting only a *flavor* of these other approaches to intervention. Readers who are interested in further information on these approaches are referred to the bibliography at the end of the chapter.

### Developmental Approaches to Intervention

The concept of a developmental approach to intervention is fundamental to the practice of occupational therapy. Although we cannot review all of the theories that contribute to a therapist's understanding of human development, there are certain shard premises of most developmental theories that are useful in understanding developmental intervention (cf. Lockman & Hazen, 1989; Mussen, 1983; Short-De-Graff, 1988).

Development can be described as a collection of *processes*, or ways that humans evolve and mature. These processes include domains of development such as sensorimotor, psychosocial, and cognitive; as well as occupational behaviors such as self-care and play, and roles such as student and player. Each of these follows a relatively predictable pattern and has its own markers or "milestones" (e.g., standing, walking) that serve to denote achievement. Often we use these milestones to gauge an individual's progress. Developmental domains, occupational behaviors, and roles often are both complementary and interdependent. That is, the normally developing child acquires a certain amount of ability in the various domains before he or she is expected to perform an occupational behavior. For example, the child develops a certain level of fine motor and visuomotor skill before he or she is expected to self-feed. In turn, as the child practices self-feeding, he or she may develop more proficient fine motor and visuomotor skill. Similarly, most children reach a basic level of proficiency before they are expected to assume the student role. However, in the student role, the child practices both self-care tasks and motor skills and becomes more proficient at both.

Antoine, a 5-month-old infant, has just learned to crawl on his stomach. This newfound mobility of Antoine's will afford him new opportunities to explore his environment and to have new sensory experiences that will, in turn, influence his cognitive development, his play, and his social interactions. Any interruption in one developmental process is likely to have an impact on development in other areas. If Antoine had cerebral palsy and was not able to crawl, he would miss out on a variety of rich experiences, unless he was given some type of assistance. Understanding these interactions of developmental processes is an important part of our evaluation and intervention.

Although developmental processes are thought to proceed in a predictable fashion, there are always variations among individuals, or *interindividual differences.* Equally important are the *intraindividual differences*, or differences within the individual in the pattern and the rates of development in the various areas.

Because development is viewed as a process, we are interested not only in what skills a child possesses but also in how these developmental skills emerge in the child. Vygotsky (1978) introduced the concept of a "zone of proximal development" to describe the process of emerging or evolving skills. To understand a child's performance, it is necessary to observe what he or she can accomplish independently as well as what can be accomplished with some assistance; that is, a child's evolving skills. For example, neither Annie nor Diane is able to tie her shoes independently. However, if Annie's mother gives Annie verbal directions, she is able to tie an acceptable bow. Shoe-tying, then is a skill that is *emerging* for Annie; it is in her zone of proximal development. Diane, on the other hand, cannot figure out how to tie no matter what kind of assistance her mother provides. We would say that Diane is not yet "ready" to tie her shoes. Understanding the zone of proximal development can give us a sense of where a child is in the developmental process and assist us in determining what type of collaboration or intervention (e.g., motor facilitation, calling attention to salient visual features) will help the child complete the task successfully.

Another concept in development is that of *stages.* A stage is a certain period of development possessing distinct characteristics that separate it from other periods in time. In general, it is assumed in "stage theories" that we must pass through a stage, learning all of the adaptive behaviors inherent in it, before we can move on successfully to other stages. For example, in Piaget's (1952) theory of development, the infant must master the behavioral aspects of the sensorimotor period before he enters the stage of preoperational thought.

Although most people currently studying development take a more flexible view, stages do provide a means for cataloging what we know about development. They provide us with frames of reference and aid us in thinking about the ways in which a child can be expected to progress. It is important for us to appreciate developmental stages while still viewing development as a *continuous process* that occurs across the lifespan.

Most contemporary theorists view development as a *transactional* process between a child's biological or genetic endowment (nature) and the particular human and nonhuman environmental experiences (nurture) to which he or she has been exposed (Plomin, DeFries, & Fulker, 1988). This approach acknowledges that heredity and environment complement each other. The individual and the environment are seen as mutually influencing; that is, they change each other. Occupational therapists often attempt to influence development by engaging the child in environmental experiences designed to facilitate individual change.

Transactions between individuals are of particular interest in studying the processes of development. Transactions that are especially important in the development of children include those that occur between a child and his or her caregiver (e.g., parents, teachers, day-care providers) and those that occur between a child and his or her peers.

Consider the following situation: Mr. L has just arrived home from work. He takes Jamal, his infant son, out of his playpen, sits down with him, and bounces the little boy on his knee. Jamal smiles and giggles at his father. Mr. L's behavior obviously has had an effect upon his son. We also can observe the effect that Jamal has had upon his father by Mr. L's look of delight and in his repeating the activity. Additionally, Mr. L is likely to try this game again when he wants a smile from Jamal. Thus, Jamal has had an impact on his father's future behavior. If Jamal had stiffened and cried when he was bounced, his actions might have had a different effect on Mr. L.

Sensory integration is a developmental theory. As in other developmental theories, behavioral manifestations of many of the constructs of sensory integration theory, such as praxis or balance, occur at each age. However, at each age the behaviors that reflect these processes are very different. What is a practic act or challenges balance for a 2-year-old (e.g., walking across a mattress and climbing over a large pillow) may not require praxis or challenge balance in an older child. For example, Daniel is a 2-year-old child who enjoys walking up and down the scooter-board ramp and roaming over (and falling on) uneven surfaces in the clinic. His grin and consistent repetition indicate that he enjoys the postural challenges in combination with the tactile and vestibular-proprioceptive input from falling. For Daniel, this is a developmentally appropriate sensorimotor activity. When Ariana, his 8-year-old sister, enters the clinic, her behavior is very similar to Daniel's. However, Ariana's behavior is not typical of children her age and may reflect poor balance and a limited ability to figure out independently how to interact with the environment.

Sensory integration theory represents one important aspect of development. However, when we plan intervention for a child, we must simultaneously consider many aspects. For example, Blair is an 11-year-old girl who has gravitational insecurity, poor equilibrium reactions, and poor bilateral motor coordination. She had made excellent progress in direct intervention, but she still had difficulty with activities that challenged her balance. Blair really wanted to learn to ride a bicycle. All of her friends had been riding bicycles for several years, and Blair felt left out when she could not ride with them to the nearby beach or the playground. Although, from a sensory integrative perspective, Blair was not "developmentally ready" to ride her bicycle, Jane, her occupational therapist, realized that her inability to ride a bicycle was limiting her opportunities to participate in some rewarding, age-appropriate social activities. Learning this skill was important to, and developmentally appropriate for, Blair's social development; it also would likely have a positive impact on her self-esteem. Jane began to teach Blair how to ride a bicycle as a part of her intervention. At Jane's suggestion, Blair's mother bought Blair a helmet to wear when riding. Within 2 months, Blair was joining her friends on their bicycle excursions.

## Sensorimotor Approaches

Thus far, this book has focused on what sensory integration *is*. It also is important to discuss what sensory integration is *not*. In this section, we will describe approaches to direct intervention that are not the same as sensory integration, even though they may be built on many of the same premises and employ similar activities, equipment, and sensory modalities.

The term *sensorimotor* has been applied in a narrow sense to approaches to intervention, such as those developed by Rood, in which a specific sensory input (e.g., vibration), presented passively, is expected to produce a specific motor output (e.g., contraction of the vibrated muscle) (Clark, Mailloux, & Parham, 1989). Sensorimotor also is used in a more generic way to refer to a class of intervention theories, including sensory integration, that emphasize the role, first described by Piaget (1952, 1969), of active, experienced-based learning. Current theories of perception (E. J. Gibson, 1988; J. J. Gibson, 1979) and motor control (Pick, 1989; Reed, 1982; von Hofsten, 1989) propose an action system that reflects the unity of sensory intake and motor action for responding to environmentally relevant goals. The unity of sensory and motor processes is considered to be reflected *in* the observed behavior and also reflective *of* the postulated neural processes underlying the action (Reed, 1982). Ayres' (1972) formulation of sensory integration theory was firmly based in both of these sensorimotor premises.

The term *sensorimotor intelligence* is based on Piaget's (1952) assumption that children learn about their bodies and their environments through experience. (For an excellent review of Piagetian theory and its relationship to empirical studies and to other theories of cognitive development, see Harris, 1983).

Piaget (Harris, 1983; Piaget, 1952) described a sensorimotor period of development that encompasses the first 2 years of life. During the sensorimotor period, infants develop increasingly purposeful and skilled control over their motor systems (and their environments). The infant learns through his or her interaction with the objects and people in the environment. For example, a 12-month-old infant may "experiment" with dropping a toy to see how far it will go, what it sounds like, and how the child's mother will react as the toy is thrown repeatedly. Repetition and slight modifications of the action are important aspects of these "experiments."

Similarly, a child learns about his or her body through the sensory feedback generated by the movement itself. Through an expanding repertoire of increasingly complex activities, the child learns about causality, the spatial environment, objects, and the body itself.

While sensory integration is considered to be an example of a sensorimotor approach, not all sensorimotor approaches to intervention can be called sensory integration. Sensorimotor approaches frequently are used by occupational therapists, physical therapists, and physical educators working with school-aged children; they are the basis of many community-based toddler exercise programs. Typically, these intervention programs differ from sensory integration in many ways.

The most significant differences are that activities (a) do not emphasize the use of suspended equipment, and (b) usually are done with a group of children. Because they must meet needs for the whole group, the activities must be highly structured. Thus, intervention based on a sensorimotor approach often lacks the flexibility and spontaneity characteristic of intervention based on sensory integration theory, in which the focus is on client-directed activities tailored to the specific needs of the client.

For example, John propelled himself through an obstacle course during a sensorimotor group led by his teacher, as well as during therapy based on the principles of sensory integration theory, conducted by his occupational therapist. In both situations, he was able to benefit from the vestibular-proprioceptive sensory information generated from the activity itself as well as to learn about the spatial properties of the environment. However, there also were differences in John's experiences in these two situations. During his sensorimotor group, John was one of 10 children going through the obstacle course built by the teacher. He did not receive any individualized assistance in propelling himself through the obstacle course, but with practice he was able to do it faster. In contrast, during occupational therapy, John was involved in selecting the activity as well in building the obstacle course, deriving benefit from the planning as well as the execution of the activity. Moreover, his therapist, aware of John's poor antigravity extension, prepared him for the extensor demands of the scooterboard activity earlier in the session. This was done through the introduction of activities that provided for the intake of enhanced linear vestibular-proprioceptive stimulation and facilitated tonic postural extension — for example, swinging in a suspended net hammock while throwing beanbags at a target.

Programs such as Movement is Fun (Young & Kepplinger, 1988) and Sensory Motor Handbook (Bissell, Fisher, Owens, & Polcyn, 1988) outline specific activities and classroom modifications useful for therapists integrating sensorimotor intervention into school programs. Both programs also can help teachers to integrate general sensorimotor learning into the early school programs. We emphasize, again, that these adult-directed group sensorimotor activities, *while frequently beneficial*, are not sensory integration.

## PERCEPTUAL-MOTOR APPROACHES

Perceptual-motor intervention theories are based largely on the work of Kephart (1960) and Cratty (1981), whose approaches share common neuropsychological roots with Ayres' initial thinking (e.g., Hebb, 1949). They were also influenced by cognitive and educational theorists such as Piaget (1952) and Montessori (1912), who emphasized the role of sensation and experience in learning. The work of Marianne Frostig (1964) also is perceptual-motor in nature and focuses on visuomotor and visual-perceptual intervention.

According to Kephart (1971; Ball, 1971), information processing (learning) develops in predictable stages. The earliest learning occurs almost exclusively as a result of motor actions directed toward the environment. The child's perceptions of the environment are based on his or her motor experience. As the child matures, perceptions control motor behavior; that is, motor processes become less important to learning, while perceptual and cognitive processes becoming more central. Learning problems occur when the child fails to develop an adequate perceptual-motor match. Kephart (1971) hypothesized that by improving the underlying perceptual-motor deficit, learning would be improved.

The assumption that "the hand leads the eye," which is central to Kephart's theory, has been challenged. Empirical studies of this assumption have documented the occurrence of intersensory integration and visual guidance of motor actions in infants prior to coordinated motor experience and its feedback (Bushnell & Weinberger, 1987; E. J. Gibson, 1988; E. J. Gibson & Walker, 1984; Ruff, 1986a).

Current perceptual-motor theorists (e.g., Laszlo & Bairstow, 1985) have acknowledged this research. They do not emphasize the stages of perceptual-motor development. Instead, they view the theory as a "conceptual framework of interrelated motor, perceptual, and, more broadly, cognitive factors" (Laszlo & Bairstow, 1985, p. 27).

Although both sensory integration and perceptual-motor theories are concerned with underlying processes, intervention based on these two theories looks quite different (Laszlo & Bairstow, 1985). Perceptual-motor approaches use specific training activities to improve these processes. For example, if a child has a problem with proprioception (commonly referred to as kinesthesia by perceptual-motor theorists), he or she would practice specifically graded activities that are thought to require proprioception (e.g., drawing circles in the air). The goal for the child is to perform these activities correctly. In contrast, a sensory integration approach involves the use of a variety of activities that provide enhanced opportunities to take in, and use, proprioceptive information in order to enhance sensory processing. The goal for the child is to improve in functional behaviors that are reflective of the enhanced sensory processing. Sensory integration also emphasizes the role of the client in guiding activities used in intervention (see Chapter 10).

Jenna is an 8-year-old girl who has been described by her teachers as "clumsy." Her occupational therapy evaluation has indicated that Jenna has problems with balance and postural responses associated with a postural-ocular movement disorder (see Chapter 4). In perceptual-motor theory, balance training is used to improve balance. Consequently, Jenna might be presented with a series of increasingly more difficult activities to perform on a balance beam. In this way, Jenna would "learn" about balance. Mastery of walking on the balance beam would reflect improvement in her balance. This training, in turn, would be expected to improve her gross motor skills.

When viewing Jenna's difficulties through a sensory integration "frame," we also would say that she had poor balance and postural responses. However, if we used the principles of sensory integration theory to plan our intervention, we would focus on improving her ability to process vestibular-proprioceptive information in the context of activities also designed to improve her balance. A variety of activities (e.g., sitting or standing on a suspended platform swing while reaching for a ring, or popping bubbles while riding on the bolster swing) would be used. The focus of Jenna's attention during intervention based on sensory integration theory would be on getting the ring or popping the bubbles without falling off the swing, not on practicing a specific motor skill such as walking on the balance beam.

## NEURODEVELOPMENTAL TREATMENT

Neurodevelopmental treatment (NDT) is a sensorimotor approach based, as its name suggests, on both neurological principles and normal development. Neurodevelopmental treatment is an approach to assessment and intervention developed by Berta and Karl Bobath, a physiotherapist and physician, respectively. It is used widely with clients who have cerebral palsy or who have sustained cerebrovascular accidents (strokes) (B. Bobath, 1970, 1985; B. Bobath & K. Bobath, 1972; Finnie, 1974).

Like sensory integration, neurodevelopmental treatment is very much concerned with the sensory aspect of movement. When using a neurodevelopmental treatment approach, direct intervention is conducted by physically "handling" the client, that is, teaching the client to move "properly" by giving appropriate input with the hands. An important tenet of neurodevelopmental treatment is that normal movement both depends on, and results in the generation of, normal sensory feedback. During treatment, the therapist tries to ensure that the client feels what it is like to move normally by inhibiting any abnormal muscle tone and movement patterns and facilitating normal postural and movement patterns.

Desirable movement patterns should be automatic and goal-directed. Gradually, the therapist attempts to withdraw his or her physical support and provides opportunities for the client to use movements appropriately, spontaneously, and as independently as possible. For more information about therapy from a neurodevelopmental treatment perspective, see Bly (1983), Boehme (1988), and Howison (1988).

Whereas sensory integration theory emphasizes the individual's ability to intake and integrate sensory information and to *plan* movement, the neurodevelopmental treatment approach focuses on the individual's ability to *execute* normal postural responses and movement. Thus, these two approaches differ in focus.

Because of its emphasis on posture and the quality of movement, neurodevelopmental treatment provides a useful way of viewing the disordered postural mechanism and awkward movements often found in the client who has sensory integrative dysfunction. Although the problems of the client with sensory integrative dysfunction are much milder than those of the client with cerebral palsy, they frequently include hypotonia, poor postural stability, and poor equilibrium. Children with sensory integrative dysfunction often "fix" their trunks and limbs in patterns reminiscent of those observed in clients with cerebral palsy.

For example, Molly is an 8-year-old child with sensory integrative dysfunction, manifested in part by poorly developed postural reactions and hypotonia. She tends to move without trunk rotation or diagonal weight shifting. Her trunk and pelvis are stiff. The neurodevelopmental treatment approach has helped her therapist understand Molly's postural and movement problems.

Molly's treatment also has been influenced by her therapist's knowledge of neurodevelopmental treatment. However, instead of physically handling Molly to facilitate weight shifting and trunk rotation (which would have limited Molly's independent exploration), her therapist suggested a game of "dumper cars," which required more independent use of her postural mechanism. Molly climbed up a tall mountain of uneven pillows to her "car." While Molly maintained the quadruped position, the therapist tipped the car from side to side. When ready, Molly pressed the "ejection button" and was dumped into the pillows. In order to get out of the pillows, she had to use trunk rotation, diagonal weight shifts, and antigravity flexion. Instead of physically handling her, the therapist was able to manipulate environmental demands in order to elicit the desired movement patterns. If Molly had not responded with the desired movements, the therapist might also have incorporated some more traditional handling to help her initiate the desired movements.

In a complementary fashion, sensory integration theory can help us in our evaluation of children with cerebral palsy. For example, John, a 4-year-old child with mild spastic diplegia, has difficulty climbing onto a platform swing. When viewing his difficulty from a neurodevelopmental treatment perspective, John's therapist assesses the impact of his spasticity on the quality of his movement. She also observes such things as his ability to shift weight from one leg to the other and maintain his balance while climbing onto the swing. However, as his therapist views the same situation from a sensory integrative perspective, she may observe for difficulties with motor planning or signs of gravitational insecurity.

## Sensory Stimulation

When administering sensory stimulation, we view the sensory systems as key pathways through which to influence brain function. However, just as sensorimotor activities are not necessarily sensory integrative intervention, even if some of the same equipment is used, sensory stimulation also is not the same as intervention based on the principles of sensory integration, even if vestibular or tactile stimulation is administered. Unlike sensory integration, sensory stimulation techniques are passively provided to the client. They need not be presented within the context of a meaningful activity, and they do not require an adaptive response.

Some clients may actively seek out sensory stimulation. For example, for months, Sandra began each treatment session pretending she was a "dusty piece of furniture" and requesting a head-to-toe "dusting" with a furry cloth. After this light touch, she was consistently more active and able to direct her play during direct intervention.

Sensory stimulation techniques also are sometimes used with clients who have sensory modulation disorders, with the idea that increasing sensory intake may have an effect on modulation. Thus, although we do not look for specific adaptive behaviors, we are looking for a change in state that reflects a change in arousal in the central nervous sytem.

Sensory stimulation can be a useful adjunct to intervention based on the principles of sensory integration. However, a client's response to sensory input and the state of the client's nervous system are mutually interdependent. In many clients, state changes occur every rapidly. Thus, supplemental stimulation must be administered cautiously, especially with clients who are known to have poorly modulated responses to their environment (e.g., premature infants, clients with documented brain damage).

Sensory stimulation also can have a strong and cumulative effect on the client's autonomic nervous system. Therefore, it is essential to *observe the child's responses carefully*. Some of the autonomic responses that suggest overarousal include flushing, blanching, perspiring, nausea, yawning, changes in sleeping or eating patterns, and significant changes in activity level. Because the response to sensory stimulation may not be apparent immediately, it is always important to let parents know when sensory stimulation has been a part of their child's direct intervention and urge them to monitor his or her behavior after the session has ended and report any signs of sensory overload or sensory disorganization to the therapist. See Chapters 4 and 10, for a more thorough discussion of these two undesirable sequelae to sensory stimulation and for suggestions to counteract their effects if either should occur inadvertently.

## Behavioral or Learning Theory

Behavioral, or learning, theory, widely used in both education and therapy, is in many ways quite different from the other theories and approaches to intervention described above. Behavioral theorists believe that all behaviors, except for reflexes, are learned. According to Skinner (1968), who had a major impact on the development of this theory,

> extraordinarily subtle and complex properties of behavior . . . may be traced to subtle and complex features of the contingencies of reinforcement which prevail in the environment. (p. 62).

Thus, what is emphasized in behavioral theory is the impact of specific aspects of the environment on *observable* behavior. Behavioral theorists do not concern themselves with what cannot be directly observed. Unlike sensory integration and many other practice theories, no assumptions are made about functions of the central nervous system and no hypotheses are made about "changing the brain" through intervention. Behavioral theory, then, is concerned with improving specific behaviors or skills, not with remediating the underlying dysfunction. In this way, it is quite different from sensory integration theory. However, many aspects of behavioral theory are useful to us when designing a therapy program using principles of sensory integration. (For a practical reference on the use of behavioral theory, see Krumboltz & Krumboltz, 1972.)

A basic concept of behavioral theory is that of conditioning. According to this theory, there are two types of conditioning, the first of which is called *classical* conditioning. An example of classical conditioning can be seen in Michael, a 3-year-old boy with severe tactile defensiveness, who was particularly sensitive to having his feet touched. Michael was not yet walking and did not even stand. There was concern that he had some abnormality in the muscles or bones of his feet. During a clinic evaluation, the physician, physical therapist, and occupational therapist each removed Michael's shoes to examine his feet and then put his shoes back on. Michael kicked and screamed each time his feet were handled and continued to cry as his shoes were put back on his feet. For the next several weeks, Michael screamed any time he saw his shoes, and his mother could not put them on him. Apparently, he had been conditioned to associate his shoes with this particularly upsetting experience. A knowledge of tactile defensiveness, combined with a basic understanding of classical conditioning, helped the occupational therapist to explain this behavior to Michael's mother. While Michael's case is an extreme example, children with sensory modulation disorders sometimes develop associations between an activity and the distress or discomfort they feel from sensory experiences.

The second type of conditioning is *operant* conditioning. The concept of operant conditioning is largely a result of the work of Skinner (1968). Whereas classical conditioning emphasizes the importance of the stimulus to behavior, operant conditioning stresses the role of the consequences of behavior. Operant conditioning is used to increase, maintain, or decrease a given behavior. Increasing and maintaining behavior are done through the use of reinforcement, either positive or negative. An object, activity, or other stimulus is said to be reinforcing if it strengthens or increases a behavior. Reinforcers or rewards can be anything from food to a smile. A critical component is that the child performs some behavior in order to receive the reward. We assume by the performance that the reward is something the child desires or enjoys. For example, when given a psychological test, Michael initially refused to try any test items. The psychologist gave Michael a sticker and told him he could earn another one by doing the first test item. Michael then engaged in the test, completing items and receiving stickers. We might say that the stickers reinforced his test-taking behavior.

We may use our knowledge of sensory integration theory to help in determining what will be reinforcing and what will not. For example, the psychologist often used a pat on the head or on the back as a reward during testing. While this might be reinforcing to some children, Michael, being tactually defensive, probably would not have liked being touched, and this could have lessened his cooperation even further.

When increasing a desired behavior, a reward generally is given on a consistent basis. In order to maintain the behavior, however, the reward is frequently given on an intermittent, or inconsistent, basis. For example, once Michael was consistently engaging in each item in the psychological evaluation, the psychologist began giving Michael a sticker after he had performed several items. The stickers were given randomly so that Michael could not predict when he would receive one. Michael continued to try each test item, indicating that this intermittent pattern of reinforcement was sufficient to maintain his behavior.

There are times when a child's behavior is inappropriate, and we would like to decrease it. One method for decreasing an unwanted behavior is to remove any reinforcement observed to be maintaining this behavior. The process of removing a reinforcer is referred to as *extinction*. Often this unwanted behavior has been inadvertently reinforced by our response to it.

When sitting at a table, Michael frequently drummed his hands on the table or the chair. This behavior interfered with his ability to engage in fine motor activities, and Susan, his occupational therapist, wanted Michael to stop the drumming. At first, she tried telling him to stop each time the drumming began, but she found that this did not help. In fact, when she timed his drumming over a few sessions, she found that he was drumming more than ever. While she had not thought that telling Michael to stop would be reinforcing, it appeared to be resulting in an increase in his drumming. Susan then withdrew this reinforcer and no longer commented on Michael's drumming. At the same time, she engaged him in fine motor activities and gave him stickers as he participated in the activity. In this way, she was *reinforcing a behavior that was not compatible* with the one that she wanted to decrease. The combination of not responding to an undesirable behavior and reinforcing a desired, but incompatible, behavior is an effective combination.

*Punishment* is another method of decreasing a behavior. When punishment is used, the behavior is paired with a negative consequence. Although the use of punishment may be effective in decreasing dangerous behaviors, such as those in which a client injures himself or others, it is not the preferred method of decreasing behavior in most instances (Krumboltz & Krumboltz, 1972; Landers, 1989). We should be aware, however, that with children who have sensory integrative dysfunction, activities that we might assume would be rewarding may not be. They could actually result in a decrease in a desired behavior, as in the case of using a pat on the head to reward Michael for engaging in test items.

Another technique often used when decreasing unwanted behavior is referred to as "time out." In time out, a child is removed from a situation so that there is no opportunity to receive reinforcement for any behavior. Often this involves isolating the child in a special part of the room. Ideally, time out is not presented in a negative or threatening way; it should not be used as a punishment. In fact, for certain children this process actually may be reinforcing, because it allows them to sit in a quiet place without being disturbed or having demands placed on them. Consequently, these children may misbehave in order to be placed in time out. Time out is effective only when the activities from which the child is removed are more rewarding than the time-out process itself.

A technique that bears a superficial resemblance to time out is that of providing children who are easily aroused, and who have difficulty modulating sensory intake, with a quiet place away from the activities of the classroom. Some children with sensory modulation disorders need to have such opportunities available to them in order to decrease the level of sensory intake.

Another major component of behavioral theory concerns the strategies used to teach specific tasks. We often use this component when teaching self-care skills. For example, when a child is unable to perform a task, such as zipping his jacket, we might break that task into a sequence of smaller steps. For zipping a jacket these might be (a) holding the two bottom sections of the jacket near the zipper, one section in each hand; (b) hooking the two bottom sections of the zipper together; and (c) pulling the zipper tab up with one hand while holding the bottom of the jacket with the other hand. These steps are taught in sequence; when the child becomes proficient at one step, the next is added. This process is referred to as *chaining*.

According to behavioral theory, a child will learn a sequenced task most efficiently when a reverse or *backward chaining* method is used. That is, the therapist performs all but the last step, leaving that step for the child. The steps are then added, in reverse order, until the child is doing the whole task independently.

Another technique is called *shaping*, in which the desired behavior is obtained through successive approximations. For example, Timmy is unable to fasten the buttons on his shirt. We might begin by having him practice on a shirt with larger buttonholes. As Timmy becomes proficient with larger buttons, we could decrease the size of the buttons and buttonholes until he is able to fasten the small buttons on his own shirt.

In addition to these methods of task analysis, prompts and assistance frequently are used to aid in skill acquisition. Prompts and assists can be physical (such as placing the child's fingers on the zipper tab or helping the child to pull the zipper), or verbal (such as saying "pull up the zipper"). Demonstration also can be used as a prompt. To promote the ultimate goal of independence in the task, prompts and assists are *faded*, or slowly removed from the task.

When one observes a direct intervention session conducted according to the principles of sensory integration theory, it is possible also to interpret many aspects of that session according to principles drawn from behavioral theory. For example, equipment is chosen partly because the child enjoys it and will be an active participant. Thus, equipment is used that will make an activity reinforcing and increase the probability that it will be performed again. Often, particularly in a child-centered direct intervention session, the child will select an activity that he or she cannot perform independently. We then modify the activity, providing assistance or prompts as needed and grading the activity so that the child will be successful.

Another situation in which we may use behavioral theory is in the case of the child who has difficulty with modulating sensory input. Here we often introduce sensory stimulation (in the context of the activity) very gradually and provide a great amount of reinforcement for tolerating that stimulation.

Sometimes a classical conditioning paradigm is used. For example, a tactually defensive child who enjoys movement may roll in a barrel lined with various textures. In this situation, a reinforcing activity (rolling in a barrel) is paired with an aversive activity (tactile input). When enough of these types of activities are presented over a period of time, the aversive quality of the tactile input may be lessened.

While it is possible to use principles derived from behavioral theory to interpret a direct intervention session, not all aspects of the two theories are compatible from the perspective of sensory integration theory. For example, the teaching of specific skills, rather than improving underlying processes, is characteristic of behavioral theory, but not of sensory integration theory. However, there are times when it is essential for a child to learn a specific skill, such as zipping a coat zipper or tying shoelaces. Behavioral theory, which provides a wealth of information on teaching skills, would be an appropriate frame of reference to use for this aspect of an occupational therapy intervention program.

## INTEGRATING APPROACHES TO INTERVENTION

As occupational therapists, we must remember that goals and objectives for our clients should be developed before we select treatment procedures. That is, the choice of intervention approaches and types of service delivery (e.g., direct intervention, consultation) should be "driven" by the outcomes desired.

Several factors must be considered when setting goals. First, goals and objectives should reflect the functional needs of the client. That is, objectives should be statements addressing functional behaviors that the client needs to do in order to meet successfully the challenges of daily life.

Second, when setting goals, we need to consider the desires of the client. Client motivation is essential to goal achievement. Motivation for intervention depends, in part, on having goals that are important to the client.

Third, we must have knowledge of the implications of the client's specific disability for the types of improvement that may be expected. Walking independently is generally considered an important skill, but independent walking would not be an appropriate goal for a 9-year-old child with severe spastic quadriplegia. Further, there are some cases in which the client's goal is an unrealistic behavior because it is very unlikely to happen, or might only be accomplished at the expense of other essential functioning. In any event, it is important that the therapist not simply discount the client's goals and go on to formulate new ones. The reasons behind a client's goals should be explored thoroughly (and perhaps over time) in order that those goals can be replaced by other goals that fulfill, as much as possible, the client's original intents.

We also must recognize that goals are for the client and *not* the therapist. While Susie may need a splint for her hand, ordering or making a splint is not a goal for *her*. It *may* be a means by which the therapist helps Susie to meet the goal of coloring with a crayon. In short, goals and methods should not be confused.

Finally, we must understand the boundaries of the approaches to intervention that we use in order to apply them appropriately and effectively to the individual client. *When all of these factors are considered, it is rarely the case that one approach to intervention, used exclusively, will result in provision of the most effective intervention program.* Thus, it is important that we know how to combine approaches effectively.

## CASE STUDIES

The following case studies are provided as examples of ways in which sensory integration theory has been combined with other approaches to intervention. Because it is important to understand the implications of specific diagnoses when developing and implementing integrated plans for intervention, we have included children with diagnoses that are commonly seen by occupational therapists.

We begin with a child who has learning disabilities; it is for these children, primarily, that sensory integration theory and intervention procedures have been developed. Each case will open with a brief discussion of the application of sensory integration theory to individuals with a specific diagnosis. The case study then will be used to demonstrate ways in which one of the approaches to intervention that we have described can be combined with sensory integration procedures.

## Julia: Combining Sensory Integration with a Sensorimotor Approach and with Sensory Stimulation in a Child who has Learning Disabilities

A sensory integrative approach is used most commonly with a specific subgroup of clients diagnosed as having learning disabilities; most of the clinical descriptions discussed elsewhere in this book have been based on clients who have learning disabilities associated with motor incoordination and poor sensory processing of vestibular-proprioceptive and tactile information. Learning problems may result from difficulties in many different kinds of cognitive, perceptual, or motor processes (including attention, memory, language, form and space perception, fine motor control, sequencing, and organization). Increased activity level and distractibility also have been associated with learning disabilities.

Learning disabilities may affect much more than a child's ability to do his or her school work. They may affect self-esteem, locus of control, socialization, play, vocational choice, and activities of daily living [see Levine (1987) for a comprehensive review]. Although this book has emphasized the role of occupational therapists in intervention with clients who have learning disabilities, most intervention programs include multidisciplinary assessment and remediation, including not only occupational therapists, but also educators, psychologists, speech and language pathologists, and physicians. An occupational therapist's assessment and treatment of a client with learning disabilities should address not only sensory integrative dysfunction but also any educationally, psychosocially, and functionally relevant areas within the scope of traditional occupational therapy practice (Clark, Mailloux, & Parham, 1989).

Julia is a 7-year-old child with a learning disability. She currently is in a regular first grade classroom where she is receiving some special-education help in math and reading for 2 hours each day. In addition, for the past 6 months, she has been seeing an occupational therapist for direct intervention based on the principles of sensory integration theory for 1 hour each week.

No one was aware that Julia had any problems until she entered kindergarten, when her teacher reported that she had difficulty remaining seated during group activities and seemed resistive to many gross motor and fine motor activities. She repeated kindergarten, but continued to have difficulty with maintaining her attention and with participating in certain classroom activities. Because of her continued difficulty in the classroom, she was evaluated by the school psychologist, who found that Julia had average intelligence but performed much better on verbal than on non-verbal tasks. He recommended that Julia be evaluated by an occupational therapist to help clarify the problems Julia was experiencing in the classroom.

The results of Julia's evaluation suggested somatodyspraxia, which explained her avoidance of many motor activities (see Chapter 6). Interviews with Julia's parents and teachers, as well as classroom observations, indicated that Julia was tactually defensive (see Chapter 5). Direct intervention was recommended and implemented. General goals included (a) improving practic abilities, so that Julia would be more actively involved in gross and fine motor activities, and (b) decreasing tactile defensiveness, which was thought to be contributing to Julia's difficulty maintaining her attention in group activities.

Sensory integration was the primary theoretical framework used in her direct intervention. Julia especially enjoyed the fact that she could be in charge of her explorations in the treatment room. She quickly fell into a comfortable routine, with most of her time spent repeating familiar activities. The specific activities used were often more sensorimotor in nature. These activities (her favorite was a three-part obstacle course) were performed successfully, but with minimal flexibility. Any attempt made by Laurie, her therapist, to introduce modifications triggered refusals and sometimes a tantrum.

As Julia developed more trust in Laurie and became more confident in her explorations, Laurie was able to introduce more complex tasks into the obstacle courses. These, in turn, required more variability in Julia's responses and demanded that she plan and produce more complex motor behaviors.

While Julia clearly was demonstrating progress, she continued to return to familiar successful activities whenever a new child was in the treatment area or whenever she encountered a new and difficult challenge. The activity that she returned to most often was the Pogo Ball, a ball with a handle that Julia could sit on and use to bounce herself across the room. The Pogo Ball is a very difficult activity requiring good balance reactions and bilateral motor coordination and sequencing abilities. As Julia used the Pogo Ball, she received vestibular-proprioceptive input.

In order to succeed at propelling the Pogo Ball, Julia had spent days practicing at home; she was very proud of her accomplishment and very aware of the fact that she could do it better than almost any other child on Laurie's caseload. Because Julia's competence on the Pogo Ball was so well learned, it no longer required praxis, but it was a valuable *sensorimotor* experience. It also provided some valuable "kid power" that contributed to Julia's sense of self-esteem.

Because of Julia's consistent need to "show off" when other children were around, Laurie felt Julia would benefit from group sensorimotor activities in which she could improve her skills and demonstrate her accomplishments to her peers. Rather than give up Julia's individual occupational therapy sessions, Laurie decided to refer her to the adaptive physical education teacher, who would provide her with this additional group experience. Julia's parents and teacher agreed with Laurie's recommendation, recognizing this as an opportunity for Julia to improve both her social and motor skills simultaneously. Laurie met with the adaptive physical education teacher to learn about the program and to provide the teacher with information about Julia.

Although Julia's practic skills improved consistently, tactile defensiveness continued to be a problem. For this reason, Laurie decided to incorporate some *tactile stimulation* into her treatment. An intensive brushing program (see Chapters 5 and 10) was instituted over school vacation with the assistance of her mother and a day-care provider. A surgical scrub brush was used to brush her arms, legs, and back. Brushing was firm but gentle and was followed by gentle joint compression of all the large joints of each limb. This brushing was done each time there was a change in activity (e.g., getting ready to go out and play) over a 5-day period. After this initial intensive period, brushing was done only four times each day on a regular schedule (as she woke up, after lunch, after school, and just before bedtime).

The brushing seemed to have a calming effect on Julia. She frequently asked for it upon entering the classroom. Her teacher noted a decrease in her "flights" from circle or group activities soon after the initiation of the brushing program. Julia also began to tolerate tactile-based play during occupational therapy sessions, although she did not actively seek it out.

All aspects of Julia's programming seemed to contribute to her growing self-esteem and improved willingness to try new motor activities. Julia's classroom teacher noticed improvements in Julia's ability to pay attention in the classroom; she also reported that Julia had become friends with another child in her adaptive physical education group. Julia's mother reported that the most significant changes she noticed at home were Julia's increased willingness to accept help when approaching new challenges and an increased flexibility when dealing with changes in her daily routine.

## Robbie and David: Combining Sensory Integration with Neurodevelopmental Treatment with Children who have Cerebral Palsy

Cerebral palsy is a disorder of movement caused by non-progressive damage to the brain. The underlying lesion is present at, or soon after, birth and before the growth and development of the brain is completed.

The types of motor deficits seen in children with cerebral palsy are variable and range from mild spasticity or asymmetry in hand use to complete inability to control movement (Bleck, 1982). Milani-Comparetti (1982) defined the motor problem in cerebral palsy as a lack of freedom of choice in movement.

While the most noticeable problem in children with cerebral palsy is motor incoordination, the brain damage may be so widespread as to result in other associated deficits, language delays, mental retardation, seizure disorders, or secondary orthopedic abnormalities (Bleck, 1982; Bly, 1983; Robinson, 1973).

Children who have cerebral palsy also commonly are reported to have difficulty performing academic and self-care skills beyond that which can be accounted for by either their motor deficit or mental status alone. The specific cause of the functional skill deficits is unknown, and it is likely that among individuals there is considerable variability in causes. However, these sorts of difficulties sometimes are reminiscent, both in type and in quality, of those seen in children who have developmental dyspraxia.

Moreover, some children who have cerebral palsy seem to have a fear of movement and postural disturbances (gravitational insecurity) that is out of proportion to their motor deficits (Fisher & Bundy, 1989). Some children with cerebral palsy also have been described as tactually defensive (DeGangi, 1990).

It is possible that the sensory processing and motor planning deficits seen in children who have cerebral palsy may be only a result of their brain damage. However, the presence of gravitational insecurity and tactile defensiveness suggests that some children may have sensory integrative dysfunction *in addition to* their primary motor deficit. The reader is urged to interpret this suggestion cautiously, since known brain damage frequently results in both practic and sensory processing disorders.

Both Robbie and David were 7-year-old boys with moderate spastic diplegia. Their motor deficits and general developmental levels were about the same, but their functional abilities were quite different. Both boys were able to walk with crutches. Both had the lower extremity spasticity, poor postural reactions, and mildly delayed fine motor abilities typical of children with diplegia (Beck, 1982). Intelligence was within normal limits in both boys, and they were in regular first grade classrooms.

Both Robbie and David had received occupational and physical therapy services since they were quite young. The focus of both therapies was on improving motor functioning. Neurodevelopmental treatment had provided the framework for their intervention.

Although the boys had many similarities, Robbie was much more successful than David in performing the functional tasks expected of 7-year-old children. In fact, Pam, the boys' occupational therapist, decided to discontinue Robbie's direct intervention. Pam's evaluation of Robbie indicated no functional problems and no fine motor, visuomotor, or visual-perceptual deficits. Robbie had no difficulty "keeping up" in his classroom, at home, or when playing with his many able-bodied friends. His ability to keep up with his friends, in spite of his obvious physical handicap, constantly amazed observers. Pam continued to provide consultation, as needed, to Robbie's classroom teacher and physical therapist.

David, in contrast, did have difficulty performing the tasks expected of him in school and at home. David's teacher described him as disorganized and distractible. His attention span was limited. David was unable to do many things for which his motor skills were more than adequate. Tasks such as putting on and fastening his jacket, organizing his room, following simple two- to three-step commands, or getting himself ready for school in the morning sometimes seemed insurmountable.

During free play, David tended to watch the other children, initiating interactions only with adults. His play, like his schoolwork, was disorganized and lacked spontaneity. He seemed to have difficulty "figuring out what to do." He spent most of his play time engaged in a limited repertoire of familiar, solitary activities. Many of these descriptors of David's difficulties performing functional tasks are reminiscent of the descriptors of children who have developmental dyspraxia (see Chapter 6).

David also showed evidence of some gravitational insecurity. He demonstrated exaggerated fearfulness whenever his balance was challenged in any way, and he disliked having his head out of the upright position (see Chapter 4). His fear of movement during therapy often led to increasing postural fixation and spasticity as well as to behavioral refusals, rather than the desired development of more mature righting and equilibrium reactions. His progress in occupational and physical therapy was slow because of his fearfulness.

Unlike Robbie, David did need ongoing direct intervention from an occupational therapist. Because of the nature of David's deficits, Pam planned to incorporate the principles of sensory integration theory into her therapy with David. Her general goals for intervention were to decrease his gravitational insecurity and to improve his motor planning ability. She worked closely with David's physical therapist, informing him of her intent to incorporate sensory integrative procedures into David's occupational therapy program, as well as to obtain feedback regarding the effectiveness of her own intervention.

In planning her direct intervention, Pam wanted to assure that David not only increased his tolerance of movement and improved his motor planning, but that he also continued to improve the quality of his movements. Therefore, it was important to prepare David for movement using handling techniques to decrease David's spasticity and abnormal movements, and to facilitate weight shifting, equilibrium, and normal movements. She based this component of her intervention on the principles of neurodevelopmental treatment.

Enhanced opportunities to take in linear vestibular stimulation were integrated into direct intervention very slowly. The first piece of equipment Pam chose to use was the bolster swing. She selected the bolster swing because (a) it assisted David in maintaining good postural alignment (it provided hip abduction and a wide base of support for sitting), and (b) it allowed him to be in control of the duration and speed of his movement. Use of the swing provided linear vestibular input that was not frightening to David but provided challenges to his righting and equilibrium reactions (see also Fisher & Bundy, 1989).

Initially, Pam sat behind David, providing pelvic support, facilitating weight shifting and righting reactions, and grading the postural demands of the activity. She was especially aware of David's weak flexor musculature, so she carefully graded the amount of backward displacement to insure that he would not lose his balance. Pam's proximity on the swing also decreased David's fear of the movement.

As his fearfulness decreased, Pam began to introduce more motor planning demands into their activities. For example, she placed large cardboard blocks on uneven surfaces throughout the clinic. After David collected them, he would use them to build a tower that he then knocked over while swinging on the bolster swing. This activity demanded both motor planning and postural adjustments.

Initially, Pam needed to facilitate some of David's movements as he attempted to move over the uneven surfaces. Gradually, however, David seemed more able to master the postural demands by using appropriate movements, and less direct handling was needed. Pam began to incorporate activities into her treatment that demanded trunk rotation, controlled active movement into both flexion and extension, equilibrium reactions, and bilateral coordination.

Close monitoring of David's responses was important to prevent overstimulation or increased tone resulting from increased effort during motor activities. When that happened, Pam immediately decreased the demands of the activity and incorporated handling and firm touch-pressure to help David organize himself better. Sometimes she modified equipment to insure that David maintained good body positions.

David's physical therapist noted changes in David, beginning about 1 month after Pam began incorporating sensory integrative activities into her direct intervention. The physical therapist also reported that David was much less fearful and stiff during movement. In addition, as his program progressed, David's mother reported that his ability to organize and perform self-care tasks had improved somewhat.

## Ramon: Combining Sensory Integration with a Developmental Approach for an Infant at Risk

The number of infants at risk for significant developmental dysfunction is increasing as medical science has become more able to keep younger, smaller, and sicker infants alive (Bauchner, Brown, & Peskin, 1988). The "cost" of these medical advances to a premature infant's developing central nervous sytem are, as yet, unknown (Fuller, Guthrie, & Alvord, 1983; Lester, 1989). In addition to the increasing numbers of premature infants who survive, there also has been a rise in the number of full-term infants who have been exposed to circumstances that may compromise their development (e.g., prenatal drug exposure) (Hyde & Trautman, 1989).

Infants whose birth, prenatal, or perinatal history, or whose social or environmental situation has placed them at risk for developmental, learning, or emotional problems, are considered to be "high-risk" infants (Hanson, 1984; Sehnall, 1989; Sweeney, 1986). Although infants at risk all have survived extraordinary circumstances, many will not manifest persistent developmental deficits. Nonetheless, there are a number of sequelae to prematurity and other conditions associated with risk in infancy that commonly are described in the experimental literature. We will review those most closely related to sensory integration theory.

Als (1986) described the task of early infancy as balancing approach and avoidance responses to the environment. Her description is reminiscent of Ayres' (1972) concept of the organization of sensory input for use; both involve analysis of the environmental demands and stimuli and the child's changing ability to organize a response to them. Premature infants (Als, 1986; Als, Duffy, & McAnulty, in press; Lester, 1989), and other infants at risk (Jacobson, 1984) have been found to have poorly modulated state behavior. These infants are easily overaroused, frequently do not have effective ways of calming themselves (e.g., sucking or turning away), and may have prolonged autonomic effects when overstressed by events or people in their environments (Als, 1986; Lester, 1989). While most of Als' work has been with neonates, Als and associates have documented a typical disorganized response pattern that persists beyond the neonatal period in children who were born prematurely.

Premature infants also have been found to exhibit slower processing of visual information (Gorsky, Lewkowicz, & Huntington, 1987; Rose, 1983, 1988), less organized exploratory action (Als, Duffy, & McAnulty, in press; Ruff, 1986b; Ruff, McCarton, Kurtzberg, & Vaughan, 1984), and less effective coping and adaptive behavior (Williamson, 1988). Mild but specific motor abnormalities (e.g., increased tone in the lower extremities, decreased flexion, persistent postural reflexes, and delayed ambulation) also have been described (Drillien, 1972; Nelson & Ellenberg, 1982; Piper, 1988).

While biological factors account for some risks to infant development, much of the recent focus of clinical researchers has been on the interaction between biological and environmental risk factors (e.g., socioeconomic status, level of parental education, community and cultural values, family support) (Garcia-Coll, Sepkoski, & Lester, 1981; Kopp & Kaler, 1989; Sameroff & Chandler, 1975). Much effort has been directed toward predicting outcomes for infants and providing effective early intervention.

Ramon was born at 28 weeks of gestation with a birthweight of just over

1000 grams. His perinatal course was complicated by severe respiratory disease, and he required hospitalization for 125 days. His home situation was unstable, and his young, single mother had a limited support system and meager financial resources. Ramon was evaluated when he was 6 months old. Because he was born 2 months prematurely, his age was "adjusted" to 4 months. His evaluation revealed hypertonicity with delayed onset of head control and persistent scapular retraction. However, by 7 months adjusted age, his neurodevelopmental evaluation was normal and his development was in the low-average range on the Bayley Scales of Infant Development (Bayley, 1969). Ramon's mother, Ms. B, was given a home program of developmentally appropriate play experiences for him, but no direct intervention was recommended.

Ramon was evaluated again at 17 months (15 months adjusted age). At that time, he was extremely active and distractible. He had difficulty attending to activities for more than a few seconds. Ms. B reported being frustrated in her attempts to manage Ramon's activity level and disorganized behavior. Developmental evaluation revealed delays in both mental and motor areas. Ramon did not yet stand or walk, and he did not use a neat pincer grasp when picking up small objects. He did not seem to be interested in manipulating the toys used for testing.

When not sitting on his mother's lap, Ramon spent most of his time in disorganized, non-directed movement, seldom pausing for exploration or manipulation. Additional discussion with Ms. B and observations of Ramon suggested that he might be gravitationally insecure. Ms. B reported that Ramon cried whenever she or his grandfather tried to roughhouse with him, toss him in the air, or swing him. Ms. B indicated that Ramon seemed afraid when he sat independently.

Ms. B was dealing with a variety of personal and financial stresses in her life. Consequently, she had particular difficulty dealing with Ramon's disorganized behavior at home. While Ms. B was concerned about Ramon's developmented delays, her most immediate need was for assistance in managing his behavior.

Leslie, the occupational therapist, and Ms. B set two general goals for Ramon. The first was to decrease his level of arousal and increase the organization of his approach to his environment. The second was to improve his motor and adaptive skills.

Because it is not unusual for children who are born prematurely to continue to have difficulty with state regulation, Leslie was not surprised to see this problem in Ramon. She felt, however, that his high level of arousal and decreased organization were contributing to the delays in his development of motor skills. She felt that his overarousal also might contribute to his gravitational insecurity. Finally, Ramon's disorganized behavior certainly made parenting him difficult.

While Leslie used primarily a developmental approach in her direct intervention she also was influenced by her knowledge of sensory integration theory. That is, her understanding of normal development provided the framework for understanding what was an adaptive behavior for Ramon. She used sensory integration theory to guide her choice of activities for intervention. In order to decrease his level of arousal and his gravitational insecurity, she wanted to provide calming and organizing activities. To do this, she provided proprioceptive input through resistive activities such as pushing a heavy ball to his mother and crawling up a slight incline. Leslie gradually added a vestibular-proprioceptive component to the activities when she rode with him on the glider, and finally introduced the frog (see Chapter 10). Leslie noted that swaddling was particularly helpful in calming Ramon. She showed Ms. B how to use this technique at home.

As Ramon's arousal decreased to a more optimal level, Leslie and Ms. B found it easier to engage him in purposeful and organized play. Prior to each session, Leslie reorganized the treatment area to minimize distractions. Using equipment that Ramon enjoyed, she and his mother guided his activity through play and modelling, allowing him to set the pace of his exploration. With this approach, Leslie and Ms. B were able to see improvement in Ramon's organization and planning of motor activities.

As Ramon became less distractible and more organized in his approach to activities, Leslie was able to introduce some more-structured fine motor activities. Leslie did this first in a small, quiet room to minimize distractions. She used "responsive" toys, such as the busy box, which required little persistence for success, to help Ramon focus on the activity. Gradually, Ramon became increasingly capable of independent and creative interaction with more complex toys. Eventually, Leslie and Ms. B were able to introduce fine motor and adaptive games, such as formboards and stacking rings, into the more distracting environment of the gross motor room and at home.

After Ramon had received 6 months of direct intervention, Ms. B seemed more comfortable with managing Ramon's behavior. Ramon, although still highly active, was more directed in his play activities. Although his fine motor skills were still slightly delayed, he was walking, and his gross motor and language skills were developmentally appropriate. Ramon's direct intervention was discontinued, but Ms. B was urged to bring Ramon back or to seek consultation from an occupational therapist if she again became concerned.

## Adam: Combining Sensory Integration with Behavioral Theory for a Child with Mild Mental Retardation

Many children and adults who have mental retardation show symptoms similar to those exhibited by individuals with sensory processing problems (e.g., low muscle tone, defensive reactions to sensory input). In some instances, it is possible that these symptoms are in fact a result of sensory integrative deficits, and that the use of sensory integration procedures would therefore be appropriate.

With individuals who have mental retardation, however, we must consider the probability of other causes for these symptoms. When the symptoms we observe also are known to be caused by frank central nervous system damage or anomaly (such as abnormality of the cerebellum in the case of individuals with Down syndrome), or by brain lesions (such as those that result from tuberous sclerosis), incorporating some activities based on sensory integration theory into an intervention program still may be appropriate. We must keep in mind, however, that sensory integration theory was developed to explain hypothesized *dysfunction* in the central nervous system. When there is known or suspected brain *damage*, as in many instances of mental retardation (particularly when the level of retardation is severe), the theory may be stretched beyond its boundaries. However, with individuals who are mentally retarded, we may find sensory integration theory helpful in explaining *some* behaviors (e.g., tactile defensiveness, gravitational insecurity, or motor planning strategies typical of a *developmental* age younger than that of the client).

Adam is a 13-year-old boy who has mild mental retardation of unknown etiology. He has been enrolled in programs for children with special needs since he was 5. Adam is a delightful, interactive young boy who enjoys the company of both adults and other children. Recent testing indicated that language and academic skills are at a 7-to-9-year level. Adam's family recently has moved and Adam has begun attending a new school. He was referred to Ann, the school's occupational therapist, for an assessment to help in planning his program.

Adam's occupational therapy evaluation consisted of portions of the Bruininks-Oseretsky Test of Motor Proficiency (Bruininks, 1978) as well as clinical observations of vestibular-proprioceptive functioning. Additionally, his mother and teacher were interviewed to obtain information on his daily living skills and his behavior, as well as on any indications of defensive reactions to sensory inputs. Adam also was observed in his classroom.

Ann's assessment of Adam revealed several indicators of possible problems with integrating vestibular-proprioceptive information. His muscle tone appeared to be low, and he could not assume a prone extension position. His equilibrium reactions were poor for his age, and his performance on the balance subtest of the Bruininks-Oseretsky was similar to that of a 5-year-old. Ms. R, Adam's teacher, observed that Adam frequently appeared to be "tired." When standing in line, he had a slouched posture. He also had a lot of trouble sitting at his desk without either leaning on an elbow, holding his head in his hand, or putting his head down altogether. Reminders to "sit up straight" didn't seem to help.

While recognizing that there could be many causes for these observations, Ann felt they suggested the possibility that processing of vestibular-proprioceptive information was a problem for Adam. Regardless of the underlying cause, Ann was concerned that Adam's low muscle tone and poor equilibrium reactions were having an impact on his classroom behavior; she was aware that vestibular-proprioceptive stimulation could be used as a facilitation technique within a program designed to increase the strength of tonic postural extensor muscles (Fisher & Bundy, 1989).

Adam also showed evidence of dyspraxia, which seemed particularly to interfere with fine motor tasks. Despite his higher language and academic abilities, Adam's performance on the fine motor portion of the Bruininks-Oseretsky was at a 4-year level. He was totally unable to figure out how to cut with scissors. His pencil grasp was immature, and although he had learned to write his first name, he had extreme difficulty copying other letters. Whereas Ann expected that his motor planning abilities would be below the norm for his chronological age, she noted that these skills also were well below his cognitive abilities. Further compounding Adam's problem was his sitting posture during these fine motor tasks. He usually leaned on both elbows and at times put his head down, making performance far more difficult.

Of even greater concern was the fact that Adam still could not manage fasteners on his clothing. His mother noted that Adam's fingers "don't seem to work quite right," and that it was far easier to assist him with his clothes than to make him struggle with dressing independently. Ms. R was concerned because

Adam could not manage his clothing when in the bathroom. His classroom was housed in a junior high school, and Adam had told Ms. R that the other boys teased him when he was in the bathroom.

Together with Ms. R and Adam's mother, Ann formulated two general goals for Adam. Their highest priority was for Adam to dress independently, including managing fasteners. Ann recognized that his difficulty with this might be due to dyspraxia, but she also realized that it was imperative for Adam to learn these specific skills as quickly as possible. Part of her therapy program, then, consisted of teaching Adam to zip and button the fasteners on his pants. She used behavioral theory when breaking the task down into small, sequenced steps. To teach these skills to Adam, Ann used a backward chaining procedure; initially she performed all but the last step, leaving that one for Adam to do. As he mastered that step, she added on the steps of the chain, in reverse order, until he was able to fasten his pants independently. Ann also had frequent contact with Adam's mother and Ms. R so that they could carry out the same program with Adam while he was learning this skill. As Adam mastered one specific self-help skill, Ann developed a teaching program for another.

The second general goal for Adam was to improve his posture when sitting. Because she felt his low muscle tone and poor proximal stability *might* be due to a disorder in processing vestibular-proprioceptive information, she decided to try a program using sensory integration procedures to meet this goal. This portion of direct intervention included activities that emphasized linear vestibularproprioceptive stimulation, incorporated into a variety of activities that also required tonic holding against resistance. Ann checked with Ms. R on a regular basis to see if his posture in the classroom was showing any improvement.

Initially, Ann decided to use the sensory integrative procedures for the first part of each session and to end with the quieter training activity. In this way, she thought that she would be able to insure sending Adam back to his classroom quiet and calm. However, within a few weeks, Ms. R reported that Adam was coming back saying he "hated" occupational therapy and that it was boring. Ann also noted that although Adam was cooperative for the portion of the session using sensory integration procedures, he was becoming more and more resistant to practicing self-help skills. At times, he would refuse to get off the equipment or would try to "trick" Ann into some other activity.

Realizing that learning to fasten his pants was essential, but apparently not very immediately rewarding to Adam, Ann turned again to behavioral theory. She began each session with the less appealing task (from Adam's perspective), using the more pleasurable portion of the session as a reward. Ann also made a chart for Adam, which she hung on the wall in the treatment room, so that Adam could see the progress he was making on these tasks. With these changes in the sessions, Adam's attitude became much more positive.

As Adam mastered specific self-help skills and his posture began to show improvement, Ann discontinued intervening directly with Adam. She consulted with Ms. R to develop approaches that could be used with Adam in the classroom to improve his handwriting; she also suggested that he learn to use the computer for written work. Ann helped Adam's adaptive physical education teacher to incorporate activities requiring the organizing and sequencing of movements into Adam's program. Although she was not intervening directly with Adam, she remained an important member of the team, contributing to the development of his educational goals and objectives and helping his parents and teachers to develop strategies that would enable Adam to benefit fully from his educational program.

## Andy: Combining Sensory Integration with Sensory Stimulation and Behavioral Theory for a Child with Autism

Although autism was formerly thought to be a psychiatric disturbance (e.g., Bettelheim, 1959), it now is recognized to be associated with neurological impairment (Bower, 1986). Developmental abnormalities of cell structure have been found in both the cerebellum and limbic regions of the brain (Bauman & Kemper, 1985).

Some children and adults with autism display unusual responses to sensory input (Allen, 1988; Bauman & Kemper, 1985). Ayres and Tickle (1980) noted that some autistic children overreact to sensory stimuli, but others underreact to, or apparently do not register sensory stimuli. Temple Grandin (Grandin & Scariano, 1986), a woman with autism, described herself as over-reactive to many sensory inputs, particularly sound, light touch, and movement or vestibular sensations, while craving deep touch-pressure. Given the hypothesized role of the limbic system in sensory modulation disorders, it is not surprising that this is one area of the brain in which abnormalities have been found in autism.

While sensory integrative procedures may be appropriate for those who display problems with modulation of sensory inputs, we must remember that autism is associated with brain abnormalities, not merely with dysfunction. Care is required not to overstep the boundaries of sensory integration theory when applying these procedures to children and adults with autism. However, sensory integration theory can assist us in understanding the affective reactions to sensory inputs often seen in these clients. Sensory integrative procedures have been found to be most effective with children who overreact to sensory stimuli (Ayres & Tickle, 1980).

Three-year-old Andy was quite a handful for his parents to manage. He seemed to be constantly "on the go," climbing on furniture and counters, pulling things off shelves, and sometimes just running around aimlessly. He did not seem to hear his parents when they told him to stop, and he became very upset, attempting to kick and bite, if either of them tried to restrain him. At first, his parents thought that Andy might not hear them, but it was obvious that he heard other sounds. In fact, he became quite upset when he heard the vacuum cleaner, responding by holding his ears and screaming. The sound of a lawn mower provoked a similar reaction, and often one parent would take him for a ride in the car while the other mowed the lawn.

Andy loved watching television and could repeat several commercials, including reciting the words verbatim. But despite his ability to repeat what he had heard, he did not use language spontaneously. Andy never asked for a snack or toy. If he did not want to do something, he screamed, but he never said "no." In fact, he really did not interact with his parents much at all.

Another of Andy's favorite activities was going to the playground. He could swing for hours, and his favorite ride was the merry-go-round. Noting his love of spinning, his parents bought him a Sit 'N' Spin, a toy on which he could sit and spin himself around in circles. This activity kept him busy and "out of trouble" for at least part of the day.

Toys, in general, did not interest Andy. However, he did have a large collection of Matchbox cars that his grandparents had bought for him. He kept them on a shelf in his room, periodically taking them down and lining them up. He always lined them up in the same order, and he always placed them back on the shelf in that order. Once, when he came into the room after his mother had taken the cars off and was dusting the shelf, he began to scream and hit, evidently distraught that the cars had been moved. From then on, Andy's mother dusted the "car shelf" only when he was occupied in another activity.

Mealtime was particularly difficult for Andy and his family. As an infant he had had no trouble eating. However, he had resisted the transition to solid foods, and he was still very fussy about what he ate. He did not like food that was either too hot or too cold, and he tolerated only smooth-textured foods.

Getting Andy dressed and undressed also presented problems. He did not like being touched or handled and tried to pull away from his parents as they attempted to dress him. Clothes had to be washed several times before he would tolerate wearing them.

At their wits' end, Andy's parents turned to their pediatrician for help. He, in turn, referred Andy to a child neurologist and to his local school system for an evaluation and a program that might help Andy.

The members of Andy's evaluation team found him difficult to assess with standardized tests. They relied heavily on their own observations as well as on those of Andy's parents. They felt that Andy's outstanding problems were his total lack of use of language for communication with others, as well as his limited social interactions with his parents and others. In contrast, Andy's gross motor and visuomotor skills seemed age-appropriate.

Mike, the occupational therapist on Andy's evaluation team, noted many indicators of tactile defensiveness, including his resistance to being handled, and his food and clothing preferences. His overreaction to noises and his craving of movement also suggested to Mike that Andy had difficulty modulating sensory inputs.

After reviewing the results of the evaluation and examining Andy, the child neurologist diagnosed him as having autism. Andy was enrolled in a special-needs program, as a part of which he received occupational therapy services. Mike, who was the occupational therapist for this classroom, was most concerned about the effects that Andy's tactile defensiveness was having on him and his family. Together with Andy's parents and teacher, Mike formulated a general goal that Andy become more tolerant of being touched and that he be willing to eat a greater variety of foods. While Mike used his knowledge of sensory integration theory to help him explain Andy's problems, he was well aware that sensory integration was not the total answer to Andy's difficulties. Given the severity of Andy's problems and his lack of interaction with others, Mike also saw the need to employ his understanding of behavioral principles in his treatment with Andy and when consulting with his parents and teacher. Further, while Mike's long-term plan for Andy included sensory integration procedures, Andy's behavior suggested to Mike that he should begin his direct intervention with Andy by combining sensory stimulation with techniques derived from behavioral theory.

Mike knew that activities that provide firm touch-pressure are thought to reduce tactile defensiveness and that slow movement and neutral warmth might also be helpful. However, Andy avoided these types of activities, preferring rapid movement. Accordingly, Mike paired activities providing rapid movement with firm touch-pressure and neutral warmth. The movement served as a reward for Andy's tolerating other sensory inputs.

For example, Andy enjoyed swinging. A toddler swing, with back and side supports, was suspended from a hook in the ceiling of the therapy room. The swing was placed so that Andy's feet could not reach the floor; thus, he had to depend on Mike to push him. Mike sat in front of Andy and gave him a ride by pushing against his legs.

Very gradually, over a period of weeks, Mike was able to hold Andy's legs and apply some deep touch-pressure for a few seconds before giving him a push. Mike also placed a blanket in the swing and began to wrap Andy in the blanket for the swing ride, combining the movement with neutral warmth and deep touch-pressure. In a similar manner, Mike adapted various other movement activities in order to pair them with tactile inputs.

In addition to intervening directly with Andy, Mike consulted regularly with Andy's teacher and parents. The classroom chosen for Andy was small and uncluttered, with only three other students in the room. Andy's teachers were careful not to touch him unexpectedly, and they watched to make sure the other children also did not touch him. They noted that Andy was particularly fond of a large beanbag chair. By placing heavy pillows on top of him when he was in this chair, they were able to provide him with some deep touch-pressure at various times during the day. Andy's tolerance for deep touch-pressure increased over the months, and his teachers thought that he seemed more calm after spending time in the chair.

At Mike's suggestion, Andy's parents decided to dress him in sweatsuits most of the time. Andy seemed to like the softness of these clothes, and they were easy for his parents to put on and take off. They also bought a beanbag chair for his room and had him sit in it for dressing and undressing. By also establishing a routine time and place for dressing, they found that he became somewhat more tolerant of this handling.

Mike began Andy's feeding program by learning from Andy's parents about the foods he liked to eat. Andy would tolerate mashed potatoes, strained vegetables, and smooth soups (such as tomato), but his favorite foods were strained fruits that were both smooth and sweet. During the next several months, Mike and Andy's teachers and parents worked on having Andy increase his tolerance for textures. They rewarded him for eating a more textured food by giving him a spoonful of the fruit. They also began mixing lumpy fruits together with the strained fruit, gradually increasing the ratio of lumpy to strained.

By the end of 6 months, Andy was somewhat easier to manage at home, although he was still quite active and intolerant of change. He was able to eat a greater variety of foods, and mealtime was not as stressful.

In school, Andy was able to follow the classroom routine. Although he tolerated being handled only for brief periods, his teachers felt they could now begin toilet training.

More importantly, both Andy's parents and his teacher reported that they understood Andy's behaviors better. Based on this understanding, which came in part from Mike's simple explanations of sensory integration theory, Andy's parents and teacher were able to develop new and more effective strategies for interacting with, and teaching, Andy.

## CONCLUSION

This chapter has presented only an introduction to the ways that sensory integration theory is applied in combination with other theories and approaches used in occupational therapy to meet the needs of the variety of children we encounter in practice. Our evaluation and intervention are *always* based on the *functional needs* of the client, not on any one theoretical approach. To meet these needs requires knowledge, flexibility, creativity, and the collaborative efforts of the therapist, the client, and the client's caregivers.

## REFERENCES

Allen, D. A. (1988). Autistic spectrum disorders: Clinical presentation in preschool children. *Journal of Child Neurology, 3*(Suppl.), S48–S56.

Als, H. (1986). A synactive model of neonatal behavioral organization: Framework for the assessment of neurobehavioral development in the premature infant and for support of infants and parents in the neonatal intensive care environment. *Physical and Occupational Therapy in Pediatrics, 6*(3/4), 3–53.

Als, H., Duffy, F. H., & McAnulty, G. B. (in press). Neurobehavioral competence in healthy preterm and fullterm infants: Newborn period to 9 months. *Developmental Psychology.*

Ayres, A. J. (1972). *Sensory integration and learning disorders.* Los Angeles: Western Psychological Services.

Ayres, A. J. (1989). *Sensory Integration and Praxis Tests.* Los Angeles: Western Psychological Services.

Ayres, A. J., & Tickle, L. S. (1980). Hyper-responsivity to touch and vestibular stimuli as a predictor of positive response to sensory integration procedures by autistic children. *American Journal of Occupational Therapy, 34,* 375–381.

Ball, T. S. (1971). *Itard, Seguin and Kephart: Sensory education—A learning interpretation.* Columbus, OH: Merrill.

Bauchner, H., Brown, E., & Peskin, J. (1988). Premature graduates of the newborn intensive care unit: A guide to followup. *Pediatric Clinics of North America, 35,* 1207–1226.

Bauman, M., & Kemper, T. L. (1985). Histoanatomic observations of the brain in early infantile autism. *Neurology, 35,* 866–874.

Bayley, N. (1969). *Bayley Scales of Infant Development.* New York: Psychological Corporation.

Bettelheim, B. (1959). Feral children and autistic children. *American Journal of Sociology, 64,* 455–467.

Bissell, J., Fisher, J., Owens, C., & Polcyn, P. (1988). *Sensory motor handbook: A guide for implementing and modifying activities in the classroom.* Torrance, CA: Sensory Integration International.

Bleck, E. E. (1982). Cerebral palsy. In E. E. Bleck & D. A. Nagel (Eds.), *Physically handicapped children: A medical atlas for teachers,* (2nd ed., pp. 59–132). Orlando, FL: Grune & Stratton.

Bly, L. (1983). *The components of normal movement during the first year of life and abnormal movement.* Oak Park, IL: Neuro-Developmental Treatment Association.

Bobath, B. (1970). *Adult hemiplegia: Evaluation and treatment.* London: William Heinemann Medical Books.

Bobath, B. (1985). *Abnormal postural reflex activity caused by brain lesions* (3rd ed.). Rockville, MD: Aspen Systems.

Bobath, K. & Bobath, B. (1972). Cerebral palsy. In P. H. Pearson (Ed.), *Physical therapy services in the developmental disabilities* (pp. 31–186). Springfield, IL: Charles C. Thomas.

Boehme, R. (1988). *Improving upper body control: An approach to assessment and treatment of tonal dysfunction.* Tucson, AZ: Therapy Skill Builders.

Bower, B. (1986). Inside the autistic brain. *Science News, 130,* 154–155.

Bruininks, R. H. (1978). *Bruininks-Oseretsky Test of Motor Proficiency examiners manual.* Circle Pines, MN: American Guidance Services.

Bushnell, E. W., & Weinberger, N. (1987). Infants' detection of visual-tactual discrepancies: Asymmetries that indicate a directive role of visual information. *Journal of Experimental Psychology: Human Perception and Performance, 13,* 601–608.

Clark, F., Mailloux, Z., & Parham, D. (1989). Sensory integration and children with learning disabilities. In P. N. Pratt & A. S. Allen (Eds.), *Occupational therapy for children* (2nd ed., pp. 457–507). St. Louis: C. V. Mosby.

Cratty, B. J. (1981). Sensory-motor and perceptual-motor theories and practices: An overview and evaluation. In R. D. Walk & H. L. Pick (Eds.), *Intersensory perception and sensory integration* (pp. 345–374). New York: Plenum Press.

De Gangi, G. (1990, March). Perspectives on the integration of neurodevelopmental treatment and sensory integrative therapy: Part 2. *NDTA Newsletter*, 1 & 6.

Drillien, C. M. (1972). Abnormal neurologic signs in the first year of life in low-birth-weight infants: Possible prognostic significance. *Developmental Medicine and Child Neurology, 14,* 575–584.

Finnie, N. R. (1974). *Handling the young cerebral palsied child at home* (2nd ed.). New York: Dutton.

Fisher, A. G., & Bundy, A. C. (1989). Vestibular stimulation in the treatment of postural and related disorders. In O. D. Payton, R. P. DiFabio, S. V. Paris, E. J. Protas, & A. F. VanSant (Eds.), *Manual of physical therapy techniques* (pp. 239–258). New York: Churchill Livingstone.

Frostig, M. (1964). *Frostig program for development of visual perception.* Chicago: Follet.

Fuller, P. W., Guthrie, R. D., & Alvord, E. C. (1983). A proposed neuropathological basis for learning disabilities in children born prematurely. *Developmental Medicine and Child Neurology, 25,* 214–231.

Garcia-Coll, C. T., Sepkoski, C., & Lester, B. M. (1981). Cultural and biomedical correlates of neonatal behavior. *Developmental Psychobiology, 14,* 147–154.

Gibson, E. J. (1988). Exploratory behavior in the development of perceiving, acting and the acquiring of knowledge. *Annual Review of Psychology, 39,* 1–41.

Gibson, E. J., & Walker, A. S. (1984). Development of knowledge of visual-tactual affordances of substance. *Child Development, 55,* 453–460.

Gibson, J. J. (1979). *The ecological approach to visual perception.* Boston: Houghton Mifflin.

Gorski, P. A., Lewkowicz, D. J., & Huntington, L. (1987). Advances in neonatal and infant behavioral assessment: Toward a comprehensive evaluation of early patterns of development. *Developmental and Behavioral Pediatrics, 8,* 39–50.

Grandin, T., & Scariano, M. M. (1986). *Emergence: Labeled autistic.* Novato, CA: Arena.

Hanson, M. J. (1984). *Atypical infant development.* Baltimore: University Park.

Harris, P. L. (1983). Infant cognition. In M. M. Haith & J. J. Campos (Eds.), *Handbook of child psychology: Vol II. Infancy and developmental psychobiology* (pp. 689–782). New York: John Wiley & Sons.

Hebb, D. O. (1949). *The organization of behavior: A neuropsychological theory.* New York: John Wiley & Sons.

Howison, M. V. (1988). Cerebral Palsy. In H. L. Hopkins & H. D. Smith (Eds.), *Willard and Spackman's occupational therapy,* (7th ed., pp. 675–706). Philadelphia: J. B. Lippincott.

Hyde, A. S., & Trautman, S. E. (1989, December). Drug-exposed infants and sensory integration: Is there a connection? *Sensory Integration Special Interest Section Newsletter, 12*(1–2), 6.

Jacobson, J. L. (1984). Prenatal exposure to environmental toxin: A test of multiple effects model. *Developmental Psychology, 20,* 523–532.

Kephart, N. C. (1960). *The slow learner in the classroom.* Columbus, OH: Merrill Publishing.

Kopp, C. B., & Kaler, S. R. (1989). Risk in infancy: Origins and implications. *American Psychologist, 44,* 224–230.

Krumboltz, J. D., & Krumboltz, H. B. (1972). *Changing children's behavior.* Englewood Cliffs, NJ: Prentice Hall.

Landers, S. (June, 1989). Skinner joins aversives debate. *Monitor,* 22–23.

Laszlo, J. L., & Bairstow, P. J. (1985). *Perceptual-motor behavior: Developmental assessment and therapy.* New York: Praeger.

Lester, B. M. (1989, December). Relationship between vagal tone and behavioral competence in preterm and full-term infants. Paper presented at the meeting of the Society of Behavioral Pediatrics, Cambridge, MA.

Levine, M. D. (1987). *Developmental variation and learning disorders.* Cambridge, MA: Educators Publishing Service.

Lockman, J. J., & Hazen, N. L. (1989). *Action in social context: Perspectives on early development.* New York: Plenum.

Merriam-Webster (1989). *Webster's ninth new collegiate dictionary.* New York: Author.

Milani-Comparetti, A. (July, 1982). *Sensory systems influence on movement and tone.* Presentation at the 10th Annual Sensorimotor Integration Symposium, San Diego, CA.

Montessori, M. (1912). *The Montessori method.* New York: Schocken.

Mussen, P. H. (1983). *Handbook of child psychology: Vols. 1–4.* New York: John Wiley and Sons.

Nelson, K. B., & Ellenberg, J. H. (1982). Children who "outgrew" cerebral palsy. *Pediatrics, 69,* 529–536.

Piaget, J. (1952). *The origins of intelligence in children.* New York: W. W. Norton.

Piaget, J. (1969). *The mechanisms of perception.* New York: Basic Books.

Pick, H. L. (1989). Motor development: The control of action [Special section]. *Developmental Psychology, 25,* 867–953.

Piper, M. C. (1989). Impact of gestational age on preterm motor development at 4 months chronological and adjusted ages. *Child Care, Health and Development, 15,* 105–115.

Plomin, R., DeFries, J. C., & Fulder, D. W. (1988). *Nature and nurture during infancy and early childhood.* New York: Cambridge University.

Reed, E. S. (1982). An outline of a theory of action systems. *Journal of Motor Behavior, 14,* 98–134.

Robinson, R. (1973). The frequency of other handicaps in children with cerebral palsy. *Developmental Medicine and Child Neurology, 15*, 305.

Rose, S. A. (1983). Differential rates of visual information processing in full-term and preterm infants. *Child Development, 54*, 1189–1198.

Rose, S. A. (1988). Information processing in seven-month-old infants as a function of risk status. *Child Development, 59*, 589–603.

Ruff, H. (1986a). Components of attention during infants' manipulative exploration. *Child Development, 57*, 105–114.

Ruff, H. A. (1986b). Attention and organization of behavior in high-risk infants. *Developmental and Behavioral Pediatrics, 7*, 298–301.

Ruff, H. A., McCarton, C., Kurtzberg, D., & Vaughan, H. G. (1984). Preterm infants' manipulative exploration of objects. *Child Development, 55*, 1166–1173.

Sameroff, A., & Chandler, M. (1975). Reproductive risk and the continuum of caretaker casualty. In F. Horowitz (Ed.), *Review of child development research: Vol. 4.* Chicago: University of Chicago.

Senhal, J. P., & Palmeri, A. (1989). High risk infants. In P. N. Pratt & A. S. Allen, *Occupational therapy for children* (2nd ed., pp. 361–382). St. Louis: C. V. Mosby.

Short-DeGraff, M. A. (1988). *Human development for occupational and physical therapists.* Baltimore: Williams & Wilkins.

Skinner, B. F. (1968). *The technology of teaching.* New York: Meredith.

Sweeney, J. K. (Ed.) (1986). The high-risk neonate: Developmental therapy perspectives [Special issue]. *Physical and Occupational Therapy in Pediatrics, 6*(3/4).

von Hofsten, C. (1989). Transition mechanisms in sensorimotor development. In A. DeRibaupierre (Ed.), *Transitional mechanisms in child development: The longitudinal perspective.* Cambridge: Cambridge University Press.

Vygotsky, L. S. (1978). *Mind in society.* Cambridge, MA: Harvard University Press.

Williamson, G. G. (1988, September). Motor control as a resource for adaptive coping. *Zero to Three, 9*(1), 1–7.

Young, S. B., & Keplinger, L. (1988). *Movement is fun: A preschool movement program.* Torrance, CA: Sensory Integration International.

# Part *IV*

## RESEARCH

# CHAPTER 14

# Research in Sensory Integration: Empirical Perceptions and Progress

**Kenneth J. Ottenbacher, PhD, OTR**

> *The Brain constructs its systems to enclose,*
> *The study paradox of thought and sense;*
> *Momentously its tissued meaning grows*
> *To solve and integrate experience.*

*Kunitz, 1979, p. 122*

## INTRODUCTION

In his classic text *Public Knowledge: An Essay Concerning the Social Dimension of Science*, Ziman (1968) argues that consensus in establishing the scientific legitimacy of an area of clinical investigation is at the core of the research enterprise. The objective of research efforts, according to Ziman (1968), is to establish a consensus of rational as well as statistical opinion. Consensual knowledge is transformed through dissemination into public knowledge, and hopefully, public support. Consensus in establishing the scientific legitimacy of an area of clinical investigation is at the core of the research enterprise. Empirical consensus that is established through collective research is gradually translated into professional agreement and eventually evolves into public confidence in professional service. Professions, therefore, strive to provide service that is supported by scientific consensus.

The obvious question in relation to research in sensory integration is — does empirical consensus exist? If not, what can be done to improve scholarly consensus, and to promote the establishment of sensory integration research as public knowledge? The first step in evaluating the existing degree of empirical consensus is to conduct a comprehensive review of previous research. Any assessment of research, including sensory integration, must by necessity begin with an overview of previous investigations, and a determination of the consensus evidenced in past empirical efforts.

Research in sensory integration has progressed to the stage where a synthesis is possible, and several reviews and critiques have been published (e.g., Arendt, MacLean, & Baumeister, 1988; Ottenbacher, 1982; Ottenbacher & Short, 1985). For example, Ottenbacher (1982) conducted a meta-analysis of the research literature examining the effectiveness of sensory integration procedures. The meta-analysis technique provides each study with a standardized measure of outcome effectiveness. Each of these measures are then used as data for the meta-analysis. When several data-based studies addressing the same general hypothesis are available, meta-analysis is an excellent methodolgy for establishing empirical consensus (Glass, 1976; Glass, McGaw, & Smith, 1981). The quantitative synthesis by Ottenbacher (1982) focused on data-based studies that each met the following criteria: (a) investigated the effects of sensory integration as the independent (treatment) variable; (b) employed at least one operationally defined outcome measure related to one or more of the following areas: academic achievement, motor skill or reflex integration, and language function; (c) reported a comparison between at least two groups or conditions; and (d) included sufficient information to generate an effect size measure and other statistics used in meta-analysis (see Glass et al., 1981).

Of the 49 research reports originally identified as potentially relevant, 8 met all of the preceding criteria and were included in the review. The analysis of the statistical results indicated the average subject receiving sensory integration therapy performed better than 79 percent of the subjects in the control or comparison conditions not receiving sensory integration therapy. This result represents performance collapsed across all diagnostic conditions, and dependent measures. While the overall results indicate a relatively strong degree of (statistical) consensus across the studies, there were several limitations related to the interpretation of the findings. For example, there was no consistency in areas of improvement. Additionally, confounds existed in several of the subanalyses. For instance, children who were identified as "at-risk" were generally younger than children labeled as learning-disabled or mentally retarded. At-risk children were more often evaluated with measures of motor performance or reflex integration than were children in other diagnostic categories, so areas of improvement varied across studies. Another limitation included the fact that none of the studies included follow-up measures. Also, children in the control groups were generally not provided any alternative intervention. A final limitation was that only a small number of studies met the criteria for inclusion in the quantitative review.

Other reviews of sensory integration research have focused on theoretical and methodological issues as well as treatment effectiveness. These reviews have provided conflicting evidence regarding empirical consensus. Arendt, et al. (1988) recently reviewed eight studies describing the use of sensory integration procedures with persons identified as mentally retarded. Their review relied on a narrative evaluation and synthesis of the studies. Based on their descriptive analysis, Arendt and colleagues concluded that "there exists no convincing empirical or theoretical support for the continued use of sensory integration theory with that population [mentally retarded] outside of a research context" (p. 410). Other researchers who have evaluated sensory integration research studies have reported conflicting or contradictory recommendations (cf. Bochner, 1978; Densem, Nuthall, Bushnell, & Horn, 1989; Feagans, 1983; Ferry, 1981; Ottenbacher & Short, 1985; Sieben, 1977; Silver, 1975).

Previous attempts to synthesize and interpret existing sensory integration research reveal that a clear empirical consensus does not exist regarding the validity of sensory integration theory or the effectiveness of sensory integration practice

(Arendt et al., 1988; Ottenbacher & Short, 1985). Thus, the purpose of this chapter is not to reevaluate past research in search of statistical or theoretical consensus. Rather, the focus in this chapter is on the directions that future research must take if empirical consensus is to be achieved and the transition to public knowledge completed. Translating research results into professional agreement, and eventual scientific consensus, ultimately depends on establishing a clear and consistent interpretation of what therapists and researchers mean when they label an intervention program *sensory integration.*

## THE INTEGRITY OF SENSORY INTEGRATION AS AN INDEPENDENT VARIABLE

Rosenthal and Rosnow (1984) define an independent variable as an observable or measurable event manipulated by a researcher to determine whether there is any effect on another event (the dependent variable). Traditional research approaches based on definitions such as that proposed by Rosenthal and Rosnow (1984) often require that the independent variable or treatment be administered to every individual in the same standardized manner. Clearly, complex interventions such as sensory integration defy a simple definition.

One characteristic of a "simple" definition associated with many independent variables is the assumption that variation within a treatment strategy must be treated as error and minimized through experimental control or statistical manipulation. When this assumption is made, this "error" or random variability in the independent variable is often minimized by reducing the treatment to a small number of standardized and strictly controlled activities.

While this practice makes it easier to operationally define the independent variable and to control its implementation, the resulting treatment may not accurately represent the construct associated with the independent variable. Examples of this linear or reductionistic approach to defining independent variables are easy to find in the sensory integration research literature. Wells and Smith (1983), for example, reported a study entitled "Reduction of Self-Injurious Behavior of Mentally Retarded Persons Using Sensory Integrative Techniques." In this study, four subjects identified as profoundly mentally retarded and evidencing self-injurious behavior received sensory integrative treatment. In describing the independent variable the authors stated:

> We used those techniques as models in developing sensory integrative treatment programs for the subjects that included slow, repetitive vestibular stimulation and firm deep tactile stimulation. The vestibular stimulation consisted of slow gentle rocking in a nylon net hammock or rocking in a rocking chair. The tactile and deep pressure stimulation consisted of vibration supplied by a cylindrical, battery operated vibrator and hands-on massage. Each type of stimulation was delivered for approximately 5 minutes before changing to another type. The entire session lasted 30 minutes. (p. 665)

Descriptions of sensory integration such as the one included in the Wells and Smith (1983) study suggest that the treatment was more a program of controlled sensory stimulation than sensory integration as defined by Ayres (cf. Clark, Mallioux, & Parham, 1989) (see also Chapters 1 and 13). The reduction of the independent variable to one or two techniques that can be operationally described and easily implemented has obvious methodological advantages. However, the independent variable defined as the component parts of a complex intervention may then no longer be representative of the construct under investigation, that is, sensory integration.

If an independent variable is reduced to component activities and studied, then it is vital that a "fit" exist between the concepts and operations associated with the independent variable. Support for the independent variable can gradually be developed through repeated studies addressing the same hypothesis and using multiple operationalizations of the concept. When such a series of studies is planned, care must be exercised that there is good concept-to-operation correspondence in the multiple operations used to represent the independent variable. For example, in the Wells and Smith (1983) investigation, the vestibular component of sensory integration was operationally defined as gentle rocking in a net hammock or rocking in a rocking chair. In a subsequent study, vestibular stimulation may be operationally defined as circular stimulation (spinning) in a net hammock or as riding a scooter board. If each of these "multiple" operations of vestibular stimulation, as a component of sensory integration, produced positive results, then support or confidence in the construct would be strengthened.

The use of multiple operations to represent and evaluate a complex construct such as sensory integration is difficult to achieve. Sensory integration, as a construct, is more than a collection of various sensory stimulation activities. When the intervention is reduced to component parts, such as vestibular or tactile stimulation, the integrative gestalt is lost. As a therapeutic construct, sensory integration is more than the sum of its sensory parts. The argument could be made that the interaction associated with sensory integration is impossible to evaluate using the isolated activities of a complex construct. Even if the component sensory stimulation activities are found to produce positive results when individually evaluated, the collective effect remains unknown.

Studies exploring the use of controlled rotary vestibular stimulation (Clark, Kreutzburg, & Chee, 1977; Ottenbacher, Short, & Watson, 1981) are examples of investigations focusing on one sensory component often associated with sensory integration. These studies allow for precise control of the sensory input by maintaining head position, and controlling rotational speed and duration of rotation. For example, Kantner, Clark, Allen, and Chase (1976) reported a study in which a program of rotary vestibular stimulation was found to produce improved motor abilities in a 6-month-old infant with Down syndrome. The vestibular stimulation was provided in a specially adapted chair that rotated the child at a set speed (100° per second). During the rotation, the child's head position was controlled to maximize the effect of the stimulation. Although controlled vestibular stimulation activities may be a part of some sensory integrative programs, the studies using isolated vestibular stimulation, such as that reported by Kantner and colleagues (1976), provide only tangential support regarding the impact of sensory integration procedures. The studies investigating controlled rotary vestibular input are studies of sensory stimulation, not sensory integration.

To summarize, sensory integration is a multifaceted intervention approach that is difficult to reduce to component parts. To ensure the integrity of sensory integration as an independent variable requires special planning. The description of the treatment, the training of individuals responsible for implementing the intervention, and the development of procedures to monitor delivery of the treatment are vital to any successful investigation. These issues will be covered in more detail in a later section.

## CONCEPTUAL RELEVANCE AND CONSENSUS

Yeaton and Sechrest (1981) have described various standards and procedures for monitoring the strength and integrity of an independent variable. They argue that strong treatments are those most likely to produce the desired effect. Treatments, however, are not absolutely strong or weak. An intervention may be a powerful treatment for some problems but not for others.

In a recent study, Densem and colleagues (1989) provided children randomly assigned to a sensory integration program with an average of 17 treatment sessions over a period of 5 months. The 55 children participating in the study were assessed in multiple areas, including language, perceptual motor skills, reading, handwriting, self-esteem, behavioral/social adjustment, and school progress. The chance of finding statistically significant improvements across all the areas assessed in studies with multiple outcome measures is small. These studies have an exploratory component to them, which implies that the investigators are uncertain about the intended focus of the intervention. If there is not a good fit between the treatment and the selected outcome measure, then the strength of the treatment is reduced to irrelevance. Without specific knowledge of the kinds of problems likely to be modified by a given treatment, researchers run the risk of producing trivial or uninterpretable results. Yeaton and Sechrest (1981) argue that a primary task of applied research is to identify which treatment is appropriate for which problem.

One way to establish the fit between treatment and outcome measures, or conceptual relevance (Sechrest & Redner, 1979), is to base research on well-established theory. A well-developed theory provides the framework for understanding and predicting the interrelationship of independent and dependent variables, that is, for establishing conceptual relevance. When no theoretical relationship exists between variables, or when conceptual relevance has not been established through previous research, then there is no clear basis to infer the strength of treatment or, for that matter, by which the parameters of treatment strength (effectiveness) can be known. To make independent and dependent variables conceptually relevant in sensory integration research requires that the research questions posed, and the outcome measures selected, be derived from current theory. When this practice is followed, conceptual relevance will contribute to empirical consensus. Unfortunately, the conceptual relevance of some studies of sensory integration theory and intervention programs is questionable. The conceptual relevance of an investigation is low when the outcome measure targeted for evaluation is not directly related to sensory integration theory, or when the population under investigation is clearly not the one for which the theory or treatment techniques were developed (see also Chapters 1 and 13).

Even strong, conceptually relevant investigations may not produce the intended effect if the treatment is not administered appropriately. The integrity of treatment refers to the degree to which the intervention is administered as intended (Sechrest & Redner, 1979). Some treatments are obviously easier to control and administer than others. As noted in the previous section, it is simpler to administer isolated rotary vestibular stimulation than to administer a complex intervention such as sensory integration, which requires that a therapeutic balance be maintained between the activities and responses of both the client and the therapist. With any complex intervention, some problems in maintaining treatment integrity will arise. It is precisely for complex independent variables, such as sensory integration, that it is most important to have a plan to ensure treatment integrity. Such a plan should begin with clear requirements for the training of those persons who will administer the treatment. Specific protocols describing the independent variable should be developed and reviewed by experts to ensure the representativeness of the procedures. Once the study has begun, departures from prescribed treatment activities can be monitored by having observers randomly check the correspondence between actual treatment activities and those contained in the treatment protocol. These measures will not guarantee the integrity of the intervention, but they will increase the probability that the independent variable is delivered as intended. Decisions regarding efficacy of sensory integration intervention programs cannot be accurately and reliably made until investigators adequately establish that there is a clear fit between concepts and operations for the independent variable, and that the intervention is properly administered.

The issues of strength and integrity apply primarily to experimental or quasi-experimental research where the independent variable (sensory integration treatment techniques) is manipulated by the researcher. Designs associated with experimental or quasi-experimental research provide the framework for managing and manipulating the treatment under investigation. Much of the research in sensory integration, however, involves nonmanipulatable independent variables where the intent of the study is to infer association, not causation. These relational studies have an important role in refining sensory integration theory and developing consensual knowledge regarding sensory integration practice.

## ASSOCIATION AS CONSENSUS

More than 30 years ago, Cronbach (1957) identified two different approaches to knowledge development in the behavioral sciences. Cronbach referred to the first as the correlational method. In the correlational method, variance among variables or individuals is explored. The second method identified by Cronbach was the experimental approach. The object of the experimental method was to study variance among treatments. The experimental method as described by Cronbach was concerned with both general and specific treatment effects. Cronbach (1957) and others (Kiesler, 1971) have argued that both types of research need to be done. Any coherent discipline will include studies of the variance between individuals and treatments, as well as explore the interactions between various subject and treatment variables. That is, a coherent discipline would combine experimental and correlational methods. There is evidence of both approaches in sensory integrative research.

Considerable confusion exists regarding the nature of the evidence and the degree of consensus generated by correlational and experimental methods. Many sensory integration research studies are associational (correlational) in nature. This is true despite the fact that two groups are often compared in a design that superficially resembles those used in experimental or quasi-experimental studies. The difference is that in the associational studies, the independent variable is not manipulated by the researcher. For example, Conrad, Cermak, and Drake (1983) conducted a study designed to identify different forms of praxis in normal boys and boys with learning disabilities. Four different areas of praxis were evaluated in the subjects using the Praxis Test for Children (Conrad et al., 1983). The results revealed that the children with learning disabilities had significantly lower scores on two of the four areas of praxis measured by the test. This study is an example of a sample-difference design. The design produces evidence that is associational (correlational) in nature despite the fact that two groups are compared and no correlational statistic is computed. That is, Conrad and colleagues (1983) made statistical comparisons between the normal boys and the boys with learning disabilities across four areas of praxis using analysis of variance (ANOVA). The analysis revealed a statistically significant difference between the normal boys and the boys with learning disabilities on two of the four praxis assessments. This information allowed the researchers to test their original hypothesis that there would be a statistically significant difference between the performance of the two groups. This analysis answers an all-or-none, yes-or-no question associated with statistical significance. That is, is there a statistically significant difference between the two groups? Or is there no statistically significant difference between the groups?

The sample-difference design employs groups that are constructed based on their dysfunction or diagnostic label (i.e., learning-disabled vs. non–learning-disabled). Since this distinction is not manipulated by the investigator, the resulting comparison between the two groups is associational. The structure of the sample-difference approach resembles designs where the independent variable is manipulated or controlled by the investigator. The sample-difference paradigm, however, has no greater interpretative power than a traditional correlational study. In fact, by grouping subjects into two or more conditions (designated as dysfunctional and non-dysfunctional), individual variation within groups, which might legitimately relate to the dependent measure, is generally lost to error variance.

For instance, information regarding the *degree* to which membership in the learning-disabled or non–learning-disabled group was associated with performance on each of the praxis activities is lost in this all-or-none decision. Information related to the degree of relationship between variables, however, may be directly related to theoretical interpretations or predictions. As Cooper (1979) has observed, "statistical significance testing which compares an observed relation to the chance of no relation becomes less informative as evidence supporting a phenomenon accumulates. The question turns from 'whether' to 'how much' of an effect exists" (p. 1017). Answering the "how much" question is more likely to provide information of theoretical interest and result in the development of consensual knowledge. One of the advantages of correlational statistical procedures is that they provide information concerning the degree of relationship between variables.

Another method to improve the consensus associated with correlational research is to study the relationship between variables over time. One procedure to accomplish this goal is the use of the cross-lag research design. The cross-lag research design allows for the exploration of relationships between two variables over time. By examining the cross-lagged correlations associated with the design, it is possible to partially rule out some confounds or alternative explanations. Suppose, for example, a researcher is interested in studying the relationship between tactile sensitivity and aggression in learning-disabled children. The first assumption that must be made is that both tactile sensitivity and aggression can be measured in an accurate and reliable manner. Given this assumption, two correlational measures are taken for the relation between tactile sensitivity and aggression. The first is taken in 1985 and the second in 1989. Figure 14–1 presents a schematic of the design for this hypothetical study. The first question is whether the two variables covary. This question is addressed by examining the correlations labeled $r_{a1b1}$ and $r_{a2b2}$. The investigator will also want to know whether the two variables are stable (consistent). This information can be obtained by examining the correlations labeled $r_{a1a2}$ and

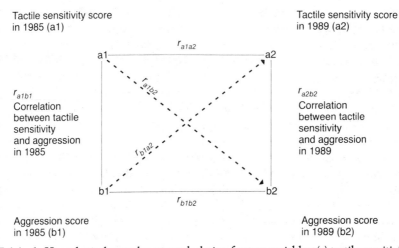

Tactile sensitivity score
in 1985 (a1)

Tactile sensitivity score
in 1989 (a2)

$r_{a1a2}$

a1 ———————————————— a2

$r_{a1b2}$

$r_{a1b1}$
Correlation
between tactile
sensitivity
and aggression
in 1985

$r_{b1a2}$

$r_{a2b2}$
Correlation
between tactile
sensitivity
and aggression
in 1989

b1 ———————————————— b2

$r_{b1b2}$

Aggression score
in 1985 (b1)

Aggression score
in 1989 (b2)

**FIGURE 14–1.** Hypothetical cross-lag research design for two variables: (a) tactile sensitivity, and (b) aggression in learning-disabled children. The dashed lines show the direction of the two cross-lag correlations, $r_{a1b2}$ and $r_{b1a2}$.

$r_{b1b2}$. If both of these correlations are high (>0.80), the researcher can conclude that the measures are relatively stable. Finally, the investigator is interested in evidence of a "causal" relationship. The cross-lag correlations provide some data regarding whether or not there is a causal relationship between a and b. One cross-lag correlation, $r_{a1b2}$, involves the relationship between tactile sensitivity in 1985 and aggression in 1989. The other correlation, $r_{b1a2}$, refers to the relationship between aggression in 1985 and tactile sensitivity in 1989. A strong correlation between a1 and b2 relative to the correlation between b1 and a2 would suggest that tactile sensitivity may be causally implicated in the relationship between tactile sensitivity and aggression. A minimal or weak correlation between b1 and a2, especially in relation to a larger correlation between a1 and b2, would strengthen the argument that aggressiveness is the dependent variable and tactile sensitivity the independent variable.

The application of cross-lag designs to correlational questions of interest to researchers in sensory integration would provide greater consensus than the currently used simple or multiple correlations. The design does require that measurements be collected over time. This requirement, however, would not be a major impediment in the many clinical environments where performance is monitored on a periodic basis as part of normal documentation.

## CONSENSUS AND SAMPLES

To accumulate scientifically useful information that builds consensus requires that samples included in research studies be clearly specified. This topic was briefly addressed in the foregoing discussion of conceptual relevance. The importance of sample specificity in developing consensual knowledge is expanded in this section. Severe difficulties arise in the accumulation of scientific information if undefined differences in sample selection and identification exist across studies.

Many studies of sensory integration theory and practice have focused on the learning-disabled population, which is notoriously heterogeneous, and has defied practical definition. The criteria for identifying children as learning-disabled can vary tremendously from one investigation to another (Kirk & Kirk, 1983). It is generally acknowledged that learning disability is not a unitary disorder (Keogh, 1983; Mykelbust, 1983) and not all children with learning disabilities have sensory integration problems. This fact is reflected in the conflicting research findings on treatment approaches for the learning-disabled population. It should be no surprise that studies using varying definitions and conflicting criteria to identify children as dysfunctional yield different or conflicting results. This occurs despite the application of similar measurement procedures and treatment techniques.

When the operational criteria specifying subject membership in a clinical population are not explicitly specified, or when criteria for sample membership lack conceptual relevance to the intervention, the problem of sample comparability is compounded. The problem of sample comparability is frequently encountered in sensory integration research. For example, Jenkens, Fewell, and Harris (1981) reported the results of a study in which sensory integrative procedures were used to enhance the motor performance of 44 children with developmental disorders. The sample consisted of 33 boys and 11 girls ranging in age from 3 to 5 years. The diagnostic labels of the children included "behavior disorders, communication disorders, health impairments, and mild and moderate mental retardation" (p. 222). No specific information was provided on the incidence of children with various diagnostic labels for any of the above categories. The heterogeneity inherent in a sample of children with such diverse and undefined conditions greatly increases within-group variability (error variance) and reduces the probability of identifying any statistically significant difference between groups or in establishing any relationship between treatment and sample (subject) characteristics.

The problem of sample validity has greatly complicated the interpretation of much of the existing research in sensory integration. If sample criteria and characteristics are not clearly defined, then study results will continue to produce confusion instead of consensus. Therefore, it is important that researchers clearly define the sample selection criteria and identify the characteristics of the subjects included in any investigation of sensory integration theory or program.

## GENERALIZABILITY AND CONSENSUS

The ability to generalize study findings is closely related to subject characteristics and to the sampling method used in a particular study. Development of empirical consensus implies that the results are generalizable. Without a convincing demonstration of their generalizability, findings in a research area cannot become public knowledge. In research texts, generalizability of research findings is discussed under the title of external validity. In fact, Campbell and Stanley (1966) originally defined external validity in the form of a question: To what populations and settings can a treatment effect be generalized? External validity, as defined by Campbell and Stanley (1966), refers to the extent to which the results of an investigation are valid or "true" for other subjects and settings.

A variety of methods have evolved to help establish the generalizability of research findings. The most powerful and widely advocated of these methods is random sampling. Random (probability) sampling suggests that the subjects in a study are randomly selected from a defined target population. The opportunity to randomly select study participants from a known target population provides statistical assurance that the sample will be representative of the population and, therefore, that the results will generalize back to other members of the parent population.

In clinical environments, however, it is usually impossible to employ a random sampling plan when conducting traditional group-comparison research studies. At best, the researcher might be able to randomly sample from some relatively small subset of the population of interest. For instance, an investigator may have access to all the learning-disabled children in one school, or even one school district. These subjects comprise the experimentally accessible population, that is, the population from which the researcher can select subjects. This population may or may not be the same as the target population (Bracht & Glass, 1968). In most cases of research in sensory integration, there is no opportunity to randomly select subjects from a target population. Researchers are rarely able to achieve any convincing degree of generalizability based on the statistical model associated with random sampling.

Another limitation in generalizing findings from traditional group comparison research is related to the problem of variability. The degree of heterogeneity among subjects in most studies of sensory integration treatment procedures is likely to be large, owing to the wide variability in subject performance levels. Random sampling of any relatively large clinical population will almost certainly result in a considerable amount of between-subject variance. This increased variability substantially reduces the probability of detecting a statistically significant "group" treatment effect (Bloom & Fischer, 1982). The argument is frequently made that single-subject research procedures that rely on analysis of within-subject variability, rather than between-subject variability, provide a viable alternative to traditional research methods (Ottenbacher, 1986). This is a particularly strong argument in areas of clinical research such as sensory integration where variability within a sample is likely to be large.

The limitations associated with random sampling in clinical research mean that investigators must often rely on alternative methods to establish the generalizability of study findings. In both group-comparison and single-subject designs, two alternative methods of developing generalizability are available: logical and empirical generalization. The use of logical generalization was originally discussed by Campbell and Stanley (1966). Logical generalizations are based on clearly developed arguments that the subjects, settings, and treatments under investigation are not idiosyncratic. Logical generalization relies on a detailed operational description of the subjects, settings, and treatments. Based on this operational description, the reader is allowed to draw conclusions as to whether the results obtained in the study would (logically) apply to other clinical samples or settings. The strength of the generalization is directly related to the degree of operational detail provided about the sample, setting, and treatment.

One clear difficulty with the method of logical generalization as applied to traditional research designs is that the description of the subjects and treatment outcomes is based on average or pooled subject performance. In most traditional studies that include a treatment and control group, the subjects are described in terms of their "mean" performance. The problem becomes obvious when the reader attempts to generalize from the "mean" treatment effect to the "individual" treatment effect.

The final method of establishing generalizability is based on replications. The systematic replication of studies is referred to as empirical generalization. Empirical generalizability is established through the accumulation of internally valid studies addressing the same research problem or question. Empirical generalizability may either be preplanned, and involve conducting a series of replication studies addressing similar questions, or else it may occur naturally. Replication strategies are most often discussed in relation to single-subject research, where generalizability cannot be established based on random sampling and the use of a statistical model (Barlow & Herson, 1984). Replication strategies, however, are important to any area of research where random sampling from a defined target population is not possible.

The practice of replication is directly related to both generalizability of research results and to the development of empirical consensus. Replications are a powerful method of establishing consensual knowledge. Sensory integration research is an area of clinical investigation where random sampling from a target population usually is not feasible. The generalizability of research findings and the development of empirical consensus in sensory integration, therefore, must rely on programs of replication. In some institutions, planned programs of replication could be connected to faculty research and thesis projects completed by graduate students. Replications should be a high priority in future sensory integration research, regardless of the design used in a particular study. As Campbell and Jackson (1979) note, "replication research not only provides the means for the building of confidence in certain research findings, but in so doing, builds confidence in a discipline" (p. 6). The establishment of public confidence in research findings is a major objective of developing an empirical consensus regarding sensory integration theory and practice. Replication studies can help to achieve this goal.

Replication alone, however, is not enough. Empirical consensus is not possible without some effort toward integration and synthesis. As Fiske (1977) has accurately noted, "science builds not on the single study but on sets of studies with similar findings" (p. 134). There is a continuing need for critical, integrative, direction-pointing scholarly reviews of sensory integration research. A recent search of several data bases (e.g., *Index Medicus, Psychological Abstracts, Cumulative Index to Journals in Education*) produced more than 300 titles when the descriptor sensory integration was crossed with therapy, treatment, or research. What does this body of literature tell us about the future of sensory integrative practice and research? It tells us that knowledge in a domain is best advanced through a scholarly interplay of theory and empirical research, as well as the synthesis of that theory and research. A thoughtful integration of the existing literature serves both to creatively organize and summarize what has been done, to point out important directions for future work, and most importantly, to build consensus.

## PERCEPTIONS AND CONCLUSIONS

Developing consensus and establishing sensory integration research as public knowledge will require a creative synthesis of past and present empirical efforts. To achieve empirical consensus, future efficacy research (regardless of design or analysis orientation) should first establish the integrity of the independent variable: sensory integration treatment programs. Once the integrity of the intervention is established, researchers should focus on maximizing the strength of the treatment by ensuring that the dependent variables are related to the theory, sensitive to changes in behavior effected by the treatment, and measured in an accurate and reliable manner. In attempting to establish an empirical consensus and to maximize the strength of the independent variable, investigators must carefully consider the sample they are studying. Strategies to generalize the results should also be considered by researchers in the planning and implementation of their investigations. Finally, and perhaps most importantly, researchers in sensory integration must realize the need for their empirical efforts to result in a consensus. Scientific consensus cannot be achieved by one investigator or one investigation. Consensus requires cooperation and collaborative effort.

Even when the above criteria are met, and the investigation appears methodologically and conceptually sound, it remains important to make a distinction between sensory integration research and sensory integration science. In the behavioral and social science literature, investigators frequently equate a particular research approach with the very essence of science (Mahoney, 1976). Certainly Science, as we understand it, cannot exist without research. But research is only one component of science, and, in fact, can produce little of lasting value unless it grows out of consensus supported by theory.

Consensual science is a complex theoretical and empirical mosaic, and research studies are only one part of this mosaic. The science of sensory integration is still in its infancy, and no single research approach has emerged as the methodology of choice in attempting to establish empirical consensus. It is not out of immaturity that a single research paradigm has failed to emerge for occupational therapy in general, or for sensory integration in particular. The absence of a unifying research paradigm is a function, rather, of a highly complex subject. Thus, the introduction and exploration of multiple empirical approaches should be encouraged and viewed as a positive development. A much greater risk for sensory integration research, to use Scriven's (1969) phrase, would be for the field to become the victim of "paradigm fixation." A diversity in research approaches ensures that important scientific questions will be addressed from multiple vantage points. The consensus derived from different empirical angles will assist in converting research findings into professional agreement and public confidence. The ultimate beneficiaries of this transition will not be the researchers, therapists, or educators, but the clients served by sensory integration theory and practice.

# REFERENCES

Arendt, R. E., MacLean, W. E., & Baumeister, A. (1988). Critique of sensory integration therapy and its application in mental retardation. *American Journal on Mental Retardation, 92,* 401–411.

Barlow, D. H., & Hersen, M. (1984). *Single case experimental designs: Strategies for study behavior change* (2nd ed.). New York: Pergamon Press.

Bloom, M., & Fischer, J. (1982). *Evaluating clinical practice: Guidelines for the accountable professional.* Englewood Cliffs, NJ: Prentice Hall.

Bochner, S. (1978). Ayres, sensory integration and learning disorders: A question of theory and practice. *Australian Journal of Mental Retardation, 5,* 41–45.

Bracht, G. H., & Glass, G. V. (1968). The external validity of experiments. *American Education Research Journal, 5,* 437–474.

Campbell, K. E., & Jackson, T. T. (1979). The role of and need for replication research in social psychology. *Replications in Social Psychology, 1,* 3–14.

Campbell, D. T., & Stanley, J. (1966). *Experimental and quasi-experimental design for research.* Chicago: Rand McNally.

Clark, D. L., Kreutzburg, J. R., & Chee, F. (1977). Vestibular stimulation influence on motor development in infants. *Science, 196,* 1228–1229.

Clark, F. A., Mailloux, Z., & Parham, D. (1989). Sensory integration and children with learning disabilities. In P. N. Pratt & A. S. Allen (Eds.), *Occupational therapy for children* (2nd ed.) (pp. 457–507). St. Louis, MO: C.V. Mosby.

Clark, F. A., & Shuer, J. (1978). A clarification of sensory integrative therapy and its application to programming with retarded people. *Mental Retardation, 16,* 227–232.

Conrad, K., Cermak, S., & Drake, S. (1983). Differentiation of praxis among children. *American Journal of Occupational Therapy, 37,* 466–473.

Cooper, H. M. (1979). Statistically combining independent studies: A meta-analysis of sex differences in conformity research. *Journal of Personality and Social Psychology, 37,* 131–146.

Cronbach, L. J. (1957). The two disciplines of scientific psychology. *American Psychologist, 12*, 671–684.

Densem, J. F., Nathall, G. A., Bushnell, J., & Horn, J. (1989). Effectiveness of a sensory integrative therapy program for children with perceptual-motor deficits. *Journal of Learning Disabilities, 22*, 221–229.

Feagans, L. (1983). A current review of learning disabilities. *Journal of Pediatrics, 102*, 487–493.

Ferry, P. (1981). On growing new neurons: Are early intervention programs effective? *Pediatrics, 67*, 38–41.

Fiske, D. W. (1977). Methodological issues in research on the psychotherapist. In A. S. Gurman & A. M. Razin (Eds.), *Effective psychotherapy: A handbook of research* (pp. 131–147). New York: Pergamon Press.

Glass, G. V. (1976). Primary, secondary and meta-analysis. *Educational Researcher, 5*, 3–8.

Glass, G. V., McGaw, B., & Smith, M. L. (1981). *Meta-analysis in social research.* Beverly Hills, CA: Sage.

Jenkins, J. R., Fewell, R., & Harris, S. R. (1983). Comparison of sensory integrative therapy and motor programming. *American Journal of Mental Deficiency, 88*, 221–224.

Kantner, R. M., Clark, D., Allen, L., & Chase, M. (1976). Effects of vestibular stimulation on nystagmus response and motor performance in the developmentally delayed infant. *Physical Therapy, 56*, 414–421.

Keogh, B. (1983). Classification, compliance and confusion. *Journal of Learning Disabilities, 16*, 25–26.

Kiesler, D. J. (1971). Experimental designs in psychotherapy research. In A. E. Bergin & S. L. Garfield (Eds.), *Handbook of psychotherapy and behavior change* (pp. 201–262). New York: John Wiley & Sons.

Kirk, S. A., & Kirk, W. D. (1983). On defining learning disabilities. *Journal of Learning Disabilities, 16*, 20–21.

Kunitz, S. (1979). *Selected poems 1928–1978.* Boston: Little, Brown.

Maxwell, S. E., Camp, C. J., & Arvey, R. D. (1981). Measures of strength of association: A comparative examination. *Journal of Applied Psychology, 66*, 525–534.

Myklebust, H. R. (1983). Toward a science of learning disabilities. *Journal of Learning Disabilities, 16*, 17–19.

Ottenbacher, K. (1982). Sensory integration therapy: Affect or effect? *American Journal of Occupational Therapy, 36*, 571–578.

Ottenbacher, K. (1984). Measures of relationship strength in occupational therapy research. *Occupational Therapy Journal of Research, 4*, 271–286.

Ottenbacher, K. (1986). *Evaluating clinical change: Strategies for occupational and physical therapists.* Baltimore: Williams & Wilkins.

Ottenbacher, K., Short, M.A., & Watson, P. J. (1981). The effects of a clinically applied program of vestibular stimulation on the neuromotor performance of children with severe developmental delay. *Physical & Occupational Therapy in Pediatrics, 1*(3), 1–11.

Ottenbacher, K., & Short, M. A. (1985). Sensory integrative dysfunction in children: A review of theory and treatment. In D. Routh & M. Wolrich (Eds.), *Advances in Developmental and Behavioral Pediatrics* (Vol. 6, pp. 287–329). Greenwich, CT: JAI Press.

Rosenthal, R., & Rosnow, R. L. (1984). *Essentials of behavioral research: Methods and data analysis.* New York: McGraw-Hill.

Scriven, M. (1969). Psychology without a paradigm. In L. Breger (Ed.), *Clinical-cognitive psychology.* Englewood Cliffs, NJ: Prentice Hall.

Sechrest, L., & Redner, R. (1979). Strength and integrity of treatments in evaluation studies. In *Evaluation Reports* (pp. 150–169). Washington, DC: National Criminal Justice Reference Services.

Sieben, R. L. (1977). Controversial treatments for learning disorders. *Academic Therapy, 13*, 128–145.

Silver, L. B. (1975). Acceptable and controversial approaches to treating the child with learning disabilities. *Pediatrics, 55*, 406–415.

Wells, M. E., & Smith, D. W. (1983). Reduction of self-injurious behavior in mentally retarded persons using sensory-integrative techniques. *American Journal of Mental Deficiency, 87*, 664–666.

Yeaton, W., & Sechrest, L. (1981). Critical dimensions in the choice and maintenance of successful treatments: Strength, integrity, and effectiveness. *Journal of Consulting and Clinical Psychology, 49*, 156–167.

Ziman, J. M. (1968). *Public knowledge: An essay concerning the social dimension of science.* Cambridge: Cambridge University.

# Index

An "f" following a page number indicates a figure; a "t" indicates a table.

**401**